AIDS and Accusation

AIDS and Accusation

Haiti and the Geography of Blame

Updated with a New Preface

Paul Farmer

UNIVERSITY OF CALIFORNIA PRESS

Berkeley / Los Angeles / London

University of California Press, one of the most distinguished
university presses in the United States, enriches lives around
the world by advancing scholarship in the humanities, social sciences,
and natural sciences. Its activities are supported by the UC Press
Foundation and by philanthropic contributions from individuals
and institutions. For more information, visit www.ucpress.edu.

Comparative Studies of Health Systems and Medical Care, 33

University of California Press
Berkeley and Los Angeles, California

University of California Press, Ltd.
London, England

Library of Congress Cataloging-in-Publication Data
Farmer, Paul, 1959–
    Aids and accusation : Haiti and the geography of blame /
Paul Farmer. — Updated with a new preface.
        p.   cm. — (Comparative studies of health systems and
    medical care)
Includes bibliographical references and index.
ISBN 978-0-520-24839-7 (pbk. : alk. paper)
1. AIDS (Disease)—Haiti. 2. Medical anthropology—Haiti.
I. Title.   II. Series.
RA644.A25F37 2006
306.4'61—dc22

                                    2005046650

Manufactured in the United States of America

15   14   13   12   11   10   11
10   9   8   7   6   5

This book is dedicated
to the memory of my father

"*If ever there were a society that ought to have ended up totally annihilated, materially and spiritually, by the trials of 'modernization,' it is Haiti.*"

Mintz (1972:7)

Contents

From Haiti to Rwanda:
AIDS and Accusations

Learning Lessons

Twenty years after initiating the research on which this book is based, and almost fifteen years after seeing *AIDS and Accusation* in print, I am pleased that my editor has asked me to write a new preface for it. The invitation has led me to reflect not so much on the book's possible impact—some suggest that academic studies rarely have significant impact on anyone but the author—as on some of the things I've learned about AIDS and related epidemics. I had already learned some of these lessons by the time this book appeared; a few I had to unlearn, and of course I have learned a host of new lessons simply by staying engaged in settings where AIDS has taken hold. I'm writing this preface from rural Rwanda, from the middle of the continent that is currently the epicenter of the global pandemic. Even a road-tested student of social conditions and infectious disease has ample occasion to keep learning in Rwanda—and perhaps to contribute something to those most affected by AIDS.

Some of the lessons I learned as a graduate student and physician in training—many of which I lay out in *AIDS and Accusation*—continue to be useful. First, I learned that AIDS, although a new disease, is deeply embedded in social and economic structures long in place and that violence, poverty, and inequality are the fault lines along which HIV spreads. Even when I wrote this book, those of us working with the disease saw that AIDS was likely to become a major killer of people living in poverty; that tuberculosis (a disease afflicting each of the young AIDS victims profiled in *AIDS and Accusation*) would likely hasten the deaths of those unfortunate enough to live in poverty and to become infected with HIV; and that much could be done, even then, to avert unnecessary suffering. The possibility for action was evident even before the development of life-saving antiretroviral medications. I learned how medical errors, bad diagnoses, and confidently expressed but incorrect claims of causality could themselves cause great suffering. Some claims came from the popular press, but many, as is clear in *AIDS and Accusation,* came from officially accredited speakers: scientific and medical authorities as well as political figures. Some authorities claimed, for example, that HIV came to the United States from Haiti—"the little Africa off the coast of Florida," according to the popular press—despite the fact that data available at the time, which I review in this book, suggested the opposite. In *AIDS and Accusation,* I characterize the Haitian epidemic as a direct subepidemic, or offshoot, of the much larger U.S. pandemic—one that is quite unrelated to the one in Africa. Technologies developed after this 1992 study characterized the genetic subtypes, or clades, of HIV and corroborate the thesis here: the Haitian epidemic is indeed caused by subtype B, the clade prevalent in the United States. AIDS did not come to Haiti from Africa, where other clades are prevalent; it came south with North American tourists. But the myth that AIDS came to the United States from Haiti prevails in the popular press and, at times, in the popular imagination.

Similarly erroneous claims about the role of stigma, a traditional topic of anthropology and other social sciences, were also common. It's true that AIDS was entangled with stigma in many ways. In rural Haiti, social responses were often tied to accusations of sorcery, a system of attitudes about the etiology of suffering with deep roots in Haiti's history as a slave colony. The modern-day accusations registered in rural Haiti were almost invariably triggered by local social inequalities. Accusing someone of sorcery is a way (maladaptive, perhaps) for the victim to transfer blame for misfortune to another person, the alleged perpetrator. But in the United States and other wealthy postslavery societies of the Americas, the stigma of AIDS combined with inveterate racism to ensure that victims of the disease would bear the blame for their own misfortune. Moreover, not only sufferers from HIV but all Haitians were branded as AIDS carriers. This variety of stigma cannot be reduced to a matter of personal concern, though I have heard hundreds of anecdotes of landlords and employers acting out of prejudice and fear and have no reason to doubt their veracity. Racism was central to the early international responses to AIDS, too, and remains a problem today, as AIDS takes its greatest toll on the continent of Africa, where the heritage of colonialism and racism weighs heavily.

In all these settings, however, accusation remained a constant, prompting the subtitle of this book: *Haiti and the Geography of Blame*. I learned that stigma, always socially constructed, works in different ways in different places and that the most important stigma in rural Haiti resulted from people's belief, correct at the time, that AIDS was an inevitably fatal disease. Stigma would later be a major barrier to the introduction of proper AIDS care when, once again, poverty and lack of access to even the most rudimentary medical care were far more likely to determine the efficacy of AIDS screening and prevention efforts than were purely clinical issues. In rural Africa as in rural Haiti, stigma is less a barrier to providing AIDS care than it is the reflection and result of a complete lack of decent health care for the poor. Stigma is a symptom of this grotesque failure but is often used as an excuse for further inaction. How often do we read, in the popular press, that stigma, rather than poor-quality services, slows HIV screening? Even today, a fundamental misunderstanding of stigma continues to hamper effective responses to the pandemic.

Among the other central lessons laid out in this book is the fact that the mechanisms by which poverty and other social injustices, such as racism and gender inequality, hasten the advance of HIV and tuberculosis are knowable. Indeed, we can understand them by linking a geographically broad and historically deep analysis both to ethnographic knowledge and to an understanding of the epidemiology of infectious disease. The more that social inequalities constrain individual agency, the faster HIV spreads. Also, at the time I wrote this book, the epidemic was changing rapidly before my eyes, as were social conditions in Haiti, so a processual approach, one alive to change, seemed to be the right way to understand a new disease rooted in long-standing conditions. This book closes with a call for an "anthropology of human suffering."

Perhaps these ideas sound like exactly the sort of thing a graduate student would write in a doctoral thesis, and *AIDS and Accusation* is indeed a revised and shortened dissertation. But although I could have presented these insights more elegantly, they remain valid. As some of us turn our attention, however tardily, to the poorer reaches of Africa, we learn that social conditions shape not only the epidemic itself but also social responses to it. I dared to make a few predictions at the end of this book, fairly obvious ones at the time, and I can say without triumph that they have come true. Here is how I concluded *AIDS and Accusation:*

> [I]f a disaster is to be averted in rural Haiti, vigorous and effective prevention campaigns must be initiated at once. And although such efforts must begin, the prospects of stopping the steady march of HIV are slim. AIDS is far more likely to join a host of other sexually transmitted diseases—including gonorrhea, syphilis, genital herpes, chlamydia, hepatitis B, lymphogranuloma venereum, and even cervical cancer—that have already become entrenched among the poor.

Alas, HIV, unknown in rural Haiti in 1983 (the date of my first visit to the village I call Do Kay in this book) and indeed in most parts of the world, including rural Africa, did become the world's leading infectious cause of adult death. Tuberculosis, a completely curable disease, has now dropped to second place, and is, as in Haiti, the leading cause of death among Africans living with AIDS.

I certainly take no pleasure in pointing out that a geographically broad and historically deep examination of the nascent pandemic in the 1980s showed that this disaster would occur unless vigorous and fundamentally structural interventions took place. Of course, nothing of the sort happened. Not until better treatment for these diseases was put in place and integrated with AIDS prevention did the Haitian epidemic begin to come under control. As I write this, the Haitian epidemic is at last shrinking, a major victory for public health in one of the most poverty-stricken countries on the planet.[1]

I've spent much of the past two decades studying these infectious killers. To be frank, however, I was never asked, in Haiti or in any of the other places in which we work (more on who "we" are in a second), to do much in the way of *studying* suffering. In fact, I cannot remember a single such invitation from patients or their families. Instead, we were inundated in Haiti and elsewhere with a different sort of request: to *do* something to allay the awful suffering associated with these infectious diseases and with the host of other problems—hunger, malaria, death during childbirth, mistreatment at the hands of the powerful or less impoverished—that people afflicted with the new disease, AIDS, had long faced.

Partners In Health, a nongovernmental organization seeking to put into practice the conviction that health care is a human right, was born in the village of Do Kay and is rooted in the experiences and years of work described in *AIDS and Accusation*. To make a long story short—and these past two decades have felt very long—the years described in the processual ethnography in this book led me to contemplate some hard choices. On the one hand, a life of careful scholarship requires all one's attention, and no graduate student can afford to lose deep respect for careful scholarship; indeed, every graduate student has been the direct beneficiary of one or more mentors who have dedicated their lives to careful scholarship and teaching. On the other hand, one can choose a life of service and make common cause with people struggling under heavy burdens of poverty, AIDS, tuberculosis, malaria, and other causes of "stupid deaths," to use the Haitian term. At the time of this book's publication, this latter choice seemed both geographically and pragmatically remote from a research university like Harvard, an institution that had already afforded me an excellent education and was now prepared to offer the promise of a rewarding teaching career.

I've called these choices "hard." They do not have the gravity of those made each day by people living in poverty and facing the threat of disease and hunger and violence. But these decisions, mine and my coworkers', felt hard at the time and still do. Anyone who has spanned the worlds of the rich (any first-world university qualifies as such) and the poor (of which Haiti and Rwanda are extreme examples) knows exactly what I mean.

Of course, no one wants to make choices that will restrict one's contributions, least of all a young physician whose doctoral thesis was transformed into a book well received by students and colleagues. But I feared, even as I finished correcting the proofs of *AIDS and Accusation,* that I would not be able to do a good job in both these arenas. I was completing an internship in internal medicine and, when not in Haiti, working well over eighty hours a week in a Harvard teaching hospital. During the same time, Partners In Health and its Haitian sister organization, Zanmi Lasante, had founded a large clinic in Do Kay and were working to build a proper hospital. I also knew that none of the people we served in Haiti would ever read my book, even upon its later translation into French, the language of Haiti's colonizers but not the language of our patients and neighbors.

I've since learned that many young scholars, especially medical anthropologists who, in their study, gaze down steep gradients of class and privilege, face similar dilemmas upon returning from fieldwork. But not many scholars are also physicians, though other avenues of service are open to them. The hard choices I made were to some extent made for me by the dreadful conditions in rural Haiti, conditions that are similar to those here in rural Rwanda. So I chose to serve primarily as a physician and activist on behalf of the destitute sick. Unexpectedly, I found that, thanks to my former teachers and current colleagues at Harvard Medical School, I could, if at times barely, remain engaged in both scholarship and direct service to the people described in this book. The ethnographic and bibliographic research that went into *AIDS and Accusation* served me well, certainly, in helping to provide decent medical care in Haiti. It also led me to new research questions and helped me teach hundreds of medical students and physicians, which I have done with great satisfaction since joining the faculty of Harvard Medical School upon graduating in 1990. One of the questions I hear most often from medical students is a simple and honest one: what can we do?

What Is To Be Done?

Partners In Health was, to some extent, born of the opportunity to study and reflect upon an emerging epidemic that collided with other catastrophes long in the making in central Haiti. My colleagues and I have worked there since the first months chronicled in this book; we·have also grown and had the privilege of caring for more than a million patients in places as far-flung as Peru, Siberia, Chiapas, Guatemala, inner-city Boston, and now rural Rwanda.[2] Our choices about where to work were responses to a constant nagging voice, with a distinctly Haitian accent as I hear it, that says, "Don't just study our suffering—do something to allay it."

But, as my students ask, do what, exactly? This question is difficult but not impossible to answer. At the end of the period I describe in this book, no effective antiretroviral therapies existed to treat AIDS. But much could be done to prevent HIV transmission, so we launched "culturally appropriate prevention campaigns," which are described elsewhere.[3] And each of the opportunistic infections that afflicted those with AIDS, often killing them, could be countered with therapies known to be effective. In Haiti, as in Africa, the main such infection is tuberculosis. So the response to "do what?" in that instance was to start an effective tuberculosis control program in rural Haiti. That's precisely what we did. As a result, we saw cure rates go from less than 50 percent to close to universal cure among patients for whom all social barriers to obtaining care—from hunger to user fees, lack of water, and lack of transportation—were removed. Scholarship also had work to do in this area, since we encountered no shortage of silliness—again, immodest claims of causality—among people attempting to explain, without alluding to the concept of neglect, why so many people died in places like Haiti from an eminently treatable disease such as tuberculosis.[4] The ranking explanation among Haitian and certain non-Haitian health professionals was that the peasants believed in sorcery and thus had no confidence in biomedicine. We learned, instead, that rural Haitians had no access to biomedicine and that they did just fine, regardless of their views on disease etiology, once we fixed the dysfunctional tuberculosis program. What needed to change was not the cultural beliefs of the patients but rather the quality of the tuberculosis program—and with it, perhaps, the cultural beliefs of part of the medical community.

Even as I was completing this book, my colleagues and I were publishing, in medical journals, our experiences of setting up a community-based program to bring *all* tuberculosis patients to cure.[5] A significant number of these tuberculosis patients were also infected with HIV, but we found that they, too, did well once they received treatment for their tuberculosis, enjoying cure rates almost as high as those for patients not co-infected with HIV. But eventually, even after their tuberculosis was declared cured, patients infected with HIV would fall ill and die of other opportunistic infections or become ill again with tuberculosis. What could we do for them?

By 1995, ample evidence existed that antiretroviral "drug cocktails"—ARVs—could transform the formerly fatal affliction of AIDS into a manageable chronic disease. But although these drugs rapidly transformed the epidemic in the United States, cutting mortality dramatically and almost wiping out mother-to-child transmission and thus pediatric AIDS, the drugs were nonexistent in the poor world where AIDS was having its greatest impact. People knew that treatment existed, but the drugs were unavailable to those who couldn't pay top dollar for them. Although we were never swayed much by arguments that prevention alone was the only "sustainable" intervention in settings riven by poverty, we were unable to acquire ARVs until 1998. Too little, too late, we thought, but we pressed on.

When our small organization decided to import these medications to treat the sickest AIDS patients in central Haiti, the cost of the drugs exceeded $1500 per patient per year—even though we benefited from concessional prices and some donated medicines. This amount was and remains roughly six times the per capita income there. But while we, and many of our patients in Haiti, despaired about lagging behind, we discovered that Partners In Health was probably the first group working in the poorest parts of the world to introduce modern AIDS care as a public good—free of charge to the patient, as is tuberculosis care.[6] We based our policy on a simple premise: these people are sick, we're health care providers, and these medications are part of the same global economy that, after all, created Haiti as a slave colony to provide Europe with sugar, coffee, and other tropical produce. But we also reasoned that if AIDS had become the leading infectious cause of adult death in Haiti, it was also a public-health challenge (to Haiti and to the rest of the world), and authorities needed to view prevention and treatment as a public good, not merely as commodities that only those with resources could purchase.

The introduction of antiretroviral therapy to a squatter settlement in rural Haiti—in a sense the epilogue to the story told in *AIDS and Accusation*—provoked radically different responses in different quarters. Rural Haiti largely greeted our efforts with gratitude and even cheers, and the growing number of people within Partners In Health were confident that we were doing the right thing, even though paying for the drugs initially accounted for about 90 percent of all program costs. But in circles often mistakenly called "the international community," including some people with an avowed interest in the health of the poor, cheering was not forthcoming. These parties greeted the use of ARVs in places like rural Haiti or Africa with skepticism—deeming such projects wasteful and neither "sustainable" nor "cost-effective" in the paradigms of our day—and sometimes even derided the treatment programs as irresponsible. I am still struck, some twenty years after I learned to listen to patients and to people living in poverty, that such criticisms come not from the intended beneficiaries but rather from people with backgrounds more akin to mine. The critics at the time were professionals from North America or Europe or officials in poor countries who had been trained in the affluent world. They had accepted, as rural Haitians would not, the notion that the poor world would remain poor and that people so unfortunate as to be born into poverty were out of luck when it came to receiving expensive but effective AIDS therapy.

This view changed as underfunded prevention strategies failed in much of the poor world, as new infections continued to multiply (in more or less the manner predicted in this book), and as AIDS mortality continued to climb. Many millions died unattended long after wealthy nations had shown that ARVs could suppress HIV in their patient populations; millions more are dying today wherever AIDS is prevalent but AIDS treatment is not. The need for urgent interventions is certainly evident to anyone who spends time in places like Haiti or Rwanda. Many others have tried to document "the race to treat AIDS," as one writer termed the phenomenon, and I won't try to do so here.[7] But I will say that Partners In Health continued to share its experiences in integrating AIDS prevention and care with the medical and health-policy "community" in articles and in countless presentations and conferences—it would be impossible to tally the number of conferences held during those long years of inaction. Moreover, by 2001 the "we" of Partners In Health was growing quickly, in part because so few other groups were pursuing a social-justice agenda in introducing the highest possible standard of care for people living with both AIDS and poverty, and in part because the project was expanding rapidly—"scaling up"—in central Haiti. In every village we visited, we met people dying of AIDS, but we also met plenty of people anxious to serve as *accompagnateurs* who could help the afflicted by giving them their pills and social support each day.[8] When effective therapy became available, stigma, the topic of much of *AIDS and Accusation* and the factor that many policy makers believed was a barrier to effective care in Africa and Haiti, began to decline. Tens of thousands of people came to our clinics to be tested, knowing that they would receive care if we found them to be sick. In scaling up the effort we had launched in Do Kay, we learned that one can deliver high-quality health care in rural central Haiti, which lacks both paved roads and electricity and whose public-health system long ago faltered and collapsed.

Indeed, Haiti and Haitians, who suffered greatly from social responses to the new and then-untreatable disease with which they were initially identified, can also claim to have led the charge against AIDS. They have launched some of the poor world's first integrated prevention-and-care programs. Over the past few years, these efforts have not gone unnoticed. The policy makers who had earlier declared that prevention alone would have to suffice in settings as poor as Haiti had to modify their positions, not so much because the model in Haiti proved to be effective but because models that ignored treatment proved to be ineffective. In 2003, a new funding mechanism, the Global Fund to Fight AIDS, Tuberculosis, and Malaria, allowed Haiti to ramp up long-standing efforts to prevent new infections and to improve care for the sick; U.S. federal funds eventually followed. Even as some poor nations seemed ready to concede defeat in the struggle against AIDS, Haiti could point to real victories. Laurie Garrett, writing in the *New York Times* in July 2004, noted that "a new Global Fund report shows that of the 25 projects supported by the fund for more than a year, 80 percent have already either achieved or even surpassed their five-year goals. As chaotic as it is, Haiti surpassed its 2006 targets after only a year of Global Fund support."[9] A more detailed article in the *New York Times,* based on reporting from Do Kay, announced in its title "Rural Haitians are Vanguard in AIDS Battle."[10]

Here in Rwanda, in the rural reaches of the world's poorest continent, some responses to the idea of integrating AIDS prevention and care were much the same as the global authorities' initial responses to the idea of treating AIDS in Haiti. Once again, we heard claims that stigma would prevent Rwandans from coming to clinics to be tested, but these claims were not supported by data. In Africa, as in Haiti, AIDS is stigmatized because it is a fatal wasting disease, but stigma did not prevent thousands of Rwandans from seeking care once it was finally available. In Rwinkwavu, a town said to consist mostly of former exiles and people displaced by the 1994 genocide, hundreds have undergone screening for HIV infection in the past few months alone. Many of the people we found to be infected are now on proper therapy, again with the help of *accompagnateurs.* Indeed, veterans of the Haiti scale-up effort, which has long been led by a dynamic and experienced Haitian physician, came to rural Rwanda to help train *accompagnateurs* and nurses to build a similar project in the Rwandan countryside.

Haiti and Rwanda are about the same size, and both countries crowd more than eight million people into a mountainous area about the size of Maryland. Most inhabitants, in both places, are or have been peasant farmers. However, when we began work in Rwanda, I quickly realized the lack of cultural similarities between rural Rwanda and rural Haiti; indeed, my Haitian colleagues needed translators to speak with the rural Rwandans, who spoke Kinyarwanda and not French. The similarities of note were of the structural sort: deep poverty, a history of postcolonial violence, and about the same burden of disease (with AIDS, tuberculosis, malaria, and hunger heading the list).

Although the Haitian AIDS epidemic is unrelated to the African pandemic in the direct ways that the popular press asserted in the 1980s, the two epidemics do have striking parallels. The first AIDS case in Rwanda was detected in 1983, while the first cases were properly documented in Haiti in 1981, at the same time as the first cases in the United States.

Rates of infection are about the same in both places. Tuberculosis is also the ranking opportunistic infection in Rwanda. And here, as in Haiti, great local enthusiasm exists for scaling up an integrated AIDS prevention-and-care program.

Given my training in anthropology, I know better than to claim that I have any knowledge of Rwandan culture until I'm conversant in the language and have spent at least a couple of years here. But I'm already convinced that a "geographically broad and historically deep" approach to learning will teach us about the relationship between AIDS (as well as other epidemics) and heavy-handed colonialism, poverty, violence, and genocide. I'm convinced, too, that the more we learn, the more we will see how Rwanda fits into a transnational web of meaning and social process, as does Haiti. Granted, Haiti's trials at the hands of the outside world have lasted about five times longer than those that Rwanda has endured; granted, too, Haiti's indigenous population was exterminated completely after the Europeans arrived in 1492, and almost all Haitians today are descendants of kidnapped Africans. But I've little doubt that significant connivance by the great powers was required to arm Rwanda prior to the 1994 genocide; I'm confident that growing social inequality in a field of great social scarcity played a role in both the violence and the spread of HIV here. And in Rwanda, as in Haiti, poverty will constitute the most daunting barrier to the establishment of effective AIDS prevention and care.

Grappling with the New Myths and Mystifications about AIDS in Africa

Here in rural Rwanda and in central Haiti, I still encounter little demand for book-length studies of AIDS or social responses to it. But that need is real, and I'm grateful to have had the chance, at least once, to spend several years working to unravel the complex skein of meaning and social process and epidemiology. Allow me to close these reflections by returning to the role of scholarship and by considering some of the analytic challenges facing those who will confront the so-called new AIDS—new because, as noted in *AIDS and Accusation,* the epidemic changes rapidly, as do social responses to it, as does, we now know, the virus itself. Once again, we need processual studies, and these studies must be properly biosocial because one of the reasons the epidemic in Africa is changing is the fact that ARVs are at last becoming available here where the need is greatest. I still believe that perhaps only anthropology has the scope to understand this complex disease, but ethnographic studies will be accurate only if anthropologists work with others familiar with the pathophysiology and epidemiology of AIDS and of other infectious pathogens. Ethnographic studies will be accurate only if they rest on a sound knowledge of history and political economy.

Many studies similar to *AIDS and Accusation,* with AIDS in Africa as their topic, have been published recently, but much remains to be done. Surely, enterprising graduate students in medical anthropology would find a rich subject in the myths and mystifications swirling around Africa today, during this period that should be the postantibiotic era but isn't yet. Across the continent, most of the people infected with HIV are not "living with AIDS," to use the American catch phrase. They are dying of AIDS.

Yet Africans everywhere know that medications exist to treat AIDS and tuberculosis (and, indeed, malaria and each of the pathologies mentioned in this book). So we see in Africa, as in Haiti, accusations and blame, myths and mystifications. If Haitians have any rivals in their degree of subjection to racist and ridiculous commentaries, or to immodest claims of causality from experts who should know better, they exist here on this continent.

We can identify some of the most pernicious myths and half-truths, especially those serving to explain inaction. People say that the medications are too expensive, which is true. But is this statement the beginning of a conversation or the end of one? In Haiti and elsewhere, the introduction of generic ARVs has lowered the price of a three-drug cocktail from about $10,000 per patient per year (the U.S. price tag for branded pharmaceuticals) or $1,500 per patient per year (the concessional price we paid in 1998) to less than $150 per patient per year. And the prices are still dropping. Surely this welcome and vertiginous drop should make economists and public-health specialists who claim that treatment is not cost-effective a little more humble. How can we make confident claims about cost-effectiveness when both the cost and the "effectiveness" of our interventions change so rapidly?

Even if we agree that AIDS care is a right, there are significant challenges. We need to understand that as long as these medications remain commodities on the open market, they will be available only to those who can afford them. Regardless of how low the costs go, there will always be those who cannot pay. For those interested in health as a human right, selling ARVs will always pose problems.

Experts point out that the poorer parts of Africa lack the public-health infrastructure to treat AIDS. This statement too is true. But, again, is it the end of a discussion of the disastrous impact of divesting from public health, or is it the beginning of one about building or rebuilding such infrastructures in the places that need them most? In Haiti, we've shown that investing in integrated AIDS prevention and care can strengthen faltering public-health systems and improve women's health, tuberculosis and vaccination programs, and primary care.[11] If recent statements about the lack of health-care infrastructure are the beginning of a long-overdue conversation, we will soon realize that one of the most important components of such infrastructure — personnel — is readily available. Unemployment is high in the places that need AIDS treatment the most, and many people can be trained to be *accompagnateurs* or community health workers; their engagement will ensure that the quality of long-term care is sustained and improved. An honest discussion about the "brain drain" that sucks trained medical personnel out of Africa to more affluent settings in Europe and North America would also be welcome.[12]

Meanwhile, some people complain that AIDS-related stigma in Africa is overwhelming. This statement too is true. But, as we learned in Haiti, stigma is not often a barrier to actual AIDS treatment; rather, proper AIDS treatment, and indeed quality medical care for any affliction, is simply unavailable to the poor. Social barriers are, in truth, economic barriers, and these barriers will not be addressed by patient education or other attempts to change the patients rather than to change their social conditions. Empty clinics and testing centers suddenly fill up when user fees are dropped and quality services become available to the poor.

Poverty is also at the heart of many of the problems facing those who seek to prevent mother-to-child transmission of HIV. We have been assured, often by "experts," that the highest standard of care — ARVs during pregnancy and avoidance of breastfeeding after parturition — is impossible in Africa for the obvious reason (that children who do not breastfeed are at risk of gastroenteritis if clean water is unavailable) but also because bottle-feeding will stigmatize mothers. Our experience in rural Rwanda has already taught us that, as real as the challenges of clean water are, little evidence exists that stigma will prevent us from launching ambitious programs that prevent babies from ingesting HIV-positive breast milk. In fact, we discovered quickly that some poor women borrowed their neighbors' children or claimed to be infected with HIV in order to receive the meager assistance — powdered milk, a kerosene stove to boil water, and a modest stipend for school fees — that our "AIDS program" offers in the Rwinkwavu area. The challenges to efforts to prevent mother-to-child transmission of HIV are, rather, of a different order: avoiding stock-out of formula; reaching the poorest women; increasing access to reliably clean water.

Debates about what is to be done in Africa rage on. Some authorities continue to tell us to focus solely on prevention in the poorest countries, as if treatment and prevention somehow contradict each other. In fact, plenty of evidence is emerging that good treatment can strengthen prevention efforts.[13] Others have admonished us to focus solely on tuberculosis, which, unlike AIDS, is a curable disease. But these two chronic infectious diseases are tightly intertwined in Africa, and we focus on only one at the peril of our patients and the public at large. HIV-infected patients with tuberculosis will one day fall ill again, sometimes with a second case of tuberculosis (whether from relapse or from reinfection), and they will continue to expose those around them to this airborne disease, rendering tuberculosis control more and more difficult. This dynamic explains why rates of tuberculosis have skyrocketed across much of Africa during the past decade.

Other experts raise the spectre of resistance to ARVs in Africa in order to slow down introduction of the medications. But any student of social behavior knows that this ploy is as wrongheaded as it is unethical. Throughout the world, people living with HIV want to stop dying of AIDS; their loved ones want them to survive. These families will sell their scant belongings to buy ARVs in a haphazard, off-and-on way. Intermittent access to these drugs is one of the quickest ways to fan an epidemic of drug-resistant HIV, as we have learned in the United States and elsewhere. Again, removing AIDS care from the market and putting it into the public domain—a public good for public health—is the smartest and most humane way to slow the emergence of acquired drug resistance, a problem with almost every infectious disease for which a treatment is available. And if AIDS is not the ranking public-health threat in much of Africa, what is?

I have described just a few of the major analytic challenges now before us, and few of them have been addressed in a properly biosocial fashion. If today one cannot easily argue that ARVs cannot be used in the poorest parts of the world—a major victory for the afflicted and those who stand in solidarity with them—confused debates nonetheless continue to waste precious time. We should brace ourselves for the next great wave of debate, which will undoubtedly focus on what the modern world owes the destitute sick. If AIDS care becomes a right rather than a commodity, some people believe we will open a Pandora's box. Others, including me, believe that we have no more excuses for ignoring the growing inequality that has left hundreds of millions of people without any hope of surviving preventable and treatable illnesses. These hundreds of millions are the same people who entered the new millennium without access to clean water, primary education, proper housing, and decent jobs. Taking on AIDS forcefully would allow us to start a "virtuous social cycle," long overdue, a process that might begin with one disease but end with a lot less inhumanity directed towards others with whom we share this fragile planet.

Rwinkwavu, Rwanda
September 2005

1. UNAIDS/World Health Organization, *AIDS Epidemic Update 2005* (Geneva: World Health Organization, 2005), available online at http://www.who .int/hiv/epiupdate2005/en/.

2. For a description of Partners In Health, see chapter 1 of *Infections and Inequalities* (Farmer 1999); see also www.pih.org.

3. We have described these programs in optimistic terms, probably in large part because obtaining financing was so hard in the early days. See, for example, Farmer (1997) and Farmer and Kim (1997); for a more critical review of these programs, see Farmer and Walton (2000). Note that the later essay, though published in 2000, was written just as we were beginning to scale up ARV therapy in central Haiti, an effort that led quickly to improved prevention outcomes.

4. These "immodest claims of causality" for tuberculosis and AIDS care are the chief topic of *Infections and Inequalities* (1999).

5. See Farmer et al. (1991).

6. The concept of "public goods for public health" is explored in Kim et al. (2003).

7. See, for example, Anne-Christine d'Adesky's (2004) engaging account of the spread of HIV to the poorest parts of the world and her description of attempts, including ours, to introduce proper AIDS care as a human right.

8. *Accompagnateurs* are almost always neighbors of patients—some of them patients themselves—who accept responsibility for supervising daily care and support for people suffering from AIDS or tuberculosis; they are trained by Partners In Health staff and are the cornerstone of our projects in Haiti, Peru, Boston, Rwanda, and elsewhere. This strategy for treating AIDS in areas now termed "resource-poor settings" is described in a number of papers in the med-

ical literature. See, for example, Farmer et al. (2001a), Farmer et al. (2001b), and Behforouz et al. (2004).

9. Laurie Garrett, "Bragging in Bangkok," *New York Times,* 16 July 2004, p. 21.

10. Celia Dugger, "Rural Haitians Are Vanguard in AIDS Battle," *New York Times,* 30 November 2004, p. 1.

11. See Walton et al. (2004).

12. We've also sought to address this issue in considering the social barriers to proper care for AIDS and other epidemic diseases; see Walton et al. (2005). For more on burnout among African physicians in a Kenyan teaching hospital, which admits hundred of patients dying of AIDS and tuberculosis but cannot care for them properly, see Raviola et al. (2002).

13. See, for example, Blower and Farmer (2003).

SUPPLEMENTAL BIBLIOGRAPHY

Behforouz, Heidi, Paul Farmer, and Joia Mukherjee
2004   From Directly Observed Therapy to *Accompagnateurs:* Enhancing
        AIDS Treatment Outcomes in Haiti and in Boston. *Clinical Infec-
        tious Diseases* 38(S5):S429-S436.
Blower, Sally, and Paul Farmer
2003   Predicting the Public Health Impact of Antiretrovirals: Preventing
        HIV in Developing Countries. *AIDScience* 3(11): www.aidscience
        .org/Articles/AIDScience033.asp.
d'Adesky, Anne-Christine
2004   *Moving Mountains: The Race to Treat Global AIDS.* London: Verso.
Farmer, Paul
1997   Ethnography, Social Analysis, and the Prevention of Sexually
        Transmitted HIV Infection. In *The Anthropology of Infectious Dis-
        ease,* M.C. Inhorn and P.J. Brown, eds., pp. 413–38. Amsterdam:
        Gordon and Breach.
1999   *Infections and Inequalities: The Modern Plagues.* Berkeley: Univer-
        sity of California Press.
Farmer, Paul, and David Walton
2000   Condoms, Coups, and the Ideology of Prevention: Facing Failure
        in Rural Haiti. In *Catholic Ethicists on HIV/AIDS Prevention,*
        J.F. Keenan, L. Sowle-Cahill, J. Fuller, and K. Kelly, eds., pp.
        108–19. New York: Continuum Publishing Group.
Farmer, Paul, Fernet Léandre, Joia Mukherjee, Marie Sidonise Claude, Patrice
Nevil, Mary Catherine Smith Fawzi, Serena Koenig, Arachu Castro, Mercedes
Becerra, Jeffrey Sachs, Amir Attaran, and Jim Yong Kim
2001   Community-Based Approaches to HIV Treatment in Resource-
        Poor Settings. *Lancet* 358(9279):404–9.
Farmer, Paul, Fernet Léandre, Joia Mukherjee, Raj Gupta, Laura Tarter, and Jim
Yong Kim
2001   Community-Based Treatment of Advanced HIV Disease: Intro-
        ducing DOT-HAART (Directly Observed Therapy with Highly
        Active Antiretroviral Therapy). *Bulletin of the World Health Organi-
        zation* 79(12):1145–51.
Kim, Jim Yong, Aaron Shakow, Arachu Castro, Chris Vanderwarker, and Paul
Farmer
2003   Tuberculosis Control. In *Global Public Goods for Health: Health Eco-
        nomics and Public Health Perspectives,* R. Smith, R. Beaglehole, D.
        Woodward, and N. Drager, eds., pp. 54–72. New York: Oxford
        University Press for the World Health Organization.
Raviola, Guiseppe, M'Imunya Machoki, Esther Mwaikambo, and Mary Jo
DelVecchio Good
2002   HIV, Disease Plague, Demoralization and "Burnout": Resident
        Experience of the Medical Profession in Nairobi, Kenya. *Culture,
        Medicine, and Psychiatry* 26(1):55–86.

Walton, David, Paul Farmer, Wesler Lambert, Fernet Léandre, Serena Koenig, and Joia Mukherjee
  2004   Integrated HIV Prevention and Care Strengthens Primary Health Care: Lessons from Rural Haiti. *Journal of Public Health Policy* 25(2):137–58.
Walton, David, Paul Farmer, and Rebecca Dillingham
  2005   Social and Cultural Factors in Tropical Medicine: Reframing Our Understanding of Disease. In *Tropical Infectious Diseases: Principles, Pathogens, and Practice* (2nd ed.), R. L. Guerrant, D. H. Walker, and P. F. Weller, eds., pp. 26–35. Edinburgh: Churchill Livingstone.

Preface to the First Edition

When he was merely a persecuted priest, Haitian President Jean-Bertrand Aristide wrote of the "unending goodness" of poor Haitians "in unimportant matters as well as [in] the gravest issues." In a setting of near-total illiteracy, it is difficult to claim that a scholarly book could be a grave issue. I must therefore thank my Haitian hosts for helping me to attend to what could only seem to be a relatively unimportant matter—a book written in English. That a non-Haitian physician/anthropologist would find himself writing a book about AIDS in Haiti is largely an accident of what might be clumsily termed historically produced social arrangements. The evolution of these arrangements and their relation to AIDS are subjects treated in considerable detail in this study, which attempts to examine current ethnographic and epidemiologic data from a historical perspective. This approach has generated some disagreement about the place of historical materials in a consideration of a thoroughly modern epidemic.

During the editorial process, the non-Haitian readers of this book felt that the history section, Part IV, could be radically abridged or cut out altogether. Haitian readers felt these chapters should stay. In the end, preserving the historical chapters became something of a sticking point, as a central thesis of the book is that the world pandemic of AIDS and social responses to it have been patterned by the social arrangements described in the historical chapters. But there was a second, more important reason for keeping these chapters: if there has been, among my informants, any consensus about the meaning of AIDS, it has been that the biological and social effects of this new scourge have to be examined in the light of past misfortunes. In many ways, then, this study is largely a *juxtaposition* of a recent and still unfolding process—the AIDS epidemic—and a sympathetic reading of the historical trajectory of the Haitian people.

A second prefatory note concerns Haiti and the origins of AIDS. As a U.S.-trained physician, it is clear to me that, even today, many health professionals have distorted views about AIDS and Haiti. These distortions are even more grotesque among the lay public, as many North Americans still believe that AIDS came to the United States from Haiti, and not vice versa. My rebuttal to this frequently encountered view about the provenance of HIV, which is informed by clinical and historical evidence, may come as unwelcome news to some. The virus itself is unwelcome, all the more so for being mysterious in its origin. The reader will, I hope, understand that my purpose in charting the social as well as biological movements of this virus is not in the least to add to the cycles of accusation and counteraccusation chronicled here. It is nonetheless important to set the record straight by correcting widely held misperceptions about AIDS and Haitians. What data exist do not support the thesis that HIV reached North America from Haiti.

Questions will arise, inevitably, about the methodologies underpinning this study. The analysis presented here was based on years of participant-observation, the central methodology of ethnographic fieldwork. Not all readers will be interested in the methodological and ethical questions posed by fieldwork conducted among the very poor and in the midst of an epidemic, and I have to a large extent relegated such discussion to journal articles and book chapters (for example, Farmer 1990a, 1991a). Other major methodological issues discussed concern the means by which it is possible, through serial interviews, to trace emerging meanings of AIDS (Farmer 1990c). Broader statements about AIDS and the constitution of an anthropology of suffering have also been elaborated (Farmer 1988a, Farmer and Kleinman 1989), as has an extended discussion of the significance of AIDS vis-à-vis the subfield of medical anthropology (Farmer and Good 1991). Further, as physician-anthropologists concerned with the prevention and treatment of infectious disease, we have discussed these ethnographic data in the context of pragmatic efforts to prevent HIV transmission (Farmer and Kim 1991; Farmer, Robin, Ramilus, and Kim 1991).

Finally, I must acknowledge the debts accrued in the course of conducting this research and writing this book. I risk a hackneyed gesture by beginning a long list of acknowledgments with a solemn thank-you to the people of "Do Kay." It is difficult to find words to express the admiration I feel for those who have suffered with dignity and still remain warm to one who represents, after all, the source of no small amount of their travail. Formal acknowledgment is due the MacArthur Foundation, whose generous support made it possible for me to pursue training in both medicine and anthropology. I am also grateful to Harvard Medical School, which twice subventioned my research in rural Haiti. Less formal, more affectionate thanks to Fritz and Yolande Lafontant, who encouraged me when scholarly questions seemed somehow unimportant. Quite simply, this book would not have been written without them. Similarly, Thomas White not only supported Pròjè Veye Sante, the preventive health project in which I worked, but also offered moral support and technical assistance.

Peggy and Jennifer Farmer and, especially, Ophelia Dahl shared some of these fieldwork experiences with me. Ophelia helped me to understand a great deal about Haiti and I will always be grateful to her. Jean François and Lernéus Joseph have spent years working on Pròjè Veye Sante, and have themselves become proficient ethnographic fieldworkers. I thank, too, the many others who work on Pròjè Veye Sante. I will never forget our three coworkers felled by preventable or treatable diseases: Acéphie Lamontagne, Michelet Joseph, and Marie-Ange "Ti Tap" Joseph.

Several Haitian physicians have my respect and admiration. For their long years of fraternity and hope, I thank Ramilus St. Luc, Simon Robin, Ernst Calixte, and Maxi Raymonville. I am grateful to Marie-Marcelle Deschamps and Jean Pape, who have contributed to the international scientific community's understanding of AIDS. Even better, they have alleviated, with few resources and under poor conditions, the suffering of hundreds of their compatriots with AIDS.

More broad-ranging counsel was given by Steven Nachman and Haun Saussy. I am fortunate indeed to have their advice, and the rigor of their scholarship stands as a challenge to those of us who become sloppy when the heat is on. Allan Brandt, Leon Eisenberg, John Hines, Mariette Murphy, Jeffrey Parsonnet, Pauline Peters, Camille K. Rogers, Ricardo Sanchez, and Madeleine Wilson have provided insightful commentary on material presented here. Stylistic advice was given by Jennifer Farmer and, especially, Carla Fujimoto and Jenny Hall. Stanley Holwitz of the University of California Press encouraged me to transform my doctoral dissertation into a book.

Several Haitianists or Caribbeanists have commented on the ethnographic or historical portions of this book. Catherine Maternowska has been a supportive yet critical reader for years. Bicultural Ruth Berggren helped me to decipher key passages from difficult interviews, as did Jenny Hall. Rosemarie Chierici, *manman poul*, attempted to remove any errors that might embarrass me. Laennec Hurbon and Orlando Patterson offered encouragement and advice. I am also grateful for the insights provided by the members of the American Anthropological Association's Task Force on AIDS, most notably Shirley Lindenbaum, and to the AIDS and Anthropology Research Group.

It is an honor to acknowledge a great debt to Arthur Kleinman. His students know him as the principal architect of a community of scholars that take seriously the study of the social construction of illness—without losing sight of the sufferers. I am also indebted to Leon Eisenberg and members of the Department of Social Medicine at Harvard Medical School, where Kleinman and Eisenberg have created a haven for an eclectic group of physicians and social scientists. Byron Good and Mary-Jo DelVecchio Good are in a category apart. They have been for many of us exemplars of scholarship who count as their family the intellectual community they have helped to build. Sally Falk Moore accorded me encouragement when it was much needed, and also lent a certain theoretical legitimacy to a fieldwork style that was mandated as much by medical school as by intellectual concerns. I have also benefitted enormously from the friendship of Joan Gillespie and Rosemarie Bernard. Most of all, I thank Jim Yong Kim, who shares a concern not only for the theoretical issues posed by anthropology and medicine, but also for the moral dilemmas that face any North American academic who would venture into the "Third World." These are the members of my intellectual community.

I could not speak of community without reference to Roxbury, Massachusetts, and Do Kay, the two settings in which I have, with brief exception, spent the last decade. Jack, Mary, Katherine, Lucy, and Carola in the States, and Papa Frico, Mamito, Flore, Jeje, Ram, Simon, Poteau, Thérèse, Paulette, Marcelin, and Carnest in Haiti have made living in two places a feasible proposition. I now look to Tom, Jim, Jenny, Cathy, Todd, Guitèle, Jody, and others from Partners in Health, who have been in both places, to help me to live up to the exacting standards set by my own family. This book is dedicated to Virginia Farmer, to Katy, Jim, Jeff, Jen, Peggy, and, especially, to the memory of our father.

1

Introduction

The Exotic and the Mundane

At about 6 A.M. on June 26, 1982, Solange Eliodor expired in Jackson Memorial Hospital in Miami. When not in the hospital, the twenty-six-year-old Haitian refugee spent her final year in a rickety boat, which reached the shores of Florida the previous July, and in prison, as the reluctant ward of the U.S. Immigration and Naturalization Service (INS). The Dade County Medical Examiner denied that the young woman showed any signs of tuberculosis—"She didn't have it. Period."—although the INS had initially maintained otherwise. The medical examiner also said that "there was no sign the woman suffered a blow to the head," an allegation raised by the director of the Haitian Refugee Center. Other Haitians interned in the Krome Avenue INS detention facility may have been dealt blows to the head, but Solange Eliodor was not one of them. The verdict was toxoplasmosis of the brain, a parasitic infection that, though common, is usually rendered harmless by immune defenses. The woman's death merited a headline in the June 30 edition of the Miami *Herald*: "Krome Camp Detainee Died from Infection Transmitted by Cats."

The details of the entire grisly story—the flight from Haiti in a boat, INS detention, the newspaper headline, the mistaken accusations of both tuberculosis and a blow to the head—are of a piece with a single, if complicated, narrative. Early in the AIDS pandemic, a number of

1

Haitians, including Solange Eliodor, fell ill with opportunistic infections characteristic of the new syndrome. Some of the ill Haitians lived in urban Haiti; some had emigrated to the United States or Canada. Unlike most other patients meeting diagnostic criteria for AIDS, the Haitians diagnosed in the United States denied homosexual activity or intravenous drug use. Most had never had a blood transfusion. AIDS among Haitians was, in the words of North American researchers, "a complete mystery." In 1982, U.S. public health officials inferred that Haitians *per se* were in some way at risk for AIDS, and suggested that unraveling "the Haiti connection" would lead researchers to the culprit. In a sample of the melodramatic prose that came to typify commentary on Haitians with AIDS, one reporter termed the incidence of AIDS in Haitians "a clue from the grave, as though a zombie, leaving a trail of unwinding gauze bandages and rotting flesh, had come to the hospital's Grand Rounds to pronounce a curse" (Black, in Abbott 1988: 254–255).

The Haitian cases and subsequent "risk-grouping" spurred the publication of a wide range of theories purporting to explain the epidemiology and origins of AIDS. In December 1982, for example, a physician with the U.S. National Cancer Institute was widely quoted as announcing that "we suspect that this may be an epidemic Haitian virus that was brought back to the homosexual population in the United States."[1] This theory, although unbolstered by research, was echoed by other physicians and scientists investigating (or merely commenting on) AIDS. In North America and Europe, other commentators linked AIDS in Haiti to "voodoo practices." Something that went on around ritual fires, went the supposition, triggered AIDS in cult adherents, a category presumed to include the quasi-totality of Haitians. In the October 1983 edition of *Annals of Internal Medicine,* for example, physicians affiliated with the Massachusetts Institute of Technology related the details of a brief visit to Haiti and wrote, "It seems reasonable to consider voodoo practices a cause of the syndrome."[2]

Why, precisely, would it be "reasonable to consider voodoo practices as a cause of the syndrome"? Did existing knowledge of AIDS in Haiti make such a hypothesis reasonable? Had voodoo been previously associated with the transmission of other illnesses? Careful review of the scholarly literature on AIDS and on voodoo would lead us to answer these three questions with "No reason," "No," and "No." The persistence of these theories represents, in fact, a *systematic misreading* of existing epidemiologic and ethnographic data. But ideas about the Haitian cult seemed to resonate with emerging notions about AIDS. Such a resonance might have been predicted decades earlier: "Certain exotic words are charged with evocative power," wrote Alfred Métraux in 1959. "Voodoo is one. It usually conjures up visions of mysterious deaths, secret rites—or dark saturnalia celebrated by 'blood-maddened, sex-maddened, god-maddened' negroes" (Métraux 1972: 15).

Although further acquaintance with the syndrome made it difficult to posit a Haitian origin for AIDS, armchair theorists were reluctant to let go of voodoo altogether. The *Journal of the American Medical Association* published a consideration of these theories under the fey title, "Night of the Living Dead." Its author asks, "Do necromantic zombiists transmit HTLV-III/LAV during voodooistic rituals?" Tellingly, he cites as his source not the by then substantial scientific literature on AIDS in Haiti, but the U.S. daily press:

Even now, many Haitians are voodoo *serviteurs* and partake in its rituals (*New York Times*, May 15, 1985, pp. 1, 6). (Some are also members of secret societies such as Bizango or "impure" sects, called "cabrit thomazo," which are suspected to use human blood itself in sacrificial worship.) As the HTLV-III/LAV virus is known to be stable in aqueous solution at room temperature for at least a week, lay Haitian voodooists may be unsuspectingly infected with AIDS by ingestion, inhalation, or dermal contact with contaminated ritual substances, as well as by sexual activity. (Greenfield 1986:2200)

Social scientists were also seduced by the call of the wild. In a heroic effort to accommodate all the exotic furbelows available in the American folk model[3] of Haitians, the following scene is depicted by Moore and LeBaron (1986:81, 84): "In frenzied trance, the priest lets blood: mammal's [sic] throats are cut; typically, chicken's [sic] heads are torn off their necks. The priest bites out the chicken's tongue with his teeth and may suck on the bloody stump of the neck." These sacrificial offerings, "infected with one of the Type C oncogenic retroviruses, which is closely related to HTLV," are "repeatedly [sic] sacrificed in voodoo ceremonies, and their blood is directly ingested by priests and their assistants." The model is completed with the assertion that "many voodoo priests are homosexual men" who are "certainly in a position to satisfy their sexual desires, especially in urban areas."

Similarly lurid scenarios were taken up in the popular press, which drew upon readily available images of voodoo, animal (and even human) sacrifice, and boatloads of "disease-ridden" or "economic" refugees. Such articles had a considerable impact on Haiti, which once counted tourism as an important source of foreign currencies. But the AIDS association affected Haitians everywhere, especially those living in the United States and Canada. Gilman (1988a:102) might not be exaggerating when he suggests that "to be a Haitian and living in New York City meant that you were perceived as an AIDS 'carrier.'" Many of the million or so Haitians living in North America complained that speculations about a Haitian origin of AIDS had led to a wave of anti-Haitian discrimination.

What gradually became known about the new syndrome in Haiti seemed to have far less impact on popular and professional "AIDS discourse" than did preexisting conceptions of the place. The link between AIDS and Haiti seemed reminiscent of a North American folk model of Haitians. The contours of the model are suggested by a recent study of Haitians living in New York. It recalls the image Haitians found waiting for them when, in the 1970s, many emigrated to the United States: "Haitians were portrayed as ragged, wretched, and pathetic and were said to be illiterate, superstitious, disease-ridden and backward peasants" (Glick-Schiller and Fouron 1990:337). Historical study shows that Haiti has long been depicted as a strange and hopelessly diseased country remarkable chiefly for its extreme isolation from the rest of the civilized world. This erroneous depiction fuels the parallel process of "exotification" by which Haiti is rendered weird. According to a journalist writing in 1989 in *Vanity Fair,* "Haiti is to this hemisphere what black holes are to outer space." Or consider the epithet given Haiti by a U.S. news magazine: "A bazaar of the bizarre."[4] Over the past decade, AIDS has been incorporated into that folk model so that, now, AIDS is every bit as necessary as any of the preceding referents.

Fieldwork in Haiti, 1983–1990

This study is based in large part on fieldwork in rural Haiti. Although both the folk model about Haitians and the nature of AIDS-related discrimination against them could best be studied in North America, an interest in AIDS in Haiti mandated research on the island. HIV did not only affect Haiti indirectly, through the prejudices of North American scientists, employers, landlords, and tourists. In 1983, the country was in the first years of its own substantial AIDS epidemic. The featured topic of that year's conference of the Haitian

Medical Association was "the new syndrome." It was not clear at that time just what was causing AIDS, but many experts were already betting on a retrovirus that attacked the immune system, eventually rendering its host vulnerable to infectious agents. At the conference, several Haitian clinicians presented case material that put the quietus on any doubts whether or not the syndrome seen in Haiti was the same as that encountered in the urban United States. Clinical presentations, suggestive of immune deficiency and subsequent opportunistic infection, were often strikingly similar in these very disparate settings.

What was more striking, however, was the accusatory tone of much of the symposium. Blame and counterblame were a prominent part of these usually sober scientific gatherings. Haitian researchers claimed that North American physicians and scientists had erroneously painted Haiti as the source of the worldwide AIDS pandemic. The Haitian scholars asserted that such a hypothesis reflected North American racism, and countered that the syndrome had been brought to Haiti by tourists from the United States—and not *vice versa*, as had been claimed. Haitians were not "mysteriously" at risk for AIDS, they argued, documenting the role of international homosexual prostitution, bisexuality, and a contaminated blood supply in shaping the contours of the Haitian epidemic.[5]

The debates in Port-au-Prince soon made it to the front page of the *New York Times,* where the president of the Haitian Medical Association attacked the "unscientific and racist attitude" of epidemiologists from the U.S. Centers for Disease Control.[6] He was seconded not only by his colleagues on the island, but by hundreds of Haitian community leaders living in North America. Several deplored an epidemic not of AIDS, but of AIDS-related discrimination against Haitians. There were reports of American mothers who would not permit their children to attend school with Haitian-born students; of families "with black skin and French names" evicted from rented housing; of Haitian cab drivers who had learned to maintain that they were from Martinique or Guadeloupe (ironically, islands with higher AIDS attack rates than Haiti); of endless quests for jobs for which Haitian applicants were "just not right." Accusation, it was fast becoming clear, was a recurrent theme in debates born of the AIDS pandemic.

A similar dynamic would later be played out in the village of Do Kay, where the majority of the ethnographic research presented in this study was conducted. A community of fewer than 1,000 people, Do Kay stretches along an unpaved road that cuts north and east into

Haiti's central plateau. By the end of the summer of 1983, a careful survey had revealed that no one in Do Kay had AIDS. In fact, when I initiated research there the word *sida,* as AIDS was termed, was just beginning to work its way into the rural Haitian lexicon.[7] In Do Kay, illnesses are usually the topic of much discussion; *sida* was not. Some villagers had never heard of the disorder already held to be responsible for the ruin of the once important urban tourist industry; others had only vague ideas about causation or typical clinical presentation.

But HIV, the silent precursor of AIDS, was probably already present in Do Kay. If villagers were then aware of but uninterested in *sida,* interest in the illness was almost universal a scant three years later. By 1987, one of the villagers was dying from AIDS, and another was gravely afflicted. Further, ideas about the disorder and its origin had changed drastically. This was only to be expected. If no collective representation of *sida* existed in 1983, when the subject elicited little interest and no passion, it is not surprising that some sort of consensus began to emerge when what was at stake was nothing less than the life or death of a fellow villager. There resulted a profusion of illness stories; active debate about what constituted the key features of *sida,* its course, and its causes was suddenly the order of the day. These narratives substantially shaped nascent understandings of *sida,* and helped to place a new disorder in the context of much older understandings of sickness and misfortune.

And there had been plenty of sickness and misfortune in the area around Do Kay. Indeed, the advent of a new and fatal disease was, in the words of one who lives there, "the last thing." The last thing, that is, in a long series of trials that have afflicted the region's rural poor. When people from Do Kay speak of *sida,* it is quite often in the same breath as other afflictions, past and present, that have rendered life in rural Haiti a precarious enterprise. It is almost a cliché now to note that Haiti is "the poorest country in the hemisphere," and "one of the twenty-five poorest in the world." An officially reported per capita annual income of $315 in 1983 misrepresented the situation in the countryside, where it hovered around $50. Expert opinion on Haiti has long been given to grim assessments and dour predictions.

With each passing year, it seemed in rural Haiti that simple survival was becoming increasingly difficult. The years between 1983 and 1990 were dramatic ones in which to be doing fieldwork there. The advent of HIV was often upstaged, first by the popular revolt that in 1986 helped to bring down the Duvalier family dictatorship, in place for thirty years, and then by vicious efforts to repress an embryonic popular movement. The years following 1985 have been punctuated by six *coups d'état,* several politically motivated massacres, and the striking irruption of the previously silent poor. These years have been rife with the Machiavellian pronouncements of a diverse cast of characters including unreconstructed Duvalierists, returning exiles, and representatives of the United States embassy. As will become clear in the following chapters, these "large-scale" events and commentaries regularly impinged upon the lives of those living—and dying—in Do Kay.

Framing Analysis in Medical Anthropology

Caribbean ethnography has for decades been replete with reminders of the local effects of large-scale change, and Do Kay offers an extreme (if inapparent) example. During the rainy season, the journey from Port-au-Prince can take several hours, adding to the impression of isolation. That impression, however, is misleading. The village owes its existence to a project conceived of in the Haitian capital and drafted in Washington, D.C. Do Kay is actually a settlement of refugee peasant farmers displaced over thirty years ago by Haiti's largest hydroelectric dam. Before 1956, the village of Kay was situated in a fertile valley, near the banks of the Rivière Artibonite. For generations, these families had farmed the broad and gently sloping banks of the river, selling rice, bananas, millet, corn, and sugar cane in regional markets. Harvests were, by all reports, bountiful; life there is now recalled as idyllic.

After the valley was flooded, the majority of the local population was forced up into the hills on either side of the new reservoir. Kay became divided into "Do" (those who settled on the stony backs of the hills) and "Ba" (those who remained down near the new waterline). By all the standard demographic measures, both parts of Kay are now exceedingly poor; its older inhabitants often blame their poverty on the massive buttress dam a few miles away, and bitterly note that it brought them neither electricity nor water.

The study of affliction in Do Kay, the unintentional by-blow of a "development project," poses sharp questions about the ways in which analysis is framed in medical anthropology. As often as not, these afflictions speak of connections to the "outside world." HIV is no exception.

There is, first of all, the obvious fact that Haiti is part of an island. A virus (in a human host) must cross water and international boundaries to reach Haiti. Second, the residents of Do Kay who had fallen ill with AIDS had each lived in Port-au-Prince, and it was likely that they had been exposed to HIV there. Third, repercussions of the debates born of the risk-grouping of Haitians were being felt throughout Haiti. Fieldwork in the Kay area revealed, to my surprise, that the North American folk model had an effect on nascent Haitian understandings of *sida*, as did, more predictably, other explanatory frameworks long in place.

In fact, the advent of AIDS highlighted many important connections between Haiti and the United States. In March 1986, one of my rural informants often spoke of a cousin working in New York. Madame Jolibois, a poor market woman, recounted that her relative was "fired because she is Haitian. . . . They said she carried AIDS, which was not true. She had a test and it was negative, her blood was fine, but still they wouldn't give her back the job."[8] The loss of this job was experienced as a hardship and a humiliation for the woman living in New York. And it had several repercussions of which the cousin's employer will never be aware. This bad news was announced to Mme. Jolibois in a letter devoid of its usual contents: U.S. dollars. Within months, Mme. Jolibois's eldest daughter was obliged to drop out of school.

This book offers a theoretical argument for the best way of approaching the study of a new sickness in a world in which the loss of a job in New York can so drastically alter the life of a girl in a Haitian village. The ties that bind Haiti to urban North America have a historical basis, and they continue to change. These connections are economic and affective; they are political and personal. One reason this study of AIDS in rural Haiti returns again and again to urban Haiti and the United States is that the boundaries separating them are, at best, blurred. The AIDS pandemic is a striking reminder that even a village as "remote" as Do Kay is linked to a network that includes Port-au-Prince and Brooklyn, voodoo and chemotherapy, divination and serology, poverty and plenty. Indeed, the sexual transmission of HIV is as eloquent a testimony as any to the salience—and complicated intimacy—of these links. Often, the links are the manifestations of the large-scale forces of history and political economy not readily visible to the ethnographer (or physician) and yet crucial to an understanding of AIDS and social responses to it. It is the task of anthropology to underscore these interconnections and seek to bring into focus the effects of large-scale forces on settings like Do Kay.[9]

But what brand of anthropology is appropriate to the task? Ethnography will have a privileged position in any effort to understand a previously undescribed phenomenon, and a solid interpretive anthropology would stand the ethnographer in good stead. Few would dispute that AIDS has been charged with peculiarly dense and often contradictory meanings. At the outset, the study of AIDS *in* Haiti called for inquiry into the complex and charged terrain of sexuality. The subject was further enmeshed in the life-and-death politics of an impoverished nation in the throes of revolutionary turmoil. An investigation of AIDS *and* Haitians also examined rapidly changing social and cultural phenomena (for example, the evolving understanding of the causes of illness in a Haitian village), as well as the more slowly changing preexisting networks of meaning (for example, North American folk models of Haiti). An interpretive approach was clearly indispensable in order to investigate what Treichler (1988b) has termed "an epidemic of signification."

But it is equally clear that a thorough understanding of the AIDS pandemic demands a commitment to the concerns of history and political economy: HIV, it shall be shown, has run along the fault lines of economic structures long in the making.[10] Among the many research questions posed by the advent of AIDS in Haiti, several are of particular importance: How does one come to be "at-risk" of exposure to HIV in Haiti? What are the means by which HIV-related disorders came to be, in the space of a decade, a leading cause of death in Haiti, especially in urban areas? Even "interpretive" questions require a historical approach. If *sida* came to be integrated into long-standing ways of understanding illness, can historical research reveal anything about the development of these understandings? Will a time-conscious approach tell us much about the ways in which health and illness are socially constructed in rural Haiti? Will it tell us about social responses—including those registered in North America—to a new and deadly disorder?

These questions are addressed in this volume, in an attempt to comprehend an essentially new phenomenon—HIV and responses to it—as it is embedded in long-standing structures of meaning in which all novelty must take shape and from which the new must take meaning. Historical perspectives, especially those attuned to political economy, are useful when attempting to address such questions:

A look through the lens of history shows the way a people—a social group, a subculture, a community, or a whole country—is laid open by the course of important economic, political, and ideological changes to new perception, new patternings of behavior and belief, new ways of seeing what is happening to them. (Mintz 1960:253)

So it is with the village of Kay, and Mintz's expression "laid open" is apt. It captures both the violence and the vulnerability that characterize the life of Haitians, especially rural and poor Haitians. It is they who are the pawns in large development schemes, such as the one that suddenly inundated the houses and fields of Kay. And it is they and their urban kin who have fallen ill with a new illness that has moved along the fault lines of an international order linking them to such far-off cities as New York and Miami.

Neither the dam nor the AIDS epidemic would exist as they do today if Haiti had not been caught in a web of relations that are economic as well as sexual. That these conditions have been important in the lineaments of the American epidemics is suggested by comparing Haiti with a neighboring island. In 1986 in Cuba, only 0.01 percent of one million persons tested were found to have antibodies to HIV (Liautaud, Pape, and Pamphile 1988:690). Had the pandemic begun a few decades earlier, the epidemiology of HIV infection in the Caribbean might well have been different. Havana might have been as much an epicenter of the pandemic as Carrefour, the nexus of Haitian domestic and international prostitution.

Ethnography and the Anthropology of Suffering

The transmission of HIV also serves as a reminder that AIDS is embodied most literally in individual experience. At this writing, three villagers from Do Kay have been mortally afflicted with AIDS. Their experiences, their words, and the words of those who lived with them are important to the ethnographic portions of this study.[11] As Kleinman and Kleinman (1989:4) have recently observed, "Anthropological analyses (of pain and passion and power), when they are experience-distant, are at risk of delegitimating their subject matter's human conditions." In seeking to attend closely to the experience of persons with AIDS, one hears Manno, a young schoolteacher who had come to Do Kay from another village in the Central Plateau. Some time after learning that he had AIDS, he said of his disorder: "They tell me there's no cure. But I'm not sure of that. If you can find a cause, you can find a cure." Manno's search for a cause was the search for the enemies who had cast a spell on him. Later his widow vowed to wreak revenge on those who had not only "sent an AIDS death" to her husband but had also zombified him for future use. "They gave him a poison," insisted Manno's wife. "To make him rise [from the grave], they had to give him poison."

One also hears the voice of Anita. Even younger than Manno and a native of Kay, she was not a victim of sorcery. In contrast to the etiologic theories advanced by Manno and his family, Anita felt that she had "caught it from a man in the city." The rest of her analysis was much more sociological, however, as she added that the reason she had a lover at a young age was "because I had no mother." Anita's mother, who had lost her land to the rising water, died of tuberculosis when Anita was thirteen:

When she died, it was bad. My father was just sitting there. And when I saw how poor I was, and how hungry, and saw that it would never get any better, I had to go to the city. Back then I was so skinny—I was saving my life, I thought, by getting out of here.

Anita was equally insistent about the cause of her family's poverty. "My parents lost their land to the water," she said, "and that is what makes us poor." If there had been no dam, insisted Anita, her mother would not have sickened and died; if her mother had been living, Anita would never have gone to the city; had she not gone to Port-au-Prince, she could not have "caught it from a man in the city."

Dieudonné was the third villager to fall ill with AIDS. His analysis recalled elements of both of those who had died before him. Like Manno, he was a victim of sorcery. Like Anita, he tended to cast things in sociological terms. Dieudonné voiced what might have been termed "conspiracy theories" on the origins of AIDS. On more than one occasion, he wondered "whether *sida* might not have been sent to Haiti by the United States. That's why they were so quick to say that Haitians gave [the world] *sida*." When asked why the United States would wish such a pestilence on Haitians, Dieudonné had a ready answer: "They say there are too many Haitians over there now. They needed us to work for them, but now there are too many over there." In an interview shortly before his death, Dieudonné observed that "*sida* is a jealousy sickness." When asked to explain more fully what he intended by his observation, Dieudonné replied,

What I see is that poor people catch it more easily. They say the rich get *sida*; I don't see that. But what I do see is that one poor person sends it on another poor person. It's like the army [firing on civilians]: brothers shooting brothers.

Dieudonné's story, like that of Manno, casts *sida* as a "jealousy sickness," and a disorder of the poor. Anita reminds us that certain events, such as the flooding of a valley, help to make people poor and jealous. Their observations and their experience of AIDS, tuberculosis, and poverty serve to affirm ethnography—based on long periods of participant-observation rather than on "rapid ethnographic assessment"—as an indispensable tool for understanding the social construction of AIDS.[12] But even an experiential approach to ethnography leads us back to a "macro" analysis: for many in Do Kay, observations about *sida* are worked into stories that relate how misfortune is manifest in the lives of individuals, communities, and even a nation.[13] Attending closely to these stories leads one to an analysis that reveals many interconnections.

AIDS and Theory in Medical Anthropology

The above discussion may seem far from the internecine debates within medical anthropology, which, as the largest subfield of the discipline, has generated its own rather arcane disagreements. Its rapid growth has not led to a unified theory, or even to agreement about what constitutes its appropriate subject of inquiry. In a recent polemic, Browner, Ortiz de Montellano, and Rubel (1988:681) bemoan medical anthropology's focus on meaning as one of the reasons why that subfield "still follows a particularistic, fragmented, disjointed, and largely conventional course."[14] Other recent assessments of medical anthropology (for example, Greenwood et al. 1988) concur about the absence of authoritative paradigms, but argue that this ferment and division is a sign of the subfield's strength.

Similar claims have been made for anthropology as a whole. Recent attempts to take the pulse of anthropology note a certain loss of faith in the paradigms that once claimed the loyalties of most anthropologists. As no grand theory has supplanted functionalism, structuralism, or other totalizing frameworks, anthropology is, for the moment at least, postparadigm. In a review of these debates, Marcus and Fischer (1986:8) qualify this disarray as "the intellectual stimulus for the contemporary vitality of experimental writing in anthropology." Of relevance to the argument advanced here is one of their chief conclusions: "An interpretive anthropology fully accountable to its historical and political-economy implications thus remains to be written" (Marcus and Fischer 1986:86).

This book is an attempt to constitute an interpretive anthropology of affliction based on complementary ethnographic, historical, epidemiologic, and political-economic analyses. Part I, "Misfortunes Without Number," offers a brief ethnographic history of Do Kay, a village mired in the deep poverty of rural Haiti. In Part II, "AIDS Comes to a Haitian Village," the advent of a new sickness is recounted as the unfolding drama it really was for the inhabitants of Do Kay, the author included. The focus here is on the lived experience of the afflicted and their families. These two sections are fundamentally descriptive, and leave unanswered many questions central to an understanding of AIDS: Were Manno, Anita, and Dieudonné representative victims of AIDS in Haiti? If so, how did they come to be at risk for exposure to HIV? If not, how do they differ from the majority of HIV-infected persons? Also unanswered are the perennial "why" questions: Why might poor Haitians have been particularly vulnerable to an epidemic of a new infectious disease? Why did the people of Do Kay respond to *sida* in the way that they did? Why do they speak of *sida* in the way that they do?

The next two sections of the book attempt to fill these explanatory lacunae by turning to other disciplines: epidemiology, history, and political economy. Cautious recourse in drawing on these disciplines is part of the "responsible materialism" of the anthropologist who would study an infectious disease that has spread throughout the world in predictable ways. Part III, "The Exotic and the Mundane: HIV in Haiti," attempts to reconstruct a socioepidemiological history of HIV in Haiti, and to answer the following questions: How did HIV come to the island, and when did it arrive? How far has HIV spread in Haiti? How is the virus transmitted in Haiti? Who is at risk for acquiring HIV infection? Why are sex differences in the incidence of AIDS diminishing, and why are "accepted risk factors" denied by more and more patients, even as the quality of epidemiological research improves? Why are other patterns of risk changing? What is the future likely to hold?

After examining the Haitian epidemic in the context of the Caribbean area, AIDS in this region may be best understood as a pandemic of the "West Atlantic system," a socioeconomic network centered in North America (see Patterson 1987). Haiti's changing role in the emerging West Atlantic system is described in Part IV, "AIDS, History, Political Economy." Committed to the analysis of historical transformations, how far back does one go? Among the conditions facilitating—or failing to prevent—rapid spread of HIV were the political arrangements in vigor at the time of its introduction. As Trouillot (1986, 1990) has shown, the rise of Duvalierism—indisputably the sociopolitical context of the present study—is to be understood as the "formalization" of a crisis that began early in the nineteenth century. What is more, the precursors of the chief variables of the contemporary equation—actors, products, modes of production—were present as early as the sixteenth century. Thus the spread of HIV across national borders seems to have taken place within our lifetime, but the conditions favoring the rapid, international spread of a predominantly sexually transmitted disease were established long ago, further heightening the need to historicize any understanding of the pandemic.

In examining nineteenth-century Haitian commerce or the Caribbean misadventures of the U.S. Marines, we are again far afield of the initial arena of inquiry. But Part IV is based on the belief that such digressions are necessary for a rich understanding of HIV in the Caribbean. Although similar readings of Haitian history can be found elsewhere, it is in juxtaposing this history with contemporary responses to AIDS that much is revealed about the true nature and origins of these responses. Part V, "AIDS and Accusation," consists of four interpretive essays drawing on both the ethnographic and historical chapters. Three essays examine the principal forms of accusation encountered in the preceding chapters: sorcery in Haitian villages, AIDS-related discrimination in North America, and "conspiracy theories" generated by Haitians in both places. A fourth essay compares the form and content of these competing social responses to AIDS. An interpretive anthropology fully cognizant of process and power can illuminate a number of phenomena, events, and patterns that remain obscure without such perspectives. The significance of such a position for medical anthropology is taken up again in the Conclusion. Although the discussion is framed to address anthropological investigations, there is much of relevance for social history, epidemiology, clinical medicine, and, especially, community-based efforts to prevent HIV infection.

Taken together, the following chapters permit certain conclusions. One of them will be advanced at the outset. Many believe that HIV is here to stay. Experience with other deadly infectious diseases suggests that, even if vaccines and effective treatments are developed, HIV infection is not likely to be eradicated. It will become, rather, a disease of the poor, of people like Anita, whose coffin cost more than her annual income. And when the illness has settled in on those social strata, research on HIV infection and its prevention will be marginalized, stimulating relatively little interest in the world's centers of medical investigation.

Although AIDS currently remains a topic of great interest in the international research community, shifts in infection rates like those just predicted have already been registered. In the United States, for example, HIV infection is becoming increasingly a condition of poor (and uninsured) city-dwellers, most of whom are people of color. In many regions, AIDS is the leading cause of death among young adults in the inner city. Among young black women living in New York state, AIDS has recently become the leading cause of death (CDC 1990). Between 1981 and 1986, deaths among women in the fifteen-to-forty-five age group increased 154 percent in New York City and 225 percent in Washington, D.C.; in low-HIV-prevalence areas like Idaho, no such increase was reported (Anastos and Marte 1989:7).[15] And as the morbidity rate among poor women continues to climb, so too does that among children: by 1988, AIDS had become the leading cause of death among Hispanic children living in New York and New Jersey; it was the number two cause of death among black children of this age group (Fuller 1991:5).

Among those already infected, poverty hastens the development of AIDS. In a recently published study of U.S. AIDS epidemic trends, an "AIDS deficit" was noted: beginning in 1987, "AIDS incidence departed abruptly" from projections based on steady, nationwide trends. But the striking deficit, attributed to antiviral therapy with zidovudine (AZT), was not seen among all groups studied:

Preliminary data suggest that groups which might be expected to have relatively good access to medical care exhibit AIDS deficits. These groups include gay men, hemophiliacs, transfusion recipients, and gay IVDUs. Most gay IVDUs are white and live outside the Northeast. Conversely, groups that might be expected to have relatively less access to medical care exhibit no appreciable deficits. These groups include IVDUs, persons infected through heterosexual contacts, and persons from a "Pattern II" country, such as Haiti. Among persons with AIDS, blacks and Hispanics constitute 80 percent of IVDUs, 71 percent of persons infected through heterosexual contact, and over 99 percent of persons from "Pattern II" countries. (Gail, Rosenberg, and Goedert 1990:305)

Among poor women, people of color, and others without easy access to appropriate care, there was no deficit; there was, rather, an AIDS surplus. "The awful theme woven through their paper," wrote Osborn (1990:295) of the study, "is the documentation that, as of 1987, it mattered more than ever who you were, who you knew, and what you earned." In Haiti, similarly, early pronouncements suggesting that AIDS-afflicted people from all economic backgrounds had to be abandoned as AIDS became, like other infectious diseases, a disorder disproportionately striking the poor.

It is my devout wish that *AIDS and Accusation* might move North Americans involved in community-based and academic responses to HIV to enlarge their own frames of analysis. Although HIV is a very cosmopolitan microbe, AIDS discourse, already so abundant as to be overwhelming, has always been provincial. Were Manno or Anita or Dieudonné to hear the North American debates triggered by AIDS they might find them elitist struggles over goods and services long denied to the poor.[16] Or they might deem such debates unreasonably abstract in the face of great suffering. Above all, these debates would suggest to them a vast distance, when, from an intracellular parasite's point of view, the distance between us is microscopic.

PART ONE

Misfortunes without Number

The country has low levels of literacy, little wage-paying employment, and high out-migration. Food production, which is drastically affected from time to time by cyclones and droughts, is further diminished by the loss of thousands of tons of soil washed into the sea each year, from deforested hillsides and flooded river plains. Over 50 percent of the deaths are among children under the age of five, with nearly 75 percent of deaths associated with or caused by malnutrition. Infectious diseases account for the majority of deaths. The major causes of childhood deaths are diarrhea, pneumonia, and tetanus; tuberculosis is the leading cause of death among adults.

Feilden et al. (1981:1)

Life for the Haitian peasant of today is abject misery and a rank familiarity with death.

Weise (1971:38)

2

The Water Refugees

The best view of Do Kay is from atop one of the peculiarly steep and conical hills that nearly encircle the village. Two deep valleys lie between this perch and the road that cuts through the village. To the left is the Peligre Reservoir, or at least that part of it not obscured by other hills. Ba Kay, several hundred feet below, is invisible from this hilltop. Viewed from the sharp outcroppings of rock protruding from the grassy crest, Do Kay looks less like a "line town" stretching along the road than a collection of tiny tin-covered huts randomly scattered on the flanks of a single, large mountainside. Scanning from the left, one first notes a cluster of houses and trees. The trees have survived because they were planted near the second of four public fountains, the first of which is hidden behind one of the hills. Looking slightly more to the right, one can make out the road, and climbing the hill to meet it, the path leading to Vieux Fonds, the very path you have taken to reach this hilltop. High above the road, atop the almost treeless mountain, sits the house of Boss Yonèl. Next door is the empty house of his oldest son, Dieudonné, dead of AIDS in October 1988. Looking lower down and further to the right, the road disappears behind a small ridge, only to reappear near the third fountain, which again is surrounded by more than its share of trees. Now the road has curved into the line of vision; on the left is the home of Marie and Pierre. Also on the left side of the road is a corner of the rusty red roof under which Anita Joseph slowly died of AIDS. On the right, the top of the bakery is visible, as is the brand new house of Pierre's parents, M. and Mme. Sonson. The large, two-story school is almost completely hidden behind a stand of trees planted in the summer of 1983. There the road is also concealed by trees and by the hill upon which the school sits, but it soon swerves, cutting once again into the field of vision.

Turning further to the right, higher on the hill, one sees the dormitory and church built during the tenure of Père Jacques Alexis of the Église Épiscopale d'Haiti. With the school, these buildings form the heart of the "Complèxe Socio-éducatif de Kay," which serves the peasant families of over a dozen villages. There is even a thatched gazebo, encircled by sea pines and often full of people meeting for one reason or another. Further to the right gleam the offices of Projè Veye Sante, the community-health project. Below that, obscured by more trees, are two long pigsties. The grunting of the pigs is quite audible, as are the sing-song voices of the invisible schoolchildren in the schoolyard.

Several other buildings make up the complex—a large clinic, a guest house, an artisans' workshop—but these are hidden by the hill, as is the house of Manno Surpris, formerly a teacher at the school. Manno was the first person on Do Kay to die of AIDS. Even further to the right, the road reappears, climbing over another of the stony, treeless shelves of lime. Plunging over the horizon, the road finally disappears into the upper portion of the central plateau.

A mere decade ago, Do Kay looked quite different from this vantage, and less than four decades ago, not a house was in sight. Writing a history of Kay poses special problems, many of which are not new to anthropology. The village is, upon cursory inspection, just another tiny settlement in the hills of Haiti. Most of its older inhabitants did not attend school; they do arithmetic with great facility, but neither read nor write. Most live in two-room houses, many with dirt floors, and cultivate plots of land that yield slowly diminishing returns. They have no tractors, electricity, or cars. Their hillside gardens are too steep for oxplows, even if they did have oxen. The people of Kay seem to be another "people without history." But the visitor who stays long enough and asks the right questions will soon discover the history lurking below the stereotype of the timeless peasant. Clues can be found in villagers' statements about themselves: "We are Kay people, but we are not from here," explained Nosant, a man in his fifties. "We are people of the valley." The apparent paradox is resolved when the speaker gestures out over the vast reservoir that lies at the base of the hills. The history of the Kay people is submerged below the still surface of this lake.

Before 1956, there was no Do Kay; the area was "a desert, a dry savanna with wind and birds and grass alone," as one of the area's first settlers described it. Most of the villagers who are now over thirty-five once lived in the valley. They were largely from an area called "Petit-Fond," a fertile and gently sloping area on either side of a stream known locally as Rivière Kay. Bursting forth from a cliff face, the largely subterranean stream joined the Artibonite River between the Rivière Thomonde and the Peligre Gorge, where the dam now stands. This small river still leaps from the bottom of the ravine, but now flows somewhat less briskly down to meet the Lac de Peligre, as the new reservoir was named. The area around the spring had long been settled, though sparsely, and it was called Kay. When the valley was flooded in 1956, much of Kay and all of Petit-Fond were submerged. Kay became divided into "Do" and "Ba." Petit-Fond became history.

Presenting a history of Petit-Fond is a legitimate, even necessary, undertaking for any anthropologist attempting to understand Kay as it is today. Even a history of the local AIDS epidemic cannot be fully understood without an appreciation of the effects the dam has had on the welfare of those who live behind it. "History" is not meant to suggest that there exists a true version of the story of the village, one that is ascertainable with careful use of accurate documents. For history varies, as has often been noted, according to winners and losers. The version presented here is that of the self-described losers. Though he was referring to an interclass struggle in a substantially different setting, Scott's (1984:205) observations are pertinent to the material gathered in Kay:

Having lived through this history, every villager is entitled, indeed required, to become something of a historian—a historian with an axe to grind. The whole point of such histories is not to produce a balanced neutral assessment of the decade but rather to advance a claim, to praise and blame, and to justify or condemn the existing state of affairs.

The substantive part of this account has been constructed from interviews: many of the older refugees were interviewed, as was Père Jacques Alexis, the catalyst for much of the recent change in Do Kay and the surrounding area. It is largely from these oral histories that I have reconstructed the history of one village's flight from the rising water and of the settlement of Kay.[1] Each narrative is profitably examined as "positioned rhetoric"—largely a rhetoric of complaint within a particular social and political context. The bounty and harmony of life in the *remembered* valley are the standard against which the present is assessed.

More accurately, the remembered valley is the weapon with which the current state of affairs is attacked. And as political change has accelerated in Haiti, the critique has become more strident.

The villagers' story is usually recounted as beginning in the mid-1950s, but the irreversible steps leading to its decline were taken considerably earlier. The "Organisme de Développement de la Vallée de l'Artibonite" (ODVA) was born of an agreement, signed in Washington, D.C., in 1949, between the Haitian government and the Export-Import Bank. Although the loans for the construction of the dam were received in August 1951, the news that the residents of the valley would be forced to relocate seemed not to have traveled far up the valley. Most of those interviewed on Do Kay claim that they were apprised of the impending inundation only a month before it occurred. To cite Nosant, who was a young man when the dam was built: "It was during the month of January that we were informed. They would be filling the valley with water, they said, and we were to move right away. . . . I think it was only a month later, in February, that they stopped up the river." All those interviewed concur that little warning was given. Valley residents did not know, said Mme. Lamandier, "until the water was upon us. We heard only rumors, which we did not believe, until a couple of months before, when they sent someone to tell us to cooperate, that our land would be flooded. This also we did not believe." A few insist that no attempt was made to inform the valley dwellers of their impending losses. Most recall, however, that the community was alerted at a public assembly. Absalom Kola put it this way:

They called an assembly to say that they would be reimbursing everyone for their gardens and land. . . . They warned us, but we all said it can't be true, it couldn't be done. We knew of nothing that could have stopped that great river. The Artibonite ran fast through the valley, and none of us believed it could be stopped.

That the residents of Petit-Fond claimed to know nothing of such an enormous project that would take years to build is striking. Construction went on only a few miles away, at Peligre Gorge, where hundreds of locals were employed at relatively high wages. Indeed, if the rural Haitian economy of the 1950s resembles the economy of today it is likely that some residents of Petit-Fond joined work crews in Peligre, although this is categorically denied by Mme. Gracia, one of the early settlers of Do Kay: "No, there wasn't anyone from Kay who went to work there. It was mostly people from Peligre or from the city

[Port-au-Prince]. There were a lot of foreigners too. No one from Petit-Fond worked there."

The area residents' disbelief in the flooding of the valley was nearly unanimous. Many of those living around Petit-Fond did not move until the day the waters "chased us off our lands," as Nosant put it. When asked why they waited until the last moment, the response most often given involves, once again, their disbelief. Absalom Kola's comments are typical:

They warned us, but we all said it can't be true; it couldn't be done. We knew of nothing that could have stopped that great river. The Artibonite ran fast through the valley, and none of us believed it could be stopped. And so on the morning they stopped it up, I watched it rise. Towards two o'clock or so, everyone was rushing around, as the water took our homeland. Everyone ran and left their mills standing. The chickens were obliged to swim; we didn't have time to gather them.

Mme. Gracia underlines the counterintuitive nature of the project: "Everyone said 'water can't climb hills.' It made sense then!" Mme. Emmanuel invokes a more moral version of disbelief: "Of course they sent word. They even came and cut a few big trees. But there wasn't a soul who believed it was true, because we saw the beautiful things we had in our gardens, the gardens of our ancestors. We were sure that no one would do such a thing." She is echoed by Mme. Lamandier:

We just stayed put; we never moved because we believed it was untrue. We saw what sort of good land we had, and how we loved it, and how we had no other land to work, and we came to believe that it just couldn't be true. You have all this and someone tells you they will take it all away . . . you just cannot believe it. But when we saw the water upon us, when even the houses began taking in water, we ran to the hills. And our houses we left to the sea.

The valley residents' disbelief could not have been universal, however, as it seems that a few landowners heeded the government's warnings, and left for nearby towns, such as LasCahobas, Thomonde, or Mirebalais. Some were said to have been reimbursed "by the state" for their lands, but most of the former valley residents interviewed stated flatly, as did Absalom Kola, that they had not:

They called an assembly to say that they would be reimbursing everyone for their gardens and land. My friend, that was a lie! They came to measure the lands, and indeed a few people did receive payment—only those who were well educated, those who had secured deeds. Our lands consisted of twenty-five *karo*.[2] This belonged to the Kola family; another twenty-five belonged to the

Pasquet family. For these lands we received nothing. And there are many others who until this very day have received nothing.

A number of reasons were cited to explain the failure to reimburse the landholders. Mme. Dieugrand, who linked her lack of reimbursement to poverty, stated that "it was the rich peasants who were reimbursed. Truly, we were all doing well back then. But some of us didn't have much land. My mother was struggling. She had no husband and seven children. That's why she got nothing." The reason most commonly invoked, however, involved a different aspect of the political powerlessness of the rural population. Although more than one informant suggested that their powerlessness was a result of their "poverty," most who spoke of political powerlessness cited lack of education, not of lack of money: "Those who were literate and who had deeds were the only ones to get paid," explained M. Kola. "And there was the problem of splitting up [jointly held] lands. If you were uneducated, though, you got nothing. If it had happened nowadays, it would be different, because our children read and write."

All who mentioned the amount of money received for the lands spoke of the government offering insultingly small sums. Mme. Gracia, the one informant who stated that she had been reimbursed, attributed her recompense to the deed: "Yes, they gave me a little—$40 for twelve *karo* [over thirty-eight acres]! Those who had the papers got a little something. Truly, there were many who didn't. But $40 wasn't a fortune back then: we were planting a lot of rice." "To those who received money, they gave such little amounts that it would have been better to receive nothing at all," observed Mme. Nosant. "If it were now, and you owned that land," offered Mme. Lamandier, "there would be no one with enough money to buy it from you. Nor would you need to sell it, because the produce from the land would net you all the money you'd need."

Some mentioned that land tenure patterns were complicated and vested power in the hands of one person. As noted above, the relatively large holdings of the Kola and Pasquet families were jointly held by family elders:

Our land was held communally (*an blok*), a land we called "eritye." Say for example your father had two *karo* that he received from his father (*sou dwa papa-l*), and his brother had two or three *karo*, but it was all one plot of land—that's called *eritye*. If you're the biggest holder, then the deed is likely to be in your keeping. When the time comes for the land to be paid for, you're the one they would turn to, you're the one who would receive the money. The other holders might get none of it. In this way, the dam turned brother against brother.

Corruption and graft also played an important part in who received reimbursement. A few "big shots" (*gran nèg*) did not fare poorly, it seems, and some of those interviewed note with bitterness that these same persons should have been advocates for the valley dwellers. The water refugees often note that "no one spoke up for us," or that "no one with power in their hands came to our defense." Some note with regret their "ignorance"—their illiteracy. "If we had had someone to speak for us," observed Sonson, "someone who could read and write, then at least we might have been reimbursed for our losses." One of the persons who might have come to the refugees' defense was Père Emmanuel Moreau, of the Église Épiscopale d'Haiti, the young priest who preceded Jacques Alexis as priest of the Mirebalais parish.[3] But Père Moreau answered the call of politics in a more fundamental way. In the year that the valley was flooded, he successfully ran for senator in his home district, and returned to the capital.[4] Alexis feels that a well-placed advocate might have altered the lot of the people of Petit-Fond:

I don't imagine that Moreau could have done anything about the dam; I don't imagine he would have wanted to. The logic was that the dam would help more people than it hurt. But what a pity that more voices were not raised against the abuse of the natives of the valley. . . . There was no [resettlement] plan and it was not long before some of those displaced by Peligre ran into new problems.

It was clear from interviews that, for many, the years following the inundation of their lands were bitter. For some refugees, reaching higher ground was not enough; their trials were not yet over: "It wasn't only the water that came after us," recalls Mme. Emmanuel, "it was also the dynamite." The department of public works, in conjunction with the ODVA and a team of U.S. engineers, had begun building a road along the hill that overlooked the reservoir. The ledge opened up by the completion of the road was known as "the terrace." The new road was to replace an older one, also drowned by the dam, that once ran from LasCahobas to Hinch. The road crews, explained Mme. Emmanuel, used explosives:

As soon as you heard them shout "Run!," then rocks would fly everywhere. They crushed rocks up there endlessly. And they would do this without looking to see if someone might be below. We couldn't stay. We were all afraid we'd be crushed by the great rocks that came crashing down with no warning. We had to go. We were the ones who came here [Do Kay] first; everyone else followed and came to join us.

Others followed Mme. Emmanuel to the stony—but safer—hills above. When asked why she came to Do Kay, Mme. Gracia replied, "Well, we didn't have anywhere else to go; we got out to avoid being drowned. We didn't have time to save our belongings. We built little lean-tos on the hill, and resigned ourselves to our losses." Some informants report a dazed feeling, and an inability to act decisively: "For a year, I couldn't do anything. I just sat there. My children were always crying. I didn't plant a thing," said Louis, who has since managed to become a moderately successful peasant. Mme. Jolibois also reports "a heaviness, a difficulty in knowing where to go, what to feed the children. Now we're used to having nothing to offer them, but back then it was a shock." Mme. Gracia's remarks echo those of her neighbors. "We had no food and little money," she recalls; "it seems as if we couldn't act. We planted nothing. So I sold the cows, one at a time, in order to feed the children." Mme. Dieugrand recalls, "We were stunned. We didn't know where to turn. We waited for God's miracles, and nothing happened."[5]

Although the land in Do Kay was by unanimous acclamation "without value," it was safer than the land by the water's edge. More than dynamite rendered it hazardous. The reservoir level was altered several times, and those who planted near the shore lost their crops when the water level was raised.[6] Also disturbing to the refugees who settled Ba Kay was the state-sponsored planting of teak trees, locally termed *bwa leta* ("state trees"), near the high watermark. These were variably justified as protection against erosion and raw material for future utility poles, but many suspected that more land would be appropriated. For these and other reasons, Mme. Emmanuel's lead was followed by quite a few families. Père Alexis states that there were only "two or three" households when he first visited Do Kay, shortly after the basin had been filled. A 1962 mapping by photogrammetric methods from 1956 aerial photography suggests, however, that there were fifteen houses on Do Kay within a year of the inundation.

One thing that is striking, in even a cursory reading of the interviews, is the refugees' almost unanimous appreciation of a central irony to their story. Each interviewee has spoken of the unfairness of a project that destroys a way of life and offers benefits only to faraway Port-au-Prince. Mme. Gracia, in response to the question "Why did they build the dam?" offered the following observation:

Well, it was in order to light up Port-au-Prince with electricity, but I get nothing out of that. Port-au-Prince has light, but I'm in darkness—and I live right next door to Peligre! It's the big shots (*gran nèg*) in Port-au-Prince who are having fun now.

She was seconded by Mme. Lamandier:

To have electricity for the city people and for the factories, that's why. The rich people, the city people bribe the bureaucrats so they can have electricity. Water makes electricity, but you need high water. So they flooded us out.

These analyses of the OVDA by former residents of Petit-Fond are scathing indeed. Mme. Emmanuel does not mince words: "I see not one speck of benefit in the water. What benefit there is goes only to the people living in the city. They all have light. Do I have things like that? It's the powerful man who gets it." A similarly dim view was offered by M. Kola, but his conclusions were tempered with a certain optimism:

Look at me now; what do I have? Poverty has come after me. I'm resigned to it. But if they were to let loose these waters and say "Here's a little plot of your old land back," I'd build a little lean-to in which to sleep, and I can promise you that I'd soon be wealthy, I and all my family. But I won't find anything now. Still, since the terrace was built, we've found a light; we've found Père Alexis, who has come to give us a bit of knowledge. Yes, there has been that to offset our loss: the sole advantage we've found has been the Alexis advantage. He has helped us raise our children; he has worked hard so that our children might be educated.

Nineteen-fifty-six was thus a traumatic year for those who had come to love the land. Mme. Emmanuel speaks, as do others, of the profound depression that followed: "My friend, everyone saw their lives ending. There were those who died of grief. This is true. My father . . . well, it is grief that killed him." She is echoed by Mme. Gracia: "We were in a bad way. Our hearts were being torn out (*se kè nou ki t'ap rache*). But we couldn't speak. Some people just plain died from the shock. And from that day on, I've never felt right again."

3

The Remembered Valley

As deforestation and erosion whittled away the hillsides on which the valley people now found themselves, it became more and more difficult to wrest sustenance from those hills. Their diminishing returns were bitterly compared to the bounty of Petit-Fond, which took on mythic dimensions.[1] The images used by the "water refugees" are often deeply affecting, as are the stories themselves. M. Kola is an eloquent representative of a generation that had grown up in the valley:

Everyone lost half of his life. Even a tiny bit of land, no more than this courtyard, would yield more than you could eat. You could never harvest all your rice, there was so much of it. You could never cut all your sugarcane in order to crush it. The bananas came faster than you could pick them. If you planted a manioc, it grew so large that you couldn't lift it from the soft earth. If you went out to plant a pot of rice, you wouldn't have room to store it all [at harvest]. And then we came here. You can work three or four *karo* of land, but you still don't have enough to eat. You plant manioc, you wait five years, and still no manioc. You plant corn, and get nothing more for your efforts than *digo*[2] cuts on your fingers. We here on Do Kay, we've grown old. And that's because we've suffered too much. We had so many pigs, two per family at least; the shoats we would sell. We all had our own cows. Now look at us, naked. You're married, say, and you have many children. You almost can't clothe them. You live on this bony soil (*tè zoklo*), and you can't make it give anything. You scrounge and save for who-knows-when, and still nothing. And then along comes three days of summer heat and your gardens wither. Down where we lived, we never even spoke of summer heat. We never had to eat milled corn, and now we'd kill for it. Back then it was rice and big plantains. My friend, look down there [gestures to reservoir]. That wasn't land we had. It was a Christ, and it's now under water. I can't speak for everyone, but leaving the valley brought nothing but pain for me. Perhaps it's only fear of the Lord that keeps me from turning to thievery.

Mme. Gracia paints a similar picture of the remembered valley: "Back then, we had a lot of rice. When June, July arrived, everyone was wading through piles of rice. Can you imagine!" Mme. Dieugrand wistfully recalled "the pots of beans, the huge bunches of bananas, the sugarcane." Although there was significant variation in the accounts of the events leading up to the "flood," the question of reimbursement, and the history of resettlement, the nostalgia for Petit-Fond was strong in each account. In Petit-Fond everyone was happy. No one was ever hungry. Sickness was rare. People lived "until their hair was white." Terms of affection, such as "mother" and even "Christ," are used when referring to the land. Other epithets recall positions of strength and security: "Ever since we left our fortress down there," sighs Mme. Jolibois, "I've been miserable." Even acknowledging the distorting effects of nostalgia, there is universal agreement that the valley was an ideal place to live as a peasant farmer. Interviews with persons who lost no land reveal a similar conviction that the valley had been exceptionally fertile.[3]

Often, the contrast is placed in stark terms of *before* and *after*. To bring home such comparisons, generational contrasts are used. Turning to Saul, one of the first villagers to attend high school, Mme. Lamandier remarked, "You would not be as you are now. You would be living in great comfort, because your father and mother would have more strength and could help you much more; you would not be where you are now, you would be much farther." Mme. Gracia mentioned selectivity of memory:

Back then, we would never have dreamed of cultivating land like this—it's just rocks. Back then, we used only hoes. My child, you see in what state we are now, but we used to be persons (*Se moun nou te ye*). But now we've fallen under the load, and the past has become even sweeter in our eyes. What we had before is what we deserve to have today.

The dehumanizing effect—"we used to be persons"—of rootlessness and of poverty is often referred to. "They took our land so that they could have electricity," said Mme. Lamandier, "and they don't even look to see whether we're people or animals." The comments of Louis have a stringent moral bite: "What was done to us was something that you don't do to God's children. If there's a storm, you bring in the cat. If there's a flood, you move the livestock. Even livestock they would have treated more kindly."

The dam's dehumanizing effects were keenly felt among families. In rural Haiti, the ideal living arrangement is called a *lakou,* a term traditionally signifying a family compound consisting of children's houses grouped around that of the *chèf lakou,* or household head. Many of the water refugees spoke at length of the dissolution of their *lakou* by the dam. "When our *lakou* was undone," said Mme. Gracia, "my father went crazy. He kept on talking about how we all had to move over to his side of the lake so we could live together as we should and honor our ancestors. He said this while sitting on a miserable pile of rocks! He was never again right in his head." These geospatial arrangements were in large part dismantled by the dam, as few if any families could regroup in arrangements of their own choosing. That residents of the valley "went crazy" after losing their land makes sense in rural Haiti. Brown (1989a:42–43) traces the contemporary matrix of kinship, land, and religion to the time of slavery:

The slaves' loss of access to family land in Africa was as great as their loss of the African family itself. Indeed, from one perspective family and land were inseparable. Prevented from visiting family graves and from leaving food offerings and pouring libations at ancestral shrines, the enslaved African had also been denied the means of ensuring the spiritual blessing and protection of the ancestors. This connection of family, land, and religion persists in rural Haiti today.

Rural Haitian family structure and peasant land tenure patterns were linked in an almost impossible obligation. As has often been pointed out, the mere passage of time weakens the ability of families to maintain such compounds:

By having in turn their own offspring, the children of the *lakou*'s founder distanced themselves from their father in order that their own children might have enough room to build around [their parents'] houses. Thus were formed what one might term sub-*lakou,* as well as a trend linking the organization of space to degree of consanguinity, given that [such arrangements] juxtaposed brothers of the second generation and first cousins of the third. (Bastien 1985:48)[4]

Even among those who did not lose all their land, the dam immediately disrupted delicately balanced competition for scarce resources and led to overt discord. As Absalom Kola put it, "The dam turned brother against brother." Stories are told in which one member of a family turned over a deed to receive compensation, and then left the valley. Many note that people were "prone to fights" as they became more and more impoverished. These quarrels, which continue to this day, are claimed by many older villagers to be the result of the dam. Life in the remembered valley, to quote Yonèl, was "one big *konbit*." [5]

We used to work hand-in-hand before the water rose. No one was trying to eat [ensorcel] anyone else. But as we sold off our livestock, just in order to have enough to eat, we became bitter, our hearts were hardened. . . . We were bitter at the sound of hungry children crying, bitter over everything. If someone succeeded in leaving all that behind, we were bitter with him too.

Other cultural institutions were weakened or altered by the loss of land and livelihood. A very detailed report published in 1956 by the Église Épiscopale d'Haiti lists several "voodoo temples" in Petit-Fond. [6] And yet a survey conducted in 1985 revealed that there was not a single temple (*houmfor*) in Do Kay and, accordingly, no *houngan* or *manbo*, as the priests and priestesses are called. The *houngan* living in Petit-Fond did not relocate with the majority of the water refugees. Mme. St. Jean, who professes faith as an *episkopal*, explained why:

The main *houngan*, the one with the most knowledge, lost a lot of prestige after the dam was built. One reason was that he told us that the dam would break. He said Clairmé would break it, because Clairmé had to be able to reach the sea. . . . When the dam was built and didn't break, he said that the *lwa* [spirits] were angry, we didn't make the right ceremonies, didn't give the right gifts—a whole lot of things. But some people were angry with [the *houngan*].

Mme. Dieugrand, a "born-again Christian" who has long been an adherent of an antivoodoo Baptist sect, recounts with a certain satisfaction the eclipse of this *houngan*'s powers:

He said he could make the water go down. It is true that he could bring the rains; it is true that he could hold (literally, *mare*, "tie") the rains. But he was talking nonsense about [the dam], and we came to see this. . . . No one came to see him anymore. He lost his power. [7]

The loss of faith transcended individual practitioners: even the *lwa* were remembered as more responsive before the dam. More than one person explained that "when the *lwa* are under the water, their powers are reduced." Others remarked that the tenacity of their newfound poverty led to a loss of faith in "old beliefs." Mme. Lamandier, for example, observed that "they got tired of holding services for the *lwa* because [the refugees] just got poorer and poorer." Still another remarked that the *lwa* were less responsive since the refugees were unable to propitiate them with "food."

The crisis in meaning posed by the loss of Petit-Fond led inexorably to bitterness, blame, and recrimination. How could the loss of "the gardens of our ancestors" be countenanced with mere resignation? Dispersion and its effects on spirituality is a central theme, not only in the Kay area, but in Haiti, generally. Further, Haitians have a long history of understanding major dislocations as coming from *human* agency. Writing of prerevolutionary Haiti, Brown (1989a:67) observes that, for the early Haitians, "natural powers such as those of storm, drought, and disease paled before social powers such as those of the slaveholder." When anger at injustice can be marshaled into social movements based on solidarity between the oppressed, Haitians have shown themselves capable of clear-sighted reprisals, such as the events that began in 1791 and led to the overthrow of slavery and the founding of the Haitian state. But when scattered peasants find themselves unable to counter the machinations of far-off or unknown oppressors, the resulting inequity is likely to give rise to accusations of sorcery.

Indeed, interviews with the water refugees suggest that interfamilial alliances, traditionally weak in family-centered Haiti, gave way in the face of new inequities. A rise in sorcery was mentioned by several of the water refugees. "People became bitter," explained Luc Joseph. "People became jealous of those who had not lost their land. They became jealous of their own past." Bitterness born of the dislocation of that period led to feuds and sorcery accusations. As shall be clear later, an understanding of sorcery is of great significance to understandings of illness causation in the Kay area today.

4

The Alexis Advantage:
The Retaking of Kay

For many older members of the Kay community, the flooding of their valley was remembered with profound sadness. Yet, happier memories were invariably invoked in reference to the arrival of the Haitian cleric Jacques Alexis. To cite Absalom Kola again: "The sole advantage we've found has been the Alexis advantage." As the villagers tell it, there seems to have been a period of relative calm after the road was completed. In many of the interviews, the next event remarked upon was the arrival, "about fifteen years ago," of Alexis. He had, in fact, arrived much earlier, but had been spending time with water refugees on both sides of the reservoir. The new road afforded him easy access to the mission in Do Kay, and he intensified his pastoral duties there.

Jacques Alexis is a priest of the Église Épiscopale d'Haiti, which was founded in the nineteenth century by an African-American pastor living in the United States. The founder dreamed of living in a country in which there was no slavery, a dream that led him and a group of black Episcopalians to Haiti. Over the past century, the church has grown slowly and has followed to a large extent the example of the Roman Catholic church, focusing on education and, to a lesser extent, medical works. Born into a middle-class Haitian family, Alexis was himself raised in this church. His departure from petit bourgeois roots resides in his belief that education is the right of *any* Haitian, "particularly," he is fond of saying, of "the Haitian peasant, the sole producer in this country of parasites." Mme. Alexis is also an educator, if one of more tempered views, and together they have founded over a dozen schools in Haiti's Central Plateau. Père Alexis initiated a school[1] in Do Kay as soon as there were enough squatters to warrant it: "The area [Do Kay] was beginning to have many families, many new children, a growing proportion of young people. That's why we thought of expanding our activities here."

"Activities," for Alexis, have always been slanted toward social programs: medical care, community organizing, small-scale agricultural projects, and, above all, school. He reserves great disdain for those priests he labels *diseurs de messe*—the "mass sayers" who fail to implement, in pragmatic fashion, the philosophies they preach. He also has little use for foreign Protestant missionaries who "spread the doctrine of resignation." They are also, by Alexis's description, "blinkered sectarians," who wield food programs, schooling, and medical care to "buy converts." He describes his own work as "completely ecumenical," and the school he founded certainly seems to bolster such a claim:

We decided to take kids of all ages for [first grade], even twenty-year-olds, as it was not their fault that there had been no school around when they were younger. School doors are not meant to be closed because someone is too old. Or because someone isn't an Episcopalian. The vast majority of these students are not Episcopalians.

The establishment of a school may seem a bit out of place given the homelessness, landlessness, and hunger of many of the water refugees. But it appears that they themselves did not feel that way. "The school was the best thing that happened to us," said Mme. Nosant. "We knew that the only way out of our problem was education." Sonson concurred: "A lot of us have wondered what would of happened if we had known how to write. If we had known how to write, perhaps we wouldn't be in this situation now. Of my children, it's Pierre who is in the best situation; he's the one who knows how to write, thanks to the priest." A few even felt that their literate children might be able to have the dam removed, but the majority dismissed this as wishful thinking.

The refugees' enthusiasm for the modest school established by Alexis, and run by his barely literate lay reader, is in keeping with what has long been known to be true for rural Haitians in general. "It is every peasant's ambition to send his children to school," notes Métraux (1960:57), "and he will make any sacrifice in order to be able to do so."[2] The reestablishment of the Petit-Fond mission school aroused immediate interest in many of the displaced families. Those on the far side of the reservoir made arrangements to send their children to Do Kay in dugout canoes. Their tenacity is in keeping with rural Haitian culture: "In remote regions without a local state school, they will club together to pay a teacher. To get to school, pupils must often walk for hours, climb *mornes* and cross torrents" (Métraux 1960:57). There are many stories of the students who wrapped their clothes and notebooks in plastic bags, strapped them to their heads, and swam across the formidable reservoir to reach Père Alexis's school.

The passion and commitment of rural parents stand in jarring and ironic contrast to the near-total illiteracy that reigns in the countryside. It is clear, however, that the barriers to the advancement of rural youth are still greater than the power of the peasants to demand their due. The stakes are high, as Lowenthal has suggested:

People of the rural areas do not remain "illiterate" *in spite* of the fact that they ensure the survival of the city folk and the export trade, but precisely *because* they do so. It is clearly in the interests of the urban higher classes to maintain the status quo, thereby limiting social mobility and impeding the growth of political consciousness among the peasantry. This reduces competition on their own class level while simultaneously defusing much of the threat of mass organization and resistance from below. (Lowenthal 1976:662)

As the 1970s progressed, more and more families sent their children to the thatch-roofed school run by Père Alexis. Supplementary classes were held under a nearby mango tree, weather permitting, because there was not enough room inside for all the students. But as the decade drew to a close, recounts Père Alexis, he and his wife were faced with certain painful realities. For three decades, they had struggled to bring schooling to the *ti moun andeyò*, "the outside children" of Haiti's hills. And although more and more children were attending school, little to no progress was being made in genuine literacy. Even less progress was made in community organization, which was recognized as a necessary prelude to social change.[3] An increasing number of children were suffering from malnutrition even as international aid to Haiti reached new heights. "Working in the Kay area, where people were landless and 'super poor,' taught us something that we should have learned long ago: being committed to schools is not enough." The Alexises made plans to expand their "development" efforts in the area surrounding the reservoir.[4]

In about 1979, Jacques Alexis began training landless peasants in carpentry, masonry, and design. A construction team was formed, and since 1980 they have built a church, a dormitory for teachers, a bakery, a clinic, a laboratory, a lunchroom, a daycare/nutrition center, a guesthouse, and pigsties. Some thirty latrines have been scattered over Do Kay, and each year more and more houses boast tin roofs and cement floors. There is no village center or "square," although the school-church-clinic complex may be taking on this function. Until March 1985, there were no retail shops or businesses in Kay. A few commodities (canned milk, local colas, small quantities of grain) could be obtained from the handful of families known to "resell." A new bakery opened in March 1985, and now serves Kay and surrounding villages. Profits from the bread, its sole product so far, are used to sustain a feeding program for undernourished children. The catalyst for all these projects has been the Alexises.[5]

The couple's long-standing commitment to education was not abandoned. Through a sister diocese in the United States, the priest was able to secure funding for a new school, a "real school," as he put it. By 1983, the new École Saint-André was finished. Père Alexis had even managed to rent a bulldozer in order to create a soccer field. Two stories tall, sitting up on a plateau over the road, the school looked faintly grandiose amid the shacks of Do Kay. The villagers were immensely proud of it, however, and school attendance swelled. In fact, many transformations took place in these years. Although they are not the subject of this study, these changes are relevant to an examination of health and change in a small village.

Perhaps the most significant change was in the size of the village. The efflorescence of new services drew many new families to the area, which had previously been considered an exceedingly inhospitable place. Between 1983 and 1989, seventy-one new dwellings were constructed in Do Kay (table 1). Some of the newcomers had come from Ba Kay: the tapping of the spring removed one of the chief reasons that water refugees remained down at the water's edge. Now that those on the hill were no longer obliged to negotiate the steep path leading down to potable water, many families wished to be closer to the school and other services inaugurated by Alexis and his coworkers.

The water refugees had erected wattle-and-daub huts, thatched with banana tree bark. These two-room huts were rarely weatherproof and did not last long. A home improvement project was initiated by Mme. Alexis, who organized the distribution of cement for floors and tin for roofs. Several homes judged "beyond repair" were quietly rebuilt under

Table 1 *Population of Do Kay*

Year	No. of Households	Total Population
1989	178	884
1988	165	835
1987	134	772
1986	129	719
1985	123	677
1984	117	632
1983	107	597

her supervision. Thirty walk-in latrines were built throughout Do Kay. Villagers dug the holes, and Père Alexis's construction crew added sturdy cement privies. Typhoid fever, which had been commonplace, virtually disappeared after 1986.[6]

An even more important change has been the advent of running water in Do Kay. Until recently, villagers were obliged to scramble down a steep hillside to a large spring eight hundred vertical feet below the level of the road. Villagers seemed to know the dangers of drinking impure water, but the temptation to store water in large pots or calabash gourds was directly proportional to one's distance from the spring. Infant deaths due to diarrheal disease were commonplace. In June 1985, the spring was capped by a team of Haitian and North American engineers working for the Église Épiscopale d'Haiti. Although none of the houses has running water, a hydraulic pump now sends water to the school and other buildings in the complex, as well as to three public fountains along the road. A marked decline in infant mortality has been recorded in subsequent years.

Another development initiative coordinated by the Alexises has not fared so well. In 1978, the appearance of African swine fever in the Dominican Republic led the United States to spearhead an epidemiologic investigation of the porcine stock in neighboring Haiti. Haitian pigs in the Artibonite Valley were found to have been infected. Curiously, however, few Haitian pigs had died. Some veterinary experts felt that this might be because the *kochon planch*, as the Haitian pig was termed, had become remarkably resistant to disease. Some peasants were sure there had been no swine fever, that the entire epidemic was a sham staged so that the North "Americans could make money selling their pigs."

North American agricultural experts feared that African swine fever could threaten the U.S. pig industry, and bankrolled PEPPADEP (Programme pour l'Éradication de la Peste Porcine Africaine et pour le Développement de l'Élevage Porcin), a $23 million extermination and restocking program. This would be no small task, as there were an estimated 1.3 million pigs in Haiti, and they were often the peasants' most important holding. The significance of the Creole pig, as it was called after its extermination, is well known to anyone who has studied the rural Haitian economy:

The peasant subsistence economy is the backbone of the nation, and the pigs were once the main components of that economy. With no banking system available to him, the peasant relied on hog production as a bank account to meet his most pressing obligations: baptism, health care, schooling, funerals, religious ceremonies, and protection against urban-based loan sharks who would grab his land at the first opportunity. (Diederich 1985:16)

The Haitian peasantry was shaken cruelly by this latest twist of fate. Years later, it became clear that PEPPADEP had further impoverished and "peripheralized" the Haitian peasantry, if such a thing were possible, and had generated an ill will whose dimensions are underlined by Abbott (1988:241): "PEPPADEP, the program to eradicate every last one of these Creole pigs, would be the most devastating blow struck [to] impoverished Haiti, but until there were actually no more pigs, the awesome consequences of PEPPADEP were neither understood nor predicted." Initiated in May 1982 (well after the abatement of any clinical disease in Haiti), the pig slaughter ended in June of the following year. By August 1984, with no pigs left, the nation was declared free of African swine fever.

It is unlikely that a single Haitian peasant celebrated this veterinary victory. Kay resident Luc Joseph refers to the slaughter of the pigs as "the very last thing left in the possible punishments that have afflicted us. We knew we couldn't have cows. We knew we couldn't have goats. We had resigned ourselves, because we at least had our pigs." "I don't know how we're going to get over this one," said Dieugrand, another of the water refugees, in the spring of 1984. "This hill is just too steep to climb." He is echoed by a Haitian economist, who observes that, although the value of the destroyed livestock has been estimated at $600 million, "the real loss to the peasant is incalculable. . . . [The peasant economy] is reeling from the impact of being without pigs. A whole way of life has been destroyed in this survival economy. This is the worse calamity to ever befall the peasant" (Diederich 1985:16). As apocalyptic as such evaluations sounded, they were soon revealed to be true:

School opening that October, the first after PEPPADEP's final eradication of the nation's pigs, revealed that [school] registration had plunged as much as 40 to 50 percent. Street vendors of cheap notebooks and pencils went hungry. The Lebanese and Syrian dry goods merchants had unsold stockpiles of check- ered cotton for the traditional Haitian school uniforms. Deschamps Printing Company's orders for Creole and French textbooks plummeted. All over Haiti children stayed at home, understanding that something was happening to them and that times were suddenly much harder. (Abbott 1988:274–275)

In Do Kay, the number of children reporting for the first week of school was down by a third, and Mme. Alexis, headmaster Maître Gérard, and mission treasurer Jésula Auguste spent days bringing uni- forms and other "classical furnishings" to the homes of the no-shows. They were all determined that not a single child would be prevented from attending school because of the pig disaster, and with Père Alexis were actively planning to restore the pigs to the peasants.

Working with USAID and the Organization of American States, the Haitian government announced a pig replacement program, act two of PEPPADEP. As "suspicious" Haitians had predicted, the replacement stock was purchased from U.S. farmers. In order to receive Iowa pigs as a "secondary multiplication center," program participants were re- quired to build pigsties to specifications and also demonstrate the avail- ability of the capital necessary to feed the pigs. This effectively elimi- nated the overwhelming majority of peasants. Père Alexis decided that helping villagers to replace their lost pigs was an undertaking that fell squarely within his mission, despite his distaste for USAID. In the space of two months, he and his team had erected a sturdy tin-roofed sty that was, as many noted, "better than the homes of Christians."[7] The priest's plan was to breed the pigs and distribute *gratis* the piglets, with the request that one piglet from each subsequent litter be returned to the project. In that way, he announced, the cycle could be continued until everyone had pigs. Since the new pigs were promised by North American agronomists to have litters of six to ten piglets, the proposal was greeted with satisfaction by the community. Dozens of villagers watched with delight as more than a score of sturdy piglets were deliv- ered in the summer of 1985.

It did not take long for this auspicious beginning to go awry. The pigs looked little like the lowslung, black Creole pigs that had populated Haiti for centuries. Although the new pigs, soon termed *kochon blan* ("foreign pigs"), were very large, they were manifestly more fragile than their predecessors. They fell ill and required veterinary intervention; they turned their noses up at the garbage that had been the mainstay of the native pigs' diet. The *kochon blan* fared well only on expensive wheat-based, vitamin-enriched feed—a commodity also sold by the government. Although public proclamations assured the people that the price of pig feed would be controlled, artificially created shortages soon led to a thriving parallel market that netted fortunes for a few in the Duvalier clique and its successors. The cost of feed each year for an adult pig ran between $120 and $250, depending on the black market.

There were, in addition to technical difficulties, dilemmas of a more cultural order. With the help of his staff, Père Alexis had decided that the first litters of pigs should go to the community councils of Do Kay and surrounding villages, where they were to be held communally. This idealistic plan was approved in a large public meeting held in Do Kay shortly after the introduction of the new livestock, and well before the arrival of the first litters. Once distributed, the pigs did very well in two or three of the ten villages with which the Kay-based staff was working. In many of the others, however, there soon were difficulties. In some settings, the pigs simply did not thrive. Villagers admitted that they were unaccustomed to caring for communally held property. In at least two villages, one member of the community council attempted to claim ownership of one or more of the pigs. In Vieux Fonds, another settlement with a large number of water refugees, machetes were drawn during the course of pig-related arguments. In a community outside the limits of Alexis's sphere of action, the priest and his coworkers were accused of "spreading communist ideas," an accusation that was to recur in 1987. Père Alexis concluded that his error had been to exaggerate the local population's enthusiasm for the idea of shared property. There would be less division, he was sure, when pigs were distributed to individual households. But the slow process of distribution meant that for well over two years, some had pigs and some did not. Others had lost their pigs to sickness or bad business deals. The setting was ripe for hard feelings related to the ownership of pigs. The next eruption of anger was expressed less directly, in *kola* accusations.

Kola is a root believed, in Do Kay at least, to be particularly noxious to pigs. When mixed with millet or corn stalks, it may be used as a pig poison.[8] If its native toxicity is deemed insufficient, many feel that *kola* may be "fixed" by an *amate,* a specialist in malicious magic. Magically enhanced *kola* is a far more efficacious poison. In this case, the poison is termed "not simple" (*pa senp*), a distinction that is invariably made when accusations of pig poisoning are brought up. Some feel that a peasant whose garden is regularly ravaged by a neighbor's pig has the right to place *kola senp* in his or her garden. Most deplore, however, the practice of magical poison; it is simply too close to sorcery. But by the end of 1986, there seemed to be a *kola* accusation for every pig death. As Ti Anne put it upon discovering that her pig had died, "We're never going to get anywhere if we can't let each other live!"

Père Alexis threw up his hands, saying, "I give up! The only way to please everyone would be to import one thousand healthy adult Creole pigs and distribute them simultaneously!" A tour of the communities surrounding Do Kay convinced him that the "white pigs" were simply not suited to Haiti. The new pigs would not eat their predecessors' fare, and the cost of wheat shorts was subject to black market control and well beyond the reach of the rural poor. The dissension and *kola* accusations discouraged him, and the priest recommended that the pig project be closed down. But Mme. Alexis was insistent that "everybody have at least one pig," and decided that henceforth she would oversee the project.

Mme. Alexis focused her distribution efforts on individual families in Do and Ba Kay, rather than working through community groups. She too met with little success. Although several poor villagers sold their pigs for handsome profits, many of the *kochon blan* did not fare well outside the complex. Some died, others simply failed to thrive. Sows came into heat infrequently and bore small litters. Less than four years after the inauguration of the pig project, Mme. Alexis also declared herself "ready to close down the project. It's a waste of time. These pigs will never become acclimated to Haiti. . . . Next they'll ask us to install a generator and air conditioning."

5

The Struggle for Health

The establishment of Clinique Saint-André as an autonomous health center may have contributed to the decline in morbidity and mortality noted above, as its staff insisted from the outset that clinical services must be linked to preventive efforts. This commitment led to the founding in 1983 of Projè Veye Sante, the preventive arm of the Kay-based health projects. Projè Veye Sante was designed to provide comprehensive preventive and primary care to inhabitants of the villages surrounding Kay, including vaccination campaigns, prenatal care, malnutrition and tuberculosis eradication programs, and AIDS prevention efforts. By August 1985, Projè Veye Sante had established satellite projects in four neighboring villages. By 1987, nine villages were being served; by 1989, sixteen villages. The area served by the Clinique Saint-André is, of course, far larger. The staff there often receives in excess of two hundred persons per day.[1]

The introduction of regular biomedical services to the Kay area did not represent the importation of a novel "health care system." The peasantry had been availing itself of such services for decades, by triaging certain kinds of illnesses to clinics in Mirebalais, Hinche, and Port-au-Prince. And yet there were inevitable clashes between various *sectors* of the health care system. An event that occurred in 1984 revealed, in a way that interviewing could not, the tensions that were present as representatives of cosmopolitan medicine began visiting Do Kay. Important to that process were the semiannual visits of small groups of foreign health professionals, largely North Americans, who came to work with the Haitians in an attempt, under the leadership of Père Alexis, to inaugurate a new clinic in Do Kay.

In January 1984, Église Saint-André was commandeered as a clinic for residents of Kay and surrounding villages. Present were Dr. Pierre, the Haitian physician then working with Père Alexis, and a few North American doctors and nurses. Early in the morning, the headmaster of the school (Maître Gérard) asked the visiting physicians to see Marie, an adolescent student who had collapsed while doing exercises on the new soccer field. When she regained consciousness, she complained of nausea and a severe headache. Her temperature was normal, and she stated that she had not "recently had a fever." The doctors found her to be quite anemic, but were unsure as to what had caused her collapse. She was given aspirin, a supply of vitamins, and tucked into the school sick bay, where she was to be seen later in the day. At noon it was discovered that Marie had declared herself "much better," and had walked home. With a long line of patients still waiting to see them, the physicians were perfectly satisfied with this response.

The next day, however, Marie slipped into a coma. Père Alexis brought her and her mother to see Dr. Pierre at the clinic in Mirebalais. Dr. Pierre examined Marie, and said very little other than "malaria." Marie, it was then revealed, had been experiencing intermittent fevers in the preceding weeks. She now presented with the symptoms of cerebral or "pernicious" malaria, and her chances of survival were estimated by Dr. Pierre to be "one or two in ten."[2] Marie was carried to the nearby house of a kinswoman, and Dr. Pierre followed with injectable chloroquine and other requisite supplies. It was agreed that she would be watched very closely.

She was not watched closely for long—not, at least, in Mirebalais. As I learned from Mme. Alexis the following day, Marie's father had "somehow rented a vehicle and driver, came in the middle of the night, and took the girl." Mme. Alexis had little else to add. But knowing Marie's family, the rest of the scenario was easy to piece together.

Marie was then eighteen years old, and lived with her parents and siblings in a house a few hundred yards down the road from the school in Kay. Though soft-spoken, she was one of Alexis's "leaders," and was active in church activities. Her mother, too, was an Episcopalian, and a regular at Père Alexis's services. Her father, however, was an irregular churchgoer, and had closer ties to Tonton Mèmè's place of worship (*houmfor*) in nearby Vieux Fonds. Tonton Mèmè was the Kay region's most well-known voodoo priest (*houngan*). Marie's father had arrived in the night, confident that doctors could not help his mysteriously felled daughter. Someone was trying to do her in, and he needed to find out who it was. As one of his friends later told me, Marie's father feared that "her illness was not simple. He thought it had an author." And he knew that only a *houngan* was going to be able to help him divine the author of her illness.

The reactions to this news ranged from dismay (on the part of the visiting physicians, who felt Marie's chances were nil without chloroquine), to weary resignation (evinced by Dr. Pierre, who also believed that Marie would not survive without chloroquine, but felt that there was nothing he could do about it), to angry anxiety (both Père and Mme. Alexis). Upon hearing the news, Père Alexis got into his pick-up truck and drove back to Do Kay, in an attempt to "wrest the girl from the clutches of a potentially fatal error." Her father refused to let anyone touch the still comatose Marie, and the priest left empty-handed and angry. A bargaining team then went to the house to ask if Marie could continue her chloroquine treatment there. A deal was struck, and Marie eventually emerged from her coma without any residual effects.

There were, however, residual effects on the community. These included a rift between Père Alexis and Marie's mother ("as one of my parishioners, she should have prevailed upon her husband to leave their daughter in the care of the physicians"), and a great deal of speculation whether it was the chloroquine or the *houngan* that had saved Marie's life. I learned of these debates in a second-hand manner. Of the dozen or so villagers interviewed about Marie's illness, only one spoke as if there was even a chance that she had been the victim of maleficence. The woman, who was an elderly relative of Marie's mother, insinuated a push and pull between opposing forces:

I'm not saying that the medicines did not help her. I'm saying that the way the thing happened suggests that it might not be God's illness (*maladi bondje*) that she had. She is well and then one minute, plop!, she's on the ground. This happens to an old lady, yes, but not a child. . . . Did Marie go to communion on Sunday? I think not, even though she always goes to communion. Could they have been trying to eat her (*manje li*)? I'm not saying that the medicines did not help her, but I'm glad she works in the sacristy. I'm glad she works with Père Alexis. A man his age should have high blood pressure, lower back pain, and problems with his eyes. But him—nothing.

The expression *manje li*, "to eat her," means to kill through magic, regardless of the specific mechanism (for example, illness, accident, even suicide).[3] The insinuation was that Marie, weakened by her inhabitual abstension from communion, was laid open to attack by a jealous rival. The rival must have engaged the services of a *bokor,* a *houngan* specializing in sorcery, who initiated the train of events necessary to *manje moun nan*—"eat the person."

It was not until 1985 that I was able to interview Tonton Mèmè himself. His *houmfor* and home, located in Vieux Fonds, stood a few yards from where his father, who had also been a *houngan,* had grown up. Two society flags, one atop a spectacularly tall mango tree, marked the house as a temple. It is usually quiet around the *houmfor,* although Mèmè's November 1 celebrations for Mèt Kafou and the *lwa bitasyon* (household *lwa*) draw hundreds of people and last for three to four days. Mèmè was among the most popular residents of Vieux Fonds. A diminutive, white-haired man, Mèmè seemed older than his fifty-seven years. "It's my work," he explained, plucking at his white hair. "There are always people here. And when we're down there," he added with a wave to his peristyle, "I neither eat nor drink nor sleep. I serve *lwa* who don't eat food."

Mèmè, his wife, and his large family live in a modest complex. It includes their house, a free-standing kitchen, a small, thatched peristyle, and a free-standing sanctum. In front of the peristyle is an impressive metal cross. It is, explained Mèmè, an *arèt,* a charm to protect the *lakou.* Inside the sanctum is an altar, which takes up a quarter of the unlit room, on top of which in 1985 were several plastic baby dolls, many bottles corked with corn cobs, cigarettes, a lighter, a deck of cards, a round yellow box for powder and a puff, and a tin box made of beer cans. The altar was presided over by a small statue of the Blessed Virgin, whose left hand touched a plastic duck, a hunting decoy. The walls were papered with pages from the magazine *Paris Match.* Several flags, the largest of which was Haitian, hung from the ceiling.[4] It is in the sanctum that Mèmè's patron spirits—Kafou and, less frequently, Tonton Bout—are consulted on the illnesses of Mèmè's clients.

Tonton Mèmè was pleased to answer questions about his profession, which brought him considerable satisfaction. These were not predominantly material: Mèmè was scarcely any less poor than his neighbors, although he did have a concrete floor. In spite of his professed overwork, Mèmè was always ready to sit someone down for instruction. The following was offered in a decidedly avuncular tone:

When a *houngan* treats someone for an illness, he attempts first to discover what [geographic] region the sickness comes from. He attempts to discover whether it was sent by a man or a woman, and why someone would wish to see [the ensorcelled person] die. But he might not know the name of the person [who sent the illness].

When asked how a *houngan* might determine these things, Tonton Mèmè explained that "the spirit (*espri*) that he serves lets him know. If (the *houngan*) needs his *lwa*, he calls it. He has a special relation with the *lwa*, when he calls the *lwa* will come, and he calls it to learn who sent [the illness]." Mèmè served two *lwa* in particular: Kafou and Tonton Bout. Kafou is a *lwa* invoked throughout Haiti, and is described in detail in the ethnographic literature. "The grand-master of charms and sorceries is Legba-Petro," notes Métraux (1972:266), "invoked under the name of Maître-Carrefour, or simply Carrefour." Tonton Bout is another story. He is not found in the literature, although local variations are well known.

Tonton Mèmè's role in Marie's near-fatal illness suggests the nature of the therapeutic systems that preceded, clashed with, and—occasionally—complemented the more newly arrived but long-consulted practitioners of cosmopolitan medicine. These dramatic struggles, it must be underlined, are not triggered by the vast majority of illness episodes. In 1985, a prospective study of twenty households in Do Kay revealed that the majority of illnesses were countered at home with the help of family or close neighbors.[5]

What sicknesses plague the inhabitants of Do Kay? There is little to suggest that the area around Kay is any different from the rest of rural Haiti. The damming of the Artibonite and the loss of land must have led to substantially increased rates of morbidity and mortality in the regions behind the Peligre dam, as the water refugees insist. Between 1983 and 1985, during the first years of Projè Veye Sante, the health surveillance project, "retrospective death reports" were collected from families in the Kay area. It appeared then that the chief causes of death among infants and children were diarrheal disease complicated by malnutrition, pneumonia complicated by malnutrition, typhoid complicated by malnutrition, and malnutrition. Neonatal tetanus and meningitis were also reported. Among adults, tuberculosis topped the list, followed by typhoid, malaria, and complications of childbirth, all of which may be aggravated by poor nutritional status.

In recent years, there have been heartening improvements, as when the capping of a major spring led to a prompt and widely appreciated decline in diarrheal disease among infants. The establishment of Projè Veye Sante led to efforts to combat malnutrition, to vaccinate children, and to bring a variety of services to the inhabitants of several villages.[6]

The effects of the founding of Clinique Saint-André are more difficult to gauge, but area residents often credit the clinic with having "saved many cases." Nonetheless, tuberculosis and other infectious diseases continue to exact a high toll on the population, and the residents of Kay are far from changing their structures of feeling[7] about illness and death:

> *Moun fèt pou mouri* ("people are born to die"), Haitians are fond of saying with a shrug of the shoulders. This proverb comments on the suffering and death that are commonplace occurrences in poverty-stricken Haiti and shows the stoic acceptance that, on one level at least, characterizes the Haitian attitude toward such a life. . . . Suffering is an expected, recurrent condition. It is not an exaggeration to say that problem-free periods in life are pervaded with an anxiety that anticipates crisis just around the corner. (Brown 1989a:40)

In the Kay region, as elsewhere in rural Haiti, suffering is indeed an expected condition. It may well be true that "we're always sick around here," as several villagers stated, and familiarity with serious illness, especially tuberculosis, certainly conditioned the response of the villagers to a previously unknown sickness. Haitian structures of feeling about suffering, in which are embedded a deep respect for the role of human agency in human affliction, were equally formative to the nascent model of *sida*. Serious illness is as often the result of injustice or malice as it is of "accident" or "fate." And as the stories of the water refugees suggest, injustice brought about by human agency is not countenanced silently.

Given that serious illnesses are commonplace in Do Kay, and that "suffering is an expected, recurrent condition," how is the fieldworker to decide which disasters are the central ones? "A central orienting question in ethnography," suggest Kleinman and Kleinman (1989:7), "should be to interpret what is at stake for particular participants in particular situations." The stakes, for the poor of Haiti, are life and death. The people of Kay recognize this and act accordingly. As will become clear in subsequent chapters, *sida* was understood through a number of interpretive frameworks that help to organize rural Haitians' readings of their world and the dangers in it. Because the boundaries of that world are far away, in Port-au-Prince or New York, the quest for an understanding of *sida* led to what might be termed a social epidemiology that underlined both local rules for living and large-scale interconnections. What is at stake is also revealed in one of their most frequently deployed responses to the question, How are you? *M'ap goumen ak lavi,* they reply: I'm fighting with life.

6

1986 and After: Narrative Truth and Political Change

The fieldwork upon which the ethnographic portions of this study are based was conducted during a tumultuous period of Haitian history. For three decades, the country was held in the viselike grip of the Duvaliers, and it was not until late 1985 that their hold on Haiti began to slip. The discontent born of the destruction of the Creole pigs fanned the anger smoldering in rural areas. Many astute observers list it as key to the movement that later ousted Duvalier:

The preliminary signs of the dictator's fall were seen simultaneously in the hunger riots of 1984 and 1985, the inability of the regime to stem the tide of boat-people reaching Florida, and the decision taken, at the instigation of U.S.-dominated foreign-aid organizations, to destroy—on the pretext of swine flu—all the Creole pigs, an essential element of the peasant economy. (Hurbon 1987b:20)[1]

Little appreciated was the contribution of another very destabilizing disaster: the advent of AIDS. Even more destructive, however, was the bad press generated by Haiti's designation as "the birthplace of AIDS." As Abbott (1988:255) has recently observed, "AIDS stamped Haiti's international image as political repression and intense poverty never had."

The debacles of contemporary Haiti—the incarceration of Haitian refugees, the destruction of Haiti's pigs, AIDS, the maintenance of the Duvalier regimes, the appalling poverty—are in fact not really "Haitian" problems at all, but *international* ones. Prior to the fall of Jean-

Claude Duvalier, their true significance as such was not widely appreciated outside of Haiti. The vast majority of North Americans were utterly oblivious to their own government's involvement with Haitian livestock. Only a minority of U.S. citizens not living in southern Florida were aware of the Reagan administration's harsh interdiction policies toward Haitian "boat people," and even fewer knew that the Duvalier dictatorships' chief source of foreign exchange had long been the United States government or U.S.-controlled multinational aid. Few North Americans knew of these issues, and fewer still construed them as anything other than "Haiti's problems." But virtually the entire Haitian population saw these issues in a much larger context, as became apparent after the collapse of the Duvalier regime.

On February 7, 1986, Jean-Claude Duvalier and his entourage left Haiti in a U.S. cargo plane.[2] The hope this awakened in 1986 gave way in late 1987 to great disappointment, as Haitians came to see that they were left with "Duvalierism without Duvalier." The military governments that took over the state apparatus were closely allied with the dictatorship, and the passing years brought no genuine change for the Haitian poor. But events of this era were experienced by all who lived in Do Kay. *Sida* came into the lives of rural Haitians at the same time they were experiencing the first nationwide political turmoil in decades, and these political changes came to have an effect on the manner in which this new sickness was perceived (see Farmer 1990b).

In fact, those who have done anthropological fieldwork both before and after *le 7 février,* as it is termed, will appreciate the significance of the changes of the past few years. In pre-1986 Haiti, the ethnographer quickly learned that politics and even recent history were subjects not to be broached directly.[3] In Kay, even close friends declined to discuss politics among one another. Searching for fear in their silence, one easily discerned it, but it seemed then to be only one of several important disincentives. The villagers also affected apathy, resignation, and—especially—ignorance. They seemed to know little about the last thirty or so years of Haitian politics, in spite of their impressive knowledge of the revolution that led to the founding of their country.

The student of Haitian history knows that the peasantry has at crucial conjunctures displayed a keen awareness of social, political, and cultural forces. The record is replete with accounts of jacqueries and peasant movements, local revolts, and organized resistance. Less well documented is what Scott (1985:xvi) terms the "small arms fire in the class war." He describes everyday forms of peasant resistance as the prosaic but constant struggle between the peasantry and those who seek to extract labor, food, taxes, rents, and interest from them. Most forms of this struggle stop well short of outright collective defiance. Here I have in mind the ordinary weapons of relatively powerless groups: foot dragging, dissimulation, desertion, false compliance, pilfering, feigned ignorance, slander, arson, sabotage, and so on.

Evidence suggests that the collective silence surrounding the key issues observed in Kay was less a conscious mechanism than "an effective and calculated strategy of resistance to the economic and political demands of the State and accompanying commercial interests" (Lowenthal 1976:665). After a couple of years in village Haiti, however, it seemed safe to conclude that the inhabitants of the Kay region were simply not as interested as I in things political. The struggle there, it seemed, was not seen as political; the struggle was for survival.

As late as the summer of 1985, Duvalier appeared to be permanently affixed to his presidential throne. Riots had taken place the previous summer, initially caused by police brutality against a pregnant woman, but also reflecting the general despair and pervasive hunger. Some foreign observers predicted that protest would spread from provincial cities to the hinterlands, but the people of Kay apparently had not heard of the riots. What they did hear was that a referendum would be held in July. The ballot was a sham, however, engineered to lend the appearance of political pluralism to the dictatorship—and the U.S. State Department, for which the referendum was staged, asked for little more.[4] Still, many Haitians gritted their teeth and voted. With the subtlety one had come to expect of the Duvaliers, the Ministry of Information announced that 99.8 percent of the voters had approved the referendum, which granted (among other things) continued carte blanche to the *président-à-vie*. Although most of the adults I knew had abstained (making it difficult to believe government reports of record turnout), those who went to the polling places voted yes. "Of course we voted yes," responded one friend wearily.

The referendum offered, stated Minister of the Interior Roger Lafontant on government radio, "a resounding lesson to all those who have not grasped that Haiti belongs to Duvalier and Duvalier belongs to Haiti."[5] Many had followed these developments on Radio Soleil, the Catholic station and sole surviving independent voice. Even though its criticisms had been elaborately veiled, the station was shut down a few days before the referendum and its manager was deported. These events became known through what is termed *teledjol,* which might be loosely translated as "teletrap"—the grapevine. Afterwards, the people of Kay turned back to their gardens and children and churches. Rural Haiti seemed stalled in a well-balanced mixture of fear, apathy, and preoccupation with day-to-day survival.

The movement that began a few months later dispelled the impression of stasis. Although there had been sporadic explosions of discontent in the years before 1985, it was not until autumn of that year that any coherent rebellion emerged. In November an obscure antigovernment protest in the city of Gonaives became the focus of national rage when government forces shot and bayoneted three schoolboys. Over the protests of the children's families, their bodies were buried in an unmarked grave at an undisclosed time: the regime wished to prevent the children's funerals from becoming antigovernment protests. That was the beginning of the end for Duvalier, who tried to placate the families by sending them condolences and envelopes stuffed with money. "The mourners spat at one and refused the other," reports Abbott (1988:295). "'You want to pay for killing our children?' a mother shouted. 'Do you think they are pigs?'" Students throughout the country "went on strike," and after Christmas simply refused to return to school until Duvalier was gone.

Popular uprisings spread throughout the provincial cities during the first week of January, finally reaching Port-au-Prince. Haitian military and paramilitary forces fired on crowds, who replied with rocks and flaming barricades. The commercial sector joined the students, and the country became entirely paralyzed. A bloodbath seemed likely, but was postponed by Duvalier's departure. He, his family, and much of their wealth left battered Haiti on February 7 in a U.S. cargo plane.

What had happened? Certainly, there had been a popular rebellion. But once again, the appearance of a "purely Haitian political event" was illusory. The fall of Duvalier was no more exclusively Haitian than any of the other events in contemporary Haiti:

Two series of events occurred on February 7, 1986: first, the departure of Duvalier; second, *the takeover of the state machinery by a group of apparently disparate individuals*: civilians and career army officers, Duvalierists and former opposition figures, past backers of repression and former human rights leaders. Missing from the dominant version, or at best viewed as secondary, are the negotiations—the tacit and explicit understandings between Haitian and U.S. politicians, in Haiti and the United States, local and foreign military and intelligence personnel, ambassadors, power brokers, and bureaucrats—that led to, and tied together, the two sets of events. (Trouillot 1990:224–225)

The U.S. government claimed it had played a major role in removing Duvalier; the leaders of the rebellion claimed that the Reagan administration, staunch supporters of Latin American tyranny, were simply grandstanding. Both sides were correct.

It was shortly thereafter that far-reaching changes in the political culture of Haiti became most evident. One of the first slogans to gain currency after Duvalier's fall was *baboukèt la tonbe*. A literal English equivalent would be "the bridle has fallen off," but the phrase would be better rendered as "the muzzle is off." One journalist recalled "the feeling of a million people talking all at once and all of a sudden" (Wilentz 1989:63). New (and sometimes short-lived) newspapers were peddled on the street corners of Port-au-Prince; banned radio stations were reopened, political tracts littered the streets, new labor unions began flexing their muscles. Most striking of all was the seeming unanimity with which the Haitians undertook the process they termed *dechoukaj*, "the uprooting." Members of the Duvaliers' militia were publicly persecuted and even killed; Papa Doc's hated red and black flag was replaced with its red and blue predecessor; a statue of Christopher Columbus—symbol of foreign imperialism—was uprooted and dumped into the Bay of Port-au-Prince, and the public square it had graced was rebaptized "Place Charlemagne Péralte," in honor of the leader of the armed resistance to the U.S. military occupation of Haiti (1915–1934).

The new Haitian government, the Conseil National de Gouvernment (CNG), did not care for *dechoukaj*. This is hardly surprising, since *dechoukaj* was mostly aimed at Duvalierists, and the CNG was becoming increasingly devoid of non-Duvalierists. Before long, it was a military junta composed of the only kind of high-ranking officers Haiti had: Duvalierists. And so expressions of popular discontent were met in proper Duvalierist fashion: "By the end of its first year in office the CNG, generously helped by the U.S. taxpayers' money, had openly gunned down more civilians than Jean-Claude Duvalier's government had done in fifteen years" (Trouillot 1990:222).

Although the majority of state-sponsored violence was in the capital, the changes overtaking Haiti were also registered in provincial towns like Mirebalais, the parish seat of Père Alexis. As the muzzle was removed, political discourse took on enormous significance in the lives of many of its citizens. Père Alexis's sermons, too, became less allegorical and often strayed into the realm of specific rebukes. On several occasions he deplored the shooting by soldiers of unarmed protesters. Referring in 1986 to a local dance, the priest stated that he was dismayed that residents of Mirebalais could "make merry" on the same day that a score of unarmed protesters were killed by government troops: "It seems strange to me that anyone could spend their time partying when the country is on its deathbed, while our sisters and brothers are falling on the battlefield."

These changes were also felt in small villages like Do Kay. Although a full year elapsed before the adventurous were wholeheartedly joined by a majority of the villagers, the transformation seemed complete by the spring of 1987. By that time, one of the most striking phenomena in rural Haiti was the degree to which previously silent and "uninformed" villagers were conversant with the slightest details of current national events. News travels quickly in rural Haiti because villagers often go to Port-au-Prince. When Bastien (1985:128) notes that rural Haitian women tend to be extremely well informed, he is quick to add that their expertise concerns "not just the rise and fall of prices, but also national events." But there are many other important ways in which villages as "remote" as Do Kay are connected to the city, and to the United States. Research conducted in the summer of 1985 should have prepared me for the sudden *mise en relief* of these connections that would appear less than a year later. During the annual census, we asked whether or not families had relatives in Port-au-Prince or the United States. Of the 123 families then living in Do Kay, 56 had kin in the urban area, and 14 families could claim consanguinity with Haitians living in the United States. Virtually all households had moral claims on various "godparents" in the capital or abroad.[6]

Further, the nature of the links of these Port-au-Prince–based kin to the United States is also complex. Some of those from the Kay area who work in the capital do so in factories assembling North American products for reexport. For example, Mme. Sonson's son Frico went to École Saint-André until he was fifteen. When his options in Kay dried up, he left for "the city" in search of work. Through another young man from Do Kay, he found work on a chicken farm, whose manager promised to help him find a visa for *lòtbò*—"the other side," that is, of the water separating Haiti from the United States. Nothing came of this promise, and Frico soon wearied of his wages of a dollar a day. Again through a young man from Do Kay, he found a job in a factory assembling windows for a North American concern. For the next eight years, he spent his days fitting glass into metal casings.[7] He regularly sent money to his parents, and helped to put his younger siblings through school in Do Kay and in Mirebalais.

It is through affective and economic connections such as these that inhabitants of Kay experienced events in the city and, beyond that, *lòtbò*. And although the importance of such links was established before 1986, certain changes that year highlighted them: (1) transistor radios suddenly proliferated or surfaced, and men, especially, spent entire days cradling their radios, switching from one Creole news program to another; (2) community councils, drastically overhauled in other villages, were strengthened in the area around Kay, and their meetings, that once drew only a score of people, attracted in the summer of 1986 over a hundred persons; (3) new civic groups were formed, and they attended to such activities as repairing roads and planting trees. All this was worked into the daily round of gardening and marketing, but stood out nonetheless, and was a reminder that there was much more to *dechoukaj* than revenge for Duvalier-period atrocities:

The operation termed *dechoukaj* was not merely the cleaning up or eradication of the macoute network, the nighttime eye of the terror infiltrating every cranny of this society. It was above all the expression of a desire to rebuild the nation on a foundation radically different from that of despotism. (Hurbon 1987b:8)

There was, however, great anger toward the Duvaliers. Mme. Sonson, widely appreciated as one of the sweetest and most easy-going residents of Do Kay, swore that if she caught up with the Duvaliers, she would settle the score with them. She then listed a series of tortures that were worthy of the slavemasters of Saint-Domingue. Old, politically incisive proverbs were given new currency, and many humorous new phrases reflected the changes. For example, someone who was holding forth on a subject was no longer simply saying what he or she thought—that person was "holding a press conference." A villager who appeared in conspicuously nice apparel stood a decent chance of being greeted as a "presidential candidate." A young woman who was behaving in a spoiled and entitled fashion was pulling a *michelbè*—a pun on "gussied up" and the name of Duvalier's acquisitive wife. Soldiers were often called *mesyè atimojen yo,* "the tear-gas gentlemen." A thwarted child might, with the right audience, threaten her mother with *dechoukaj*. People painted "chak 4 an" ("every four years") on their houses, as well as the verb *dechouke*. In the spring of 1987, a rather good-natured skepticism about politics and politicians seemed to be the order of the day in Kay.

In the summer of 1987, when the ruling junta announced that it was dissolving a militant labor union and usurping the role of the civilian electoral council, that skepticism turned into an angry cynicism. It was, the villagers seemed to agree, a *coup d'état* by inches. When a general strike was called by a hastily formed opposition coalition, roadblocks were erected even in Kay. The strikes, at first a huge success, eventually wore the rural population down. And villagers heard, by *teledjol* and radio, that the army had opened fire on demonstrators in Port-au-Prince: more than fifty were killed in a single month. Families with sons and daughters in the city pleaded with them to be careful. Although the running of elections was restored to the electoral council and the banned union was reestablished, the cynicism and disappointment remained. Presidential hopefuls were now regarded with a good deal of suspicion, and a great deal of village rhetoric was devoted to classing the candidates as *makout, ameriken* (two substantially overlapping sets), or *pèp,* of the people. Les Frères Parent, a musical group popular in rural Haiti, had a hit single with "Watch Out for the Candidates":

Veye yo, se pou nou veye yo—
Restavèk 'Meriken

[Keep an eye on them, we must keep an eye on them—
(North) America's live-in maids]

The violent eruption of overtly political concerns continued throughout the summer and came to be reflected in all aspects of community life, especially for those tied somehow to "the city."

Another important link between Do Kay and the capital is constituted by those who work in the school and clinic. By far the area's largest employer, the school-clinic complex is dependent on regular provisions from Port-au-Prince. On August 1, 1987, Mme. Alexis and several school staff were buying supplies for the school in the market area around city hall. Meanwhile, Père Jacques was ordering medications for the clinic. Shortly thereafter he began walking the half-mile back to the center of the city, where he was to meet his wife and coworkers, when he saw a *kouri*—hundreds of panicked people stampeding away from the square behind city hall. Assuming that the military had again opened fire on a crowd, the priest began running toward the meeting place.

As he rounded the last corner before Avenue Jean-Jacques Dessalines, the city's main thoroughfare, Alexis came upon a grisly sight: a city garbage truck full of corpses had been set afire by an incensed crowd. The driver narrowly escaped with his life, as the crowd cried "Murderers!" and "The State is killing the people!" Troops and police arrived and began firing automatic weapons. Soon many were wounded and three bystanders lay dead, including a market woman, slumped over her basket of cabbages. No one from Kay was injured, perhaps because, as Mme. Alexis put it, "We beat it as soon as we heard the gunfire." Everyone was, however, shaken and revolted that, to quote Père Alexis, "the government would insolently parade its victims before us."

The government radio station later explained that the corpses were actually the bodies of indigent patients who had expired in the state-run General Hospital. Their remains were only being transferred, however unceremoniously, to a communal grave north of the city. Though the explanation appears to have been true, few in Kay believed it, and that night word of the "death truck" (*kamyon lanmo*) spread, it seemed, to every house. A kinswoman of one of those who had been with Mme. Alexis later remarked:

[The mayor] said they were poor people who had died in the hospital. Do you believe that? Do they usually transport the dead in garbage trucks? No, they use big ambulances. Do they usually drive an open truck full of bodies through the mud of Port-au-Prince? On the busiest morning of the week? No, they don't do that unless they want to intimidate the people.

The government was "shameless" or, even more damning, "motherless" (*san manman*). The next day was a Sunday, during which Père Jacques was scheduled to say mass in Do Kay. He recounted with emotion the scene from the day before. Even small children were listening as he closed his sermon with the following peroration:

Why shouldn't we doubt their story? Yes, they tell us that these were the bodies of the poor, those who had died in the General Hospital. Of natural causes, they said. But what is natural about death from poverty? What is natural about being pitched like offal into a truck? Being paraded through the city covered with flies? . . . And what did this poor market woman die for? Absolutely nothing, unless it was to serve as a reminder of the absolute disregard for the people's sensibilities that has long reigned in Port-au-Prince. But remember what Luke, chapter 1, promises:

He has stretched out his mighty arm
and scattered the proud
with all their plans.
He has brought down the mighty
kings from their thrones,
and the lowly he has lifted up.
He has filled the hungry with good things
and sent the rich away
with empty hands.

It was an electrifying performance, with abundant audience response. Several people wept, although there was an air of *déjà vu* about the story. Disturbingly, everything about the entire sequence of events, from the *kouri* to the killings to the sermon, was of a piece with "the new Haiti."

What, exactly, had happened in Do Kay? No important structural changes had taken place in the rural economy, just a continuation of the slow decline that had been in process for decades. And yet surely something more than an epidemic of radio-dial twirling and conscious politicization of song and discourse had come to pass. Certainly, the changes were related to allowed and disallowed discourse. But not only were the villagers talking about subjects previously forbidden, they were talking about old subjects in new ways. Hurbon links the events of 1986 and after to a change in the peasants' conceptions of their roles in a country they have so long supported:

The novelty of February 7 seems to lie in the peasants' expressed rejection of the image constructed of them, that of "savages of the interior." They claim that from now on they are full-fledged citizens, determined to defend their own interests. Since the fall of the dictatorship, all the "Duvalierist" State violence has rained down upon them, and upon the crowds of the shantytowns (products of the rural exodus) in particular. (Hurbon 1987b:19)

Something truly new was going on, and it was difficult to define. Haiti was still run by Duvalierists. State-sponsored violence still rained down upon dissenters, especially poor ones, and the disastrous economic situation had only worsened. But Haiti was rhetorically construed by the rural and urban poor as a place that could and must be different. Such rhetorical trends suggest that these changes occurred between language and the theories people hold about their world and their possibilities within that world. The shifts of the post-1986 era have been subtle, yet far-reaching. Not only were the rural people intentionally politicizing their discourse, but because "the muzzle was off" there have been subtle shifts in the *uses* of talk, discourse, and story-telling—a certain reorganization of modes of speech and thought.

These shifts have had, as we shall see, a discernible effect on the way in which illness is discussed. The political changes of the last few years, as limited as they have been in terms of tangible benefits to the peasantry, have had a significant impact on the social construction of *sida*. The illness narratives collected in Do Kay would be regarded as politically inoffensive by both the speakers and those persons most feared as oppressors.[8] And yet they reflect, through changes in narrative and rhetorical structure, the reorganization of modes of speech and thought that has occurred since 1986. Much of this reorganization has revolved around *questions of agency in suffering*. Is it the infertility of the soil, or the heartless machinations of the urban bourgeoisie that are invoked in discussions of poverty? Is infant diarrhea caused by microbes, or by microbes caused by dirty water, which in turn is caused by an irresponsible government? Is *sida* caused by sorcery, or by the bitterness that drives the poor to "send illness" on one another? The illness narratives collected in Do Kay posit several different kinds of cause. And underlying these is a series of oppositions: personal/impersonal, just/unjust, merited/unmerited, necessary/unavoidable, endurable/unendurable, inside/outside, and others not yet uncovered. Equally important categories—and somewhat different from that of cause—are local understandings of recrimination and appeal and the assignment of blame.

As we turn now to consider the Haitian AIDS epidemic in the context of a larger "West Atlantic pandemic," we will see that changes in a rhetoric of complaint have been important in the social construction of *sida* in Do Kay and elsewhere. Is AIDS caused by microbes or by poverty born of the dam? Is AIDS an infectious disease or a "jealousy sickness," related somehow to competition in a setting of great material scarcity? Is AIDS a product of North American imperialism? Can one person send "an AIDS death" to another through sorcery? Are Haitians a special "AIDS risk group"? Are "boat people" disease-ridden and a threat to the health of U.S. citizens? These questions underscore several of the West Atlantic pandemic's central dynamics—blame, search for accountability, accusation, and racism—that have shaped both responses to AIDS and the epidemiology of a new virus.

PART TWO

AIDS Comes to a Haitian Village

As new medical terms become known in a society, they find their way into existing semantic networks. Thus while new explanatory models may be introduced, it is clear that changes in medical rationality seldom follow quickly.

Good (1977:54)

7

Manno

When I lie down to sleep, the hours drag;
I toss all night and long for dawn.
My body is full of worms;
It is covered with scabs;
Pus runs out of my sores.
My days pass by without hope,
Pass faster than a weaver's shuttle.

Job 7:4–6

This cry cannot be muted. Those who suffer unjustly have a
right to complain and protest. Their cry expresses both their
bewilderment and their faith.

Gutierrez (1987:101)

Manno Surpris moved to Do Kay in 1982, when he became a teacher at the community's large new school. He was twenty-
five years old. Born in the village of Saut d'Eau,[1] Manno grew up and
received his early education in a family of peasant farmers. After having
passed his primary school exams, Manno moved to Mirebalais, a large
market town not far from Saut d'Eau. He began his secondary school
education there, but found Mirebalais "very difficult. I had no one
there, and couldn't stay on in the room I was using." Several months
after his arrival, he received word from a cousin that he could board
in her house in a poor quarter of Port-au-Prince. Manno left Mirebalais

immediately, expecting to complete his secondary education in the capital. As is often the case for rural children with such expectations, Manno did odd jobs in order to pay tuition at one of what many urban Haitians label "lottery schools" (so called because, insofar as learning is concerned, "you take your chances"). In five years, Manno finished only two more grades. Concluding that he would never be able to complete his studies, Manno moved back to Mirebalais, where he hoped to find a job.

Well before Père Jacques Alexis completed the school he was building in Do Kay, he began looking for teachers interested in working with villagers. He knew that *lycée* graduates would not be easy to recruit, and was quite happy to offer a position to Manno, who had the equivalent of an eighth-grade education. Less than a year after his arrival, he had become Père Jacques's favorite teacher, and within two years had been entrusted with a number of very public responsibilities. In addition to teaching, Manno was in charge of the new pigsty and had attended training seminars in animal husbandry. He was responsible for the maintenance of the water pump on which the community depended for all its water. As Père Jacques later recalled, "I felt that he was good-natured and dependable. But most of all, he didn't seem to be in as much of a hurry to get back to Mirebalais on Friday afternoon. He really seemed to like working in the village." Alourdes Monestime, a Kay area native working at École Saint-André, was one reason that Manno enjoyed staying in Do Kay. In 1984, their daughter was born; a year later, they began building their own house not far from the school. A second child was on the way.

It was not difficult to see that Manno was not universally popular. He was a salaried teacher; some of his other duties were also remunerative, and so he was confronted by the envy of the less fortunate. Jealousy was compounded by the fact that for the villagers he was *moun vini,* a newcomer or outsider. This resentment was made obvious when, shortly after Duvalier's departure in February 1986, Manno's half-finished house was knocked down. His house, it was widely remarked, was *dechouke*—this in spite of the fact that he had virtually no ties to any *makout* individual or institution. Although these sorts of events were common throughout Haiti, this was the only such incident in the Kay area, where *dechoukaj* otherwise consisted of graffiti alone.

The true dimensions of the sentiment against him were not clear until August 1986, when Manno beat a schoolboy for some transgression in the pigsty. The intensity of the community's reaction was surprising. The "facts" were quickly circulated by word of mouth: the schoolboy had inadvertently let several pigs escape. Manno, upon discovering this, lit into him with a length of rubber hose. The first reactions I heard were those of Mme. Kado, who remarked, "He would never have dared to beat him if the poor boy were not an orphan. He would never dare to strike one of Sonson's children." The old man who had unofficially adopted the boy upon the death of his mother was not in the village. A couple of local men were muttering about settling the score with Manno. Someone sent word to the boy's grandmother, who lived a couple of hours from Do Kay. Someone else went to look for the foster father. A couple of schoolboys began carrying their own lengths of hose "for self-defense." The crisis was defused by Mme. Alexis, who called for a meeting among the adults concerned (Manno, the child's grandmother, and the foster parent in Do Kay). With Manno's apology to the boy and his partisans, the whole affair had been ostensibly closed.

After a day or two, there was no more public grumbling about Manno. In conversing about the incident, Mme. Dieugrand noted the silence, and thought this might be due to his illness: "Poor fellow, the whole affair has left him sick." But Manno had been ill well before the incident. He had been plagued with intermittent diarrhea throughout the summer, and also by superficial skin infections. He had been treating the latter with a topical antifungal agent prescribed by one of the doctors at the Clinique Saint-André. The patches would clear up, only to reappear, usually on the scalp, neck, or face. Early in the fall, Père Jacques took Manno twice to see a dermatologist in Port-au-Prince. Manno's diarrhea had by then come and gone, and come again. His weight loss had become evident even to casual acquaintances. By December, his decline was drastic, and Manno began to cough. Père Jacques took him to Port-au-Prince again shortly before Christmas. He saw one of the country's best-known internists, and a chest radiograph and tuberculin skin test were ordered.[2]

Indeed, more than one villager suggested that Manno had fallen ill with tuberculosis. Others were of the opinion that the dermatological process was a manifestation of *move san,* attributed by some to the "bad blood" born of the beating of the schoolboy. One spoke of the effects on Manno of having his house *dechouke,* while three villagers interviewed insisted that his *move san* was the result of nearly being struck by lightning some years earlier. "It was not his wife alone that was ill with *move san,*" explained Mme. Sonson. "It was both of them. She was smart enough to have hers treated, as she had a breastfeeding baby. But Manno let it drag on and on and on and on."

By Christmas, the clinical staff of Clinique Saint-André began to whisper, among themselves, that AIDS could be the cause of Manno's problems. Nothing was said to Père Jacques. Manno was seeing an eminent physician, they reasoned; he would certainly not overlook such an obvious possibility. After the New Year, each day brought a noticeable decline in Manno's health. At the same time a rumor, very hushed, was circulating around Do Kay: Manno was the victim of some sort of evil. His illness was the intentional result of some angry or jealous rival. I heard this from an eighteen-year-old former student of Manno's. He would not say who had passed this gossip on to him, and attempted to dismiss it. "I don't believe it myself," said the student, "but that's what some people say." He also stated that he did not know who would wish to harm the teacher. When asked how he thought such an illness could have been inflicted on Manno, the youth was again rather vague: "I don't know . . . some people can do it by themselves, some go to a *bokor*."

Manno's beating of the boy and its sequelae returned to mind when the student shared the rumor. Was the putative sorcery related to the beating? When the subject was broached with Mme. Alexis, I found that she also knew of the sorcery rumor, and she had received the story from Alourdes herself. "But once a real diagnosis is given, everyone will understand that this is not a case of evil done to him," said Mme. Alexis. "That's why it's imperative that his family know the real diagnosis." She stated this in mid-January, while Manno was being evaluated by the distinguished internist. Everyone agreed that a diagnosis was needed. Manno was dying, and all the doctor's expensive tests had been negative. Père Jacques had already considered the possibility that Manno might be ill with AIDS. Madame Alexis, who had not, was shocked when it was suggested to her as a possibility. "But how on earth could he have contracted that illness? . . . He's been married for three years," she protested. "And surely he isn't homosexual?"

After two months of uncertainty, the internist referred Manno to the country's sole public AIDS clinic, which is located in Port-au-Prince and operated by a team of clinician-researchers. By the time he was referred, the clinic had closed for the weekend. It was unclear if Manno would last until Monday. He could no longer walk, was dehydrated, weighed less than ninety pounds, and was disoriented. Père Jacques suggested that Manno spend the weekend in Mirebalais, at the priest's rectory. Manno could be made more comfortable, it was decided, in one of the houses then being used as dormitories for villagers who were studying at the town *lycée*.

Manno did survive the weekend, and reported to the AIDS clinic at 9:30 A.M. on Monday. It was by then already crowded with emaciated men and women. Manno was among the sickest-looking, and he was seen almost immediately. A physician looked at Manno, and then at the X-ray taken during the previous work-up. Dr. Boyer was a young internist who had already established herself as an "AIDS doctor." Boyer had a reputation of maintaining compassion while others had "burned out." She questioned Manno in Haitian, and then turned to me and said in perfect English: "I don't understand [the referring doctor's] verdict. I read this as a clear-cut case of disseminated tuberculosis." She paused, and then added, "I'm afraid the [HIV] test will prove positive; regardless, you've got a very sick man on your hands. We'll draw the blood for the test, and start him on [antituberculous medications]."

Manno was taken back to the house in Mirebalais, where he began receiving the new drugs under the supervision of the medical staff of another clinic founded by Père Jacques; members of the Clinique Saint-André staff were also encouraged to visit Manno regularly. The sick man had been badly dehydrated and responded well to intravenous fluids. Within three days, Manno no longer looked like a dying man. He spoke easily, and seemed grateful for the visits that, only a few days before, had seemed only to confuse him. His cough persisted, but was less incessant, and he began eating. As he started to improve, he was better able to converse about his illness. In an interview conducted in the first week of February, before the results of the HIV-antibody test were known, I asked Manno what he thought had made him so sick. He looked embarrassed and troubled. "Well, I don't really know . . . I don't know." What are you most afraid of? Tears came to his eyes. He knows, then, I thought. He knows that he might have AIDS. Instead, he replied:

Most of all, I hope it's not tuberculosis. But I'm afraid that's what it is. I'm coughing, I've lost weight . . . I'm afraid I have tuberculosis, and that I'll never get better, never be able to work again. . . . People don't want to be near you if you have tuberculosis.

It was during this time that Manno spoke of the history of his sexual activity. For a thirty-year-old who was thought to have AIDS, his reported sexual activity was strikingly sparse, especially when compared to sexual histories elicited from North Americans with AIDS, or to their HIV-seronegative, age-matched controls. Manno had far fewer sexual contacts than a cohort of male AIDS patients in Port-au-Prince.[3] Manno reported sexual contact with only four persons, all of them women. None of them was involved in prostitution, although one was, he said, "a little bit free with her body." Two of these women he met in Port-au-Prince, the third in Mirebalais, and the fourth was Alourdes, whom he had met in Do Kay in 1982. Since he became involved with Alourdes about four years ago, he said, he had slept with no one else. He reported never having had sexual contact with a man or a boy; he denied use of any narcotics (indeed, he had heard of neither heroin nor marijuana, although he was familiar with the Haitian word for "illicit drug"). He had received, however, "at least a dozen" injections, usually of penicillin or injectable vitamins, by hypodermic needle. Although many of these had been administered in the preceding months, several injections dated from years ago. He had never received a transfusion; the IV fluids he had received in the past month had been administered with sterile needles.

According to the national laboratory, Manno did indeed have antibodies to HIV. Since he also had tuberculosis, he responded very well to an antituberculous regimen. On Manno's next trip to see the AIDS specialist, Alourdes went with him. She tested seronegative, and Dr. Boyer advised her to avoid unprotected sexual contact with Manno. The doctor informed both of them that Manno had AIDS, but that she would do everything in her power to help him fight off the infections to which he would likely fall prey. Getting over the tuberculosis would be the first of several trials, she predicted, urging the couple to remain in close contact with the clinic.

Manno remained in Mirebalais for over a month. Père Jacques, although disheartened by the lab results and fully aware of the usual course of the disease, spared no expense in treating Manno: prescriptions were filled promptly, well-balanced meals were prepared and delivered to the house in which he was recovering. His mother came from Saut d'Eau; Alourdes's sister came from a village near Do Kay. Everyone took turns caring for Manno. No one seemed afraid to touch him, although family members had been warned that Manno's illness was "caused by a microbe, a virus." By mid-February, Manno was going for walks, and by the end of the month had put on almost twenty pounds. He soon stopped coughing completely. By early March, he no longer looked ill at all. Père Jacques wondered whether or not Manno might return to teaching by the fall semester. Mme. Alexis was sure that he had been misdiagnosed, despite warnings from her medical coworkers that this was a common course of the syndrome.

Manno did so well, in fact, that some of his covillagers began to wonder why he had not returned to Do Kay. Although no one seemed particularly leery of Manno, he was frightened of something or someone. When Alourdes returned to her teaching post, she chose not to sleep in her house, but to stay with her mother—almost an hour's dusty walk from the school. Mme. Sonson, who counted herself a kinswoman of Alourdes, commented on this arrangement, attributing it at first to the tensions that had helped to generate Manno's *move san*. "Oh sure, his blood's spoiled (*gate*)," stated Mme. Sonson. "He has very serious, big problems, and it's no wonder his blood has gone bad." Although nine of twenty villagers consulted stated that *move san* contributed substantially to his problems, the remainder felt that Manno's blood had nothing to do with either his condition or his actions. "His problem is not *move san*," opined Mme. Charité cryptically. "Not at all *move san*, something else." For some of those informants, *sida* was at the root of Manno's problems. For many others, however, the "something else" was related to sorcery. When Père Jacques was asked why Manno might be reluctant to return to Kay, he responded candidly:

I have heard that Manno believes that he is the victim of someone's ill-will. I hope you can at least see why this sort of accusation is dangerous. It doesn't hurt anyone if you blame a microbe, but blaming someone else for your misfortunes leads to division and hatred. That's why I'm so unhappy that Manno believes he's been the victim of evil.[4]

Père Jacques's "unhappiness" may have resulted in a confrontation with Manno. In any case, Manno departed from Mirebalais surreptitiously. Père and Mme. Alexis later condemned Manno's "lack of personality." "He should at least have come by [the rectory] before leaving Mirebalais," complained Père Jacques, "but I haven't seen him at all." Manno was nowhere to be found. At the end of March, I traveled to Alourdes's mother's house at least three times; her son-in-law was never there. He was "in his own country, at his mother's," or "in Mirebalais for a couple of days." Alourdes's sister informed me that Manno had "gone to Mirebalais to vote for the new Constitution." These responses seemed legitimate, and I would have kept on believing them, but a member of Projè Veye Sante lived next door to Alourdes's mother. Community health worker Christian Guerrier was also related to Alourdes by blood—their fathers were brothers. The day after my third visit, Christian walked from his house to Do Kay, and asked if I would "interview him for my research." He explained that there was much that I did not understand:

> There's something you need to understand about Haitians, at least some of them. They believe that there are different kinds of medications for different kinds of illnesses. Some illnesses require several different kinds of medications. . . . Manno is not at his mother's house. He is in Vieux Fonds, being treated by a *houngan*. He believes that, because someone sent him the illness, it must be taken away.

Throughout our long interview, Christian spoke as if he did not believe that recourse to a *houngan* would prove useful. He used the word *fetich* several times, which has a slightly less pejorative ring to it in Haitian than it does in English. He stated that Manno's treatment might take a long time—"many days or weeks"—and that he would not return until the *houngan* had finished treating him. When asked why the treatment took so long, Christian replied cautiously: "Well, these people believe that when someone 'sends the dead' that the dead go into the body, into the chest of the sick person. It's very hard to get the dead out." "Expedition of the dead" is a model of illness causation well documented in the scholarly literature on voodoo. Métraux refers to the sending of the dead as "the most fearful practice in the black arts." His description of "expedited" illness is phenomenologically similar to untreated pulmonary tuberculosis:

> Whoever has become the prey of one or more dead people sent against him begins to grow thin, spit blood and is soon dead. The laying on of this spell is always attended by fatal results unless it is diagnosed in time and a capable *houngan* succeeds in making the dead let go. (Métraux 1972:274)

Further, Métraux's description seems to echo that of Christian: "The dead embed themselves in the organism into which they are inserted and it is very difficult to make them let go" (Métraux 1972:276).[5] Finally, Christian intimated that I might wish to confront Alourdes about her husband's whereabouts, taking care not to let her know that her cousin had revealed the true nature of Manno's absence.

There was only one bona fide *houngan* in Vieux Fonds: Tonton Mème.[6] It did not seem appropriate to drop in on him while Manno was in his care, as it was clear that Manno would be embarrassed to be seen there. An interview with Alourdes then revealed that her husband was in fact not in Vieux Fonds; Christian was mistaken or altering the facts slightly. On the other details, however, his story was confirmed, and so I followed his advice and raised the subject with Alourdes. I began by noting that "there are different kinds of medications for different kinds of illnesses. Some illnesses require several different kinds of medications." After initial surprise, Alourdes did not seem reluctant to impart more detailed information about Manno's treatment. At first, she was careful to attribute his activities to "his own beliefs" about his illness: "Manno believes that they did this to him because they were jealous that he had three jobs—teaching, the pigsty, and the water pump." Later in the same interview, however, she dropped all pretense at skepticism, noting that "the people who did this to him already know what they've done; they know what kind of illness they've sent. He won't survive: there are people who know how to send a TB death (*voye yon mò tebe*) on someone; that person gets TB."[7] She said nothing about *sida,* so it was not clear whether she meant the new disorder was unrelated to Manno's real problem, or whether someone had sent, through a similar process, a *mò sida.* When it was noted that Manno seemed to be doing quite well for a man with such a sentence over his head, Alourdes responded with a proverb: "A leaf doesn't rot on the same day that it falls into the water."

If Alourdes had succeeded in diagnosing the problem, she was reluctant to tell who was responsible for sending the dead. I pressed her, as she had already noted that Manno preferred not to speak of it, even with her:

Yes, you know the people who did this. One comes from my husband's country [hometown]; another comes from here; the third is even related to me, although he pretends that he is not. Two of them work inside [the school complex]. The one who comes from my husband's country is at the head of it. . . . He's the master of the affair, he arranged it.

One of the schoolteachers, Maître Fritz, was also from Saut d'Eau. When asked if it was indeed he, Alourdes nodded, and then quickly added that another teacher, Pierre, was a second member of the triad. She adamantly refused to name the third, stating only that "she is someone even closer." But, as the Haitian third-person singular pronoun *li* can mean either "he" or "she," not even the sex of the person was then apparent to me.

How typical of rural Haitian sorcery was this first case of magically induced *sida*? The mechanism of expedition of the dead is, as noted, classically associated with serious illnesses such as tuberculosis. In her study of tuberculosis in southern Haiti, Weise (1971:95, 98–99) notes that the disease may be "sent upon the sufferer by another human being." The actions of Manno and his family recall those prescribed in southern Haiti: "Divination is employed to detect the offending person. Even if a particular individual is not identified, attempts are made to break the evil spell." In such instances, divination, often accomplished with cards or a candle, is synonymous with diagnosis:

Diagnoses point to disruptions in relationships. . . . The cards often reveal that someone is suffering because of the "jealousy" of other persons. Jealousy is understood to be such a strong emotion that the lives of its targets can be seriously disrupted. Within the Vodou system the object of jealousy rarely escapes at least part of the burden of blame. Such an attitude reflects a society in which it is expected that anyone who has much should give much. (Brown 1989a:53)

In Manno's case, divination would probably only confirm the family's suspicions, formed by the response to the guiding question: "Who lost out when Manno was chosen for these jobs?" And the answer to this question was his fellow schoolteachers, who were passed over by Père Jacques when he sought a "right-hand man" to help with community projects. Pierre, for example, "was a *moun Kay* [a Kay person], and ought to have been awarded the work before a stranger," as his aunt put it. Several interviewed also remarked that Pierre was poorer than Manno, as was Maître Fritz. Further, many suspected that Père Jacques did not care for Fritz, which made Fritz despise Manno even more.

Since Tonton Mèmè was not professionally involved in the case, a trip to Vieux Fonds promised to clear up some of my confusion. Upon visiting Mèmè, I found that he knew nothing of "the young schoolteacher with the persistent illness," as I put it. He asked enough questions to suggest that he was put out that someone with so grave a problem had not been brought to his attention. But knowledge of the accusation seemed to be widespread in Do Kay. Mme. Alexis brought up the subject on several occasions, and continued to express her exasperation over "their persistent superstition."

I know people believe that someone can *voye yon mò pwatrine* ["send someone a chest death"], but how can they think that it's evil when they know the diagnosis? I was sure that when the family received the [HIV-antibody] test results they would abandon the notion that a person was responsible.

It was my assumption that Manno fully shared his wife's understanding of his illness. A full month elapsed, however, before I was able to speak again to Manno. While in his neighborhood for a meeting in early May, I stopped by Alourdes's mother's house. The family owned two tiny houses, built side by side with a granary between them. One of the dwellings had been emptied for Manno and his family. Alourdes's mother and a couple of children occupied the other (her father lived by himself a half-mile away, in an even smaller house). Manno was lying in bed, but he jumped to his feet in a robust manner when greeted from the yard: "Manno, I never seem to see you." He gave a nervous laugh, no different from a dozen other occasions. Although he was ill at ease, his health seemed to have returned. His handshake was firm, and he had put on at least another fifteen pounds. "Oh, you know," he replied, "I just don't seem to get down to Do Kay."

A month later, another visit revealed that Manno was, indeed, once again the picture of health. And yet external appearances were deceiving, for if Manno's medical problem had temporarily lifted, his social dilemma had not. His social network had shrunk considerably. He and his family blamed close friends for what they feared to be an inevitably fatal illness; he had abandoned his house, and alienated his and his wife's employer. By late June, when Manno's health began to give way to diarrhea and fever, I knew from Christian that Manno and his family were increasingly obsessed not with the course of the disease, but with its ultimate origin. Until he was willing to speak more candidly with me about the sorcery accusations, however, the course of his illness remained the chief focus of our regular discussions.

It was during early July that these issues were first broached. In the afternoon preceding a follow-up appointment with Dr. Boyer in Port-au-Prince, Manno was sitting under the granary, holding his sixteen-month-old son. He gave his usual embarrassed greeting, and stated that he was "fine, except for a few stomach cramps." He was still taking his medications. When asked about his impending appointment he replied, "I remembered it. I've been waiting for a bus all day." He pointed to his bundle, perched in the crotch of a tree in the yard. He eagerly accepted a ride to Mirebalais, where he could more easily catch a bus for Port-au-Prince, but needed to wait until Alourdes returned from school and could take care of the children.

Heading back down the road toward Do Kay, I had walked no more than a hundred yards or so when Manno called my name. His mother-in-law had arrived, and so he could walk back with me. In response to the comment that we hadn't had the opportunity to talk about his illness, he replied, "I know. We haven't been able to see each other." I then asked, "Tell me more about your illness; the sort of things we haven't been able to talk about for lack of privacy." His response was equally direct: "I know that I am very sick, even though I don't look it. They tell me there's no cure. But I'm not sure of that. If you can find a cause, you can find a cure." The cause, according to Alourdes, had been Fritz, Pierre, and an unnamed third person. But when I asked, "What is the cause of your illness?" Manno unhesitatingly replied, "A microbe." When silence followed this, I asked him, "Why aren't you staying in your house?" "Well, my mother-in-law suggested that we move in with her until I was feeling better." "But you've been feeling better for months now," I answered. "Yes . . . that's true," came the halting reply. "It's been suggested," I added, "that you moved out of your house because you thought someone from Do Kay was trying to harm you." Manno weighed this a bit. I began to wonder if he were short of breath, but his answer came steadily enough: "Perhaps that's what they say, but that doesn't mean it's true . . . I don't know that someone is trying to harm me, but I don't know that someone isn't. Maybe, maybe not." We were approaching Do Kay by then, and so stopped our conversation there. We made a rendezvous for the following week.

The summer of 1987 was a hard time for keeping appointments. The military junta that had taken over after Duvalier's departure had become universally unpopular: in the area around Kay, one would have been hard-pressed to find a single government supporter. When the junta again attempted to take over the elections, thousands of Haitians poured into the streets of Port-au-Prince and other cities, demanding that the junta resign. The army shot them by the dozen. On several occasions, national political upheaval paralyzed the major cities and provincial towns.[8] My meeting with Manno was cancelled by a strike that shut down most roads. Manno also missed at least two appointments at the AIDS clinic, once because gunfire in the streets outside scared away staff and patients. "Haiti," said Père Jacques acidly, "has never been a country in which to be sick and poor."

By late July, Manno again began complaining of diarrhea. His neighbor, Christian, informed me that Manno's cough had reappeared. Again owing to political problems, Manno was unable to replenish his supply of one of the antituberculous drugs. Port-au-Prince was shaken daily by demonstrations, tear gas, and automatic weapons fire, and many establishments, including pharmacies, remained closed for days at a time. By early August, Manno was vomiting, and complained of "terrible headaches." His speech seemed altered, but he claimed to be having no difficulty reading. On more than one occasion, I found him lying in bed, reading his well-worn Bible: "To give me strength, to protect me," explained Manno.

By the third week in August, Manno was gravely ill. A group of young men from Do Kay, most of them members of Projè Veye Sante, asked one night to be driven to Manno's house "for a prayer meeting." "For we have heard," one of them added, "that he and his wife are in spiritual danger." We reached the house by 9 P.M., and found them all in bed. The children were asleep on a straw mat on the floor, and it looked as if their mother was sleeping there with them. Manno was in his bed, and seemed somewhat embarrassed by our visit. Saul, especially, greeted Manno warmly, which visibly pleased the sick man.[9] When asked about his headaches, he qualified them as "no better, no worse." One of the health agents initiated a couple of songs, the Nicaean creed, a few snatches of Bible verse, and a psalm. Another community health worker prayed, asking the Good Lord to send down his "spiritual medication." There were a couple of references that were strange to my ear: he implored God to "help [Alourdes] to refrain from doing anything she'd regret." There was some mention of Lot's wife, as well as a plea to "help her to have the heart of Job." I wondered then if these intercessions were related in some way to Alourdes's rumored infidelity, or perhaps she was seen as the driving force in the quest for "magical therapy." It was later revealed that she was actively planning her revenge.

By the end of the month, Manno's breathing was labored, the painkillers no longer helped, and he had not been sleeping. He was vomiting after most meals and had lost a great deal of weight. Another prayer meeting was planned, and again I was invited. As we were pulling away from Do Kay, Pierre walked over. It was already dark. He asked if he could come, and I said yes, but with great anxiety as I anticipated the reaction of Manno and Alourdes. I would be bringing one of their alleged enemies right into their house, for Pierre was, with Maître Fritz, one of the triumvirate accused of sending sickness on Manno. Other questions arose: Who was the third person, "even closer" to Alourdes? Was he also in the jeep? Or was the accused a woman? Was Pierre oblivious to the widespread rumor that placed him among those accused of ensorcelling Manno? Clearly not, for upon getting into the jeep, Pierre informed Saul that he (Pierre) had been publicly fingered by Alourdes's family. When we reached Manno's house, Pierre was greeted in the same manner as everyone else.

Manno's decline continued. On September 12, during the course of a Projè Veye Sante meeting, Christian informed us that Manno was worse than ever. When the meeting was over, Christian asked to speak with me privately. He hemmed a bit, reporting news that he'd already imparted during the meeting. He finally explained what was on his mind, prefacing the disclosure with the disclaimer that, as I had told him about my research, perhaps I would like to interview him once again. During our conversation I discovered that I had overlooked a salient kinship tie: Christian's sister was soon to be Maître Fritz's wife! She was the third, "even closer" person accused of sending *sida* on Manno—she was Alourdes's cousin. "My sister is not a part of this," said Christian defensively. "She is not involved in magic (*li pa konn fè maji*)." He had dropped all pretense to skepticism about such matters:

They say my people helped to send a *sida* death on him. But where would we find a person dead of this sickness? We have never seen it here. . . . I am not saying that no one wishes to harm [Manno], but it's clear that whoever is doing this is someone who travels a great deal, someone who knows the ways of the city.

He had no idea, he said, who would meet such a description.

We reached Manno's house late in the afternoon. His mother was there, indicating the family's awareness that Manno did not have long to live. Also present were his brother and a cousin, neither of whom I had met before. Manno's short, labored breathing was audible from the yard. Saul and Christian remained outside during the half-hour I was in the house. Manno had great difficulty speaking, but seemed to be lucid. His eyes rolled when he spoke, and he was as thin as he had been in January. For some reason, a cock was tied to the bed, and crowed in response to the chickens outside: the noise was somehow amplified. It seemed clear then that Manno was dying, and Alourdes's father refused requests to take him to the hospital. "No, no—I'm in the middle of treating him with herbs," he answered evenly but forcefully. "I'll give him to you, but after twenty-one or so days."

Manno died the next morning. The news reached Do Kay just before midday, and a small contingent of mourners from Do Kay went immediately to the house in Ti Bwa. There were a dozen or so friends and family sitting quietly under the granary. Alourdes's mother was wailing in the doorway of her house; Alourdes was inside her mother's front room, sitting on the bed. She looked more tired than grief-stricken. Her little boy was nursing. My presence seemed to call for a retelling of the last few hours, for she began, unprompted, to hold forth about them. Manno had not slept last night, nor had she. He had asked for some cola and milk early in the morning, but vomited it almost immediately. (Alourdes's sister interjected that he had taken some soup later in the morning.) At about 10:30 or so, continued Alourdes, Manno had complained that he was almost out of breath. This must be due, he felt, to his short rations: groaning, he asked her to prepare him a plantain banana. "A few minutes later," concluded Alourdes, "when I noticed he wasn't groaning, I went back in. He had died while I was cooking the plantain."

Chairs were brought out for the new arrivals, and we sat for a while. But I thought it might be wise to go and inform Père Jacques, who was visiting a mission station on the far side of the lake. Alourdes explained that the funeral would be tomorrow; she had sent to have the coffin made, and her father was to go and make arrangements for the grave in a nearby cemetery.

In a sturdy jeep, it takes more than half an hour to reach the dam from Ti Bwa. When we were a mile or two from the dam, we saw that Père Jacques and a few of his coworkers were crossing the reservoir in a motor boat. We parked the jeep in the accustomed spot as they were clambering out of the skiff. "Is there a problem?" he called up from the water's edge. There was no reply, confirming, no doubt, his suspicion. He repeated the question at least three times before I replied, "Yes there is a problem. It's Maître Manno." Père Jacques spoke of Manno all the way back to Do Kay: "In the end, he did not have the faith that he once had. He was sure that he was the victim of magic (*maji*)." Père Jacques also recalled that Manno had been to an *houngan* early in the course of his illness. "For all you know," he added, "Manno attributed his spectacular reprieve [in February] to the efficacy of another system. For all you know, he stopped taking the doctor's medications early in the Spring."

At 7:30 P.M., during the wake, Manno's family members were in much the same positions and attire, although Alourdes had put on a scarf. There was a good deal of crying, and very little attempt at the sort of humor often seen at the funerals of older Haitians. In fact, there was nothing to do. There were no card games, no folk tales, no remi-

niscing, no eating or drinking—in short, none of the activities that traditionally help mark the passage of the dead. Shortly after presenting
our condolences, those from Do Kay made as if to leave. Alourdes told
me not to rush, that she wished to write a note to Père Jacques and
his assistant concerning the funeral arrangements. Shortly thereafter,
she handed me an unfolded piece of paper and awaited my response.
It read:

Dear Fathers Jacques Alexis and Bruno Robin:

It is our sad duty to present you with our deepest excuses. We also beg you,
dear Fathers, to come and perform the funeral service of our regretted Maître
Manno Surpris who passed away at eleven this morning. We would like to set
the funeral for ten o'clock tomorrow morning at home.

We are sure, dear Fathers, that you will be able to grant this request. Thank
you.

Signed: Madame Alourdes Surpris and family

I said that I would pass the note on to Père Jacques. Upon reaching
Kay, however, I discovered that the priest had left for Mirebalais, the
parish seat, and so gave the letter to Maître Gérard, the lay reader of
the Do Kay mission and the principal of the school that had employed
Manno. Gerard did not know when Père Jacques would be returning.

The priest did not return until well after 10 A.M., which Alourdes
took as a deliberate gesture of disapproval. Finally, as noon approached,
Gérard asked me to drive him to Ti Bwa. But we found that Manno
had already been buried, and there were no more than a dozen people
left milling about the yard. What looked to be Manno's effects were
covered by a large sheet of plastic. Maître Gérard announced that he
would offer his "ministrations at the time of death," which meant, I
soon discovered, that he would read from a Haitian version of *The Book
of Common Prayer,* and hold forth on any lessons to be learned from
the brief life of Manno Surpris. When Gérard stepped into the room
in which Manno had died, only Alourdes, carrying her son, and
Manno's mother followed him.

I was very uncomfortable when Maître Gérard called me into the
house, where he was lecturing to his polite but distracted audience.
"Man cannot hurt man," said Gérard elliptically:

Manno never hurt anyone; on the contrary, one thing he was known for was
his ready smile. So why would someone wish to harm him? It is a very bad
thing to accuse someone else of trying to harm him, a very heavy load. No,
we all know what illness he had. He had *sida.*

At this point Gérard turned to me and added, "Didn't he?" It was the first time I had heard members of the family publicly confronted with the word *sida,* though there was no one in the room who did not know of the diagnosis. It was not naming the illness that disturbed me, but the fear that Alourdes would think I had betrayed her confidence by discussing the subject with Gérard. Hoping that she knew that he had gotten his information elsewhere, I said nothing.

Perhaps Gérard understood that all present might agree that Manno had died of *sida* but that someone—and the name Maître Fritz kept surfacing—sent the illness "on him." Gérard spoke, however, as if these were mutually exclusive possibilities. He began to speak of his own wife, who had died some years before of cancer. He had done everything he could, he recounted, but some illnesses were invariably fatal. Again he turned to me and said, "Isn't that right?" At about this time, Alourdes's father came in. Gérard might as well have been speaking to a mahogany tree, for the man began whispering, in an unabashed way, the latest signs of maleficence from Maître Fritz.[10]

Many questions remained unanswered, not just for the ethnographer, but for others interested in or anxious about the new disorder. For most of those involved, however peripherally, in Manno's illness, that *sida* could be sent seemed obvious by the time of his death. But how was *sida* sent? How was it different from other sent sicknesses? Was all *sida* sent *sida*? What relation, if any, did *sida* have to blood disorders? To tuberculosis?

In an interview conducted a few weeks after Manno's funeral, Tonton Mèmè attempted to answer some of these questions:

It's a sent sickness, that is clear. And the people who sent his sickness were very close to him, worked with him. Not anyone can do this, send a *mò sida.* You have to know where to raise the dead, and send it so it hangs on. That's how it's different from other sent sicknesses. A *mò sida* wants to leave, to attack others. It must be made to stay on the person (*rete sou moun nan*). Not just anyone can do all that.

One of Mèmè's sons, a truckdriver, asked if "all the homosexuals in Port-au-Prince died from sent *sida,* and if so, who sent it?" Saul, who was also present, observed that perhaps there was more than one way to contract the illness. Mèmè rubbed his jaw thoughtfully at this suggestion. He seemed, uncharacteristically, at a loss. When asked how he would treat sent *sida,* he said he was not yet sure; he was "still studying the question." A week later, however, Tonton Mèmè observed that "if it's a *sida* death, you would treat it with magic and then roots (*rasin*).

You would call on *eskòt petro*," the rough *lwa* associated with sorcery and violence in general. Mèmè seemed distracted, and had little else to add.[11]

Wherever AIDS strikes, it seems, accusation is never far behind. In at least one Haitian village, what was observed was not at all the American-style hysteria, the refusal to care for patients, the angry parents refusing to send their children to school with children who have AIDS. Noticeably absent was the revulsion with which AIDS patients are faced in North America, in both clinical settings and in their communities. In the United States we read of employers summarily firing persons with AIDS; in rural Haiti we encounter an employer angry because his employee with AIDS is avoiding him. This striking difference cannot be ascribed to Haitian "ignorance of modes of transmission." On the contrary, those interviewed in the earlier years of the epidemic had ideas of etiology and epidemiology that reflected the incursion of the "North American ideology" of AIDS—that the disease is caused by a "microbe" and is somehow related to homosexuality. These were soon subsumed, however, in distinctively Haitian beliefs about illness causation.

The first of these frameworks made its contribution before Manno was diagnosed. Talk on the radio and elsewhere suggesting that a contaminated blood supply had contributed to the Haitian epidemic may have moved people in the Kay area to think of *sida* as a blood disorder. In 1985 and 1986 discussions of *sida*, there were frequent references to "dirty" or "spoiled" blood, and also an association with *move san*. Indeed, several villagers first thought of Manno's illness as *move san*. As Mme. Sonson commented early in Manno's illness, "He has very serious, big problems, and it's no wonder his blood has gone bad." But in the end the course of Manno's illness helped to undermine this association, as did the preexisting "social epidemiology" of severe illness. Understandings of tuberculosis and "expedition" came to lend structure to the cultural meaning taking shape during 1987.[12]

Long before AIDS came to Do Kay, one might have asked the following question: Some fatal diseases are known to be caused by "microbes" but may also be "sent" by someone. Was *sida* to be such a disease? It was, and accusations of *maji* should not have come as a surprise. They did not surprise Père and Mme. Alexis, although the latter expressed dismay that such a "false idea" could be held concurrently with "knowledge of the real cause." The Alexises knew a great deal about the accusation of malign magic, because, as Père Jacques later explained, a "very close friend of [the Surpris family], one of those accused of perpetrating this, came to me and told me the entire story." That, I surmised, was Pierre, who had worked with both Manno and Alourdes for years.

Although Père Jacques cast his analysis in terms of the familiar antinomy of voodoo and Christianity, my informants and coworkers spoke in less clear-cut terms. A series of oppositions, rather than one, seemed to guide many of our conversations: an illness might be caused by a "microbe" or by maleficence or by both. Some even spoke of the night, years ago, that Manno had been knocked out of bed by a bolt of lightning. The shock, they said, had left him "susceptible" to *sida*. Depending on who was asked, the new illness might be treated by doctors or voodoo priests or "leaf doctors" or prayer or any combination of these. The extent to which Manno believed in each of these therapeutic modalities remains unclear. He may well have been thankful for all of them.

8

Anita

Will no one teach you to be quiet—
The only wisdom that becomes you!
Kindly listen to my accusation
And give your attention to the way I shall plead.

Job 13:5–6

If these men were to be silent and listen, they would
demonstrate the wisdom they claim to possess. Those who
experience at close range the sufferings of the poor, or of
anyone who grieves and is abandoned, will know the
importance of what Job is asking for. The poor and the
marginalized have a deep-rooted conviction that no one is
interested in their lives and misfortunes. They also have the
experience of receiving deceptive expressions of concern from
persons who in the end only make their problems all the
worse.

Gutierrez (1987:24)

Anita Joseph once referred to herself as "a genuine resident of Kay," but her name did not surface in the census of 1984. The
following year, however, a study of ties to Port-au-Prince and the
United States revealed that Luc Joseph, her father, had a daughter in
"the city." She was, he reported, "married to a man who works in the
airport." Less than two years later, Anita, gravely ill, was brought back

80

to Do Kay by her father. After years of hearing almost nothing from Anita, Luc had received word that Anita was "lying in a stranger's house," laid low by a fever on her way back to Do Kay. She was pale, coughing, and "thin enough to have sharp shoulders." In April of 1987, Mme. Alexis referred her to the clinic as "someone who seems to have tuberculosis." Examination of Anita proved Mme. Alexis correct, and she became a patient of the physician then working at the clinic.

It was at about this time, too, that villagers began to speak more of *sida,* although the "AIDS fear" was not yet prominent. Several villagers were already confident, it later became clear, that Manno was ill with the disorder; radio programs dispensing information about *sida* were by then common. But stories about *sida* were rare and inspired no passion; the syndrome did not yet mean much locally. Knowledge about *sida* was not widely shared, and Anita's diagnosis of tuberculosis did not occasion a great deal of speculation about *sida.*

Anita was enrolled, at the time of her diagnosis, in a study that sought to identify determinants of the course and outcome of tuberculosis in Kay and surrounding villages. Interviews with Anita preceded any suspicion that she might have been exposed to HIV. The study addressed the *experience* of the illness, and questions about her experience of tuberculosis tended to evoke long and rather autobiographical responses. She seemed especially to enjoy the opportunity to "recount my life," and resisted any attempt to focus discussions. "Let me tell you the story from the beginning," she once said; "otherwise you will understand nothing at all."

The beginning of the story, as Anita told it, was down in the flooded valley. Her mother had been born near the banks of the small stream that cuts through Ba Kay. Anita's mother was to inherit, with her brothers, a choice piece of farmland that promised to keep them all prosperous and well fed. Luc Joseph was from a neighboring settlement, and the young woman's mother—Anita's grandmother—gave her blessing to the union. Luc paints an idyllic picture of their first years together. The dam altered their fortunes overnight, commented Luc, "spoiling our lives in a single day." Anita's mother miscarried two pregnancies shortly after the valley was flooded. It was a dispirited woman who later gave birth, up in Do Kay, to Anita.

Although many girls in the village did not go to school, Anita's mother insisted that she attend Père Alexis's then modest establishment. A visit to the school archives later revealed that Anita had been a good student, and she recalled her time there with nostalgia. It offered her a chance, she said, to learn to read, and to escape the tension of her home. As a little girl, Anita had been frightened by the arguments her parents would have during the dry seasons. By the time she was "old enough to understand," she felt that bickering was her parents' chief domestic activity:

My mother and father were always having arguments. My mother wanted to buy us shoes, my father wanted to buy seeds. My mother said yes, so my father said no. One day, when she was pregnant with [Anita's younger sister], my father yelled at her. . . . She became ill, she had *move san*. My father should have had her treated right away, but he let it drag on. Then she got very skinny.

When his wife began coughing, Luc first consulted a *doktè fey,* who prescribed an herbal preparation known to cure *move san*. But the herbalist warned the family that, should the woman begin coughing blood, they could safely assume that the illness was "not simple," and that it would require "another kind of medicine." Luc did not wait for his wife to begin coughing blood. When she failed to improve, he sold all the family's livestock—two pigs and a goat—in order to buy a "consultation" with a distinguished doctor in the capital. Tuberculosis, he told them, and the family felt there was little they could do other than the irregular trips to Port-au-Prince, and the equally irregular attempts to placate the *lwa* who might protect the woman. Anita dropped out of school to help take care of her mother, who died shortly after the girl's thirteenth birthday.

It was very nearly the *coup de grace* for her father, who became depressed and abusive. Anita, the oldest of five children, bore the brunt of his spleen. "We got poorer, and he got meaner. He began to argue with me just as he had with my mother." The idea of running away came to her suddenly:

One day, I'd just had it with his yelling. I took what money I could find, about $2, and left for the city. I didn't know where to go. I had never been to the city before, although my mother used to go there to sell [produce]. . . . I got off [the bus] in a crowded place.

The crowded place was Belair, in the northeastern part of Port-au-Prince. The neighborhood's more middle-class section runs down a hill and touches the main commercial thoroughfare of the capital. Anita found herself in the midday bustle of lower Belair, already hungry, and without a plan of action. She sat down on the curb and began to weep.

"Actually," she recalled, "I didn't really need to cry. I thought it might be a way to get someone to help me." But Port-au-Prince is a city where countless tears are shed, and it is perhaps not surprising that Anita's were not drawing more than a few guilty glances.

After "a good long time," Anita got up and began walking up the hill. Soon she had left behind the middle-class neighborhood and entered the poor quarter of Belair. Scraps of wood, unmortared cement blocks, and corrugated tin are the chief building materials in upper Belair, and there are no curbs, had Anita wished to retry her ploy for sympathy. The streets themselves give way to winding and narrow dirt "corridors" that follow no logic other than the settlement patterns of those who came to inhabit the area. Laguerre, who has conducted fieldwork in Belair, describes the neighborhood from the air:

The zinc sheet roofs on the shacks built all over the upper Belair hill look like deteriorated steps leading nowhere. The Upper Belair community . . . appears like a wild boar, sitting on its haunches, refusing to eat from the trough of slop placed in front of it, but fixing its eyes angrily on the wealthy and powerful as though ready to devour those residing in the National Palace, located about half a mile away. (Laguerre 1982:15)

These people were much more familiar to Anita, she recalled. Several spoke to her, and an old woman selling fried foods gave her some *marinad,* or fried dough, simply because she thought that Anita looked lost. Anita sat down beside the old woman and waited silently "for her to ask me something." By the time the woman at last asked Anita how she came to look so lost, it was late afternoon. By the time Anita had finished her story, which was rather commonplace by Haitian standards, it was dusk. The old woman said that Anita could stay with her for the evening, but sternly observed that there were already too many people in the house.

Because the woman "knew everybody in Belair," Anita soon had the good fortune to find a family in need of a maid. There were two women in the household, and both had jobs in a U.S.-owned assembly plant. This was unheard-of good fortune: two steady jobs under one roof in this part of upper Belair was and is unusual. The husband of one of the women ran a snack concession out of the house, further augmenting their income. Anita received a meal a day, a bit of dry floor to sleep on, and $10 per month for what sounded like incessant labor.[1] She was not unhappy with the arrangement, stating that "I was very lucky to find such a good situation. Some girls are so hungry they have to work for food alone."

Anita spoke of her first month in Belair as "very difficult. People are hard in the city; their hearts are hard. The streets are dirty. I missed my mother and my father, too." After the initial adjustment, after giving up dreams of going to school during the evenings, Anita stated that her life became much easier. She settled into a routine of "water, clothes, food." Her fetching, washing, and cooking lasted until both women who employed her were fired for participating in "political meetings," because unions were, in effect, banned in Duvalier's Haiti. Again, Anita found herself in a small house full of tension. The women soon made it clear, as Anita recalled, that she was becoming a nuisance. Anita asked to stay and forfeit her salary, but the family had already begun to make plans to emigrate to the bigger job market in the United States. It was not long before a spat flared into a fight, and Anita once again found herself on the street. This time, her tears were genuine.

Anita wandered about for two days, until she happened upon a kinswoman selling gum and candies near a downtown theater. She was, Anita related, "a sort of aunt." Anita could come and stay with her, the aunt said, as long as she could help pay the rent. And so Anita moved into Cité Simone, the sprawling slum on the northern fringes of the capital.[2] It was not at all clear, however, how Anita might help pay the rent. It was through her aunt that she met Vincent, one of the few men in the neighborhood with anything resembling a job: "He unloaded the whites' luggage at the airport." Vincent made a living from tourists' tips.

In 1982, the year Haiti became associated, in the North American press, with AIDS, the city of Port-au-Prince counted tourism as one of its chief industries. Many of those employed in that sector lost their jobs the following year. Living in an area whose unemployment rate was greater than 60 percent, Vincent could command considerable respect. He turned his attentions to Anita. "What could I do, really? He had a good job. My aunt thought I should go with him." In a conversation that took place late in her illness, Anita linked her decision to join Vincent to events that had occurred in her childhood:

When I did that [took Vincent as a lover], it was only because I had no mother. And when she died, it was bad. My father was just sitting there. And when I saw how poor I was, and how hungry, and saw that it would never get any better, I had to go to the city. Back then I was so skinny—I was saving my life, I thought, by getting out of here.

Anita was not yet fifteen when she entered her first and only sexual union.[3] Her lover set her up in a shack in the same neighborhood. Anita cooked and washed and waited for him. As tourism continued to decline, Vincent had less and less money. Competition for the attention of tourists was already intense by the time widespread political turmoil slowed all foreign travel to a trickle. On occasion, the entire airport closed, as the residents of Port-au-Prince prepared themselves for the fall of the Duvalier regime.

It was during the irruption of anti-Duvalier sentiment that Vincent fell ill. Anita recounted that "we had already spent many months together before the sickness. Things had not been going well between us, but I felt sorry for him when he was sick."[4] It began insidiously, she recalled: night sweats, loss of appetite, swollen lymph nodes. Then came months of unpredictable and debilitating diarrhea. Anita again became a nurse. She eagerly sought the advice of those reputed to know how to treat such illnesses: "We tried everything—doctors, charlatans, herbal remedies, injections, prayers. He just lay there, and got all puffy; he was coughing, too." After a year of decline, she took Vincent to his hometown in the south of Haiti. There it was revealed that the man's illness was the result of malign magic: "It was one of the men at the airport who did this to him. The man wanted Vincent's job. He sent an AIDS death to him."

The *houngan* who heard their story and deciphered the signs was straightforward. He told Anita and Vincent's family that the sick man's chances were slim, even with the appropriate interventions. There were, however, steps to be taken. He outlined the treatment as followed:

[The *houngan*] said, "This boy needs a big treatment." He said, "He needs big sacrifices. The persons who have made this expedition have themselves made big sacrifices." They made a ceremony for him. [The *houngan*] advised us to pray a great deal and told us which prayers to make and a whole bunch of old things I didn't understand.

Anita reported, however, that these instructions were understood and followed by the family. But the power of Vincent's enemies was stronger, and he succumbed within days of the treatment. "When he died, I felt spent. I couldn't get out of bed. I thought that his family would try to help me to get better, but they didn't. I thought they would put me in treatment.[5] I knew I needed to go home."

She made it as far as Croix-des-Bouquets, a large market town at least two hours from Kay. There she collapsed, feverish and coughing, and was taken in by a woman who lived near the market. She stayed for a month, unable to walk, until her father came to take her back home. Five years had elapsed since she'd last seen him. Luc Joseph was by then a friendly but broken-down man with a luckless reputation. He lived with one of his sons in a dilapidated, one-room, dirt-floor hut.[6] It was no place for a sick woman, the villagers said, and Anita's godmother, honoring twenty-year-old vows, made room in her over-crowded but dry house.

Mme. Pasquet, the godmother, was a member of Père Jacques's church, and had long been friendly with Mme. Alexis. Although Mme. Pasquet thought that Anita was ill with *move san*, she suspected that her goddaughter needed the attention of a physician, and she knew that Mme. Alexis would "make the arrangements." Within two days of Anita's homecoming, Mme. Alexis had brought the young woman to the attention of those working in Projè Veye Sante. Mme. Alexis her-self helped the emaciated young woman walk the few hundred yards that separated her godmother's house from the clinic. There Anita was promptly diagnosed as having tuberculosis, and she responded rapidly to antituberculous therapy. Within two months, she had regained her lost weight and felt healthy. Anita did well enough, in fact, to go to Mirebalais to take a job as a maid. She let no one there know that she was *pwatrine*, tuberculous, but managed to return for clinic appoint-ments in Do Kay. During one of these visits, she spoke to me of what had caused her disorder:

When in the city, I used to work in ladies' houses (*kay madam*); I was exposed to a lot of heat and a lot of cold. Perhaps it's that which has put me in the state I'm in now. If I had tuberculosis . . . truly, I might, because I was cooking, I was in and out of the refrigerator . . . it must be that work, the work of a maid, that left me ill, because I never did any other work, not agricultural, not commerce. It's working in ladies' houses that has caused me to get where I am now.

At least three of those interviewed then agreed that Anita's illness was the result of her "city work." In fact, two of these individuals ended their narratives about Anita with the same line: *chache lavi, detri lavi.*[7] A literal translation is "Look for life, destroy life," and it is a proverb usually invoked when someone dies or is gravely injured while trying to make a living (for example, when a market woman is killed in a truck accident, or when someone falls from a mango tree while culling fruit).

There was no community consensus, however, on the nature of Anita's illness. Shortly after her return to Do Kay, Ti Malou Joseph informed me that she had heard that Anita might have *sida*. The rumor was not surprising, as there was at that time a great deal of talk about

Manno's illness. Anita, Ti Malou remarked, looked like Manno had earlier that year. Anita has been in the city, and was *sida* not a city sickness? But inquiries revealed that few people believed the rumor to be true. Two villagers observed that Anita was *moun Kay,* a native of Kay, and people from Kay did not get *sida*. Others agreed that Anita did not have *sida*: she was "too innocent." The logic behind the statement was radically different from that underpinning similar statements made in North America. "Innocence" had nothing to do with such things as sexual practices (some villagers believed that Anita had led a "free life"), but rather underlined the fact that, very often, a string of bad luck signifies that one is the victim of *maji*. But sorcery is never random; it is sent by enemies. Most people make enemies by inspiring jealousy or by their own malevolent magic. Destitute and dogged by bad luck, Anita had never inspired the envy of anyone. Two persons who had previously explained to me the nature of Manno's illness queried rhetorically, "Who would send a *sida* death on this poor, unfortunate child?" It was in this sense that Anita was qualified "innocent." Since the sole case of *sida* registered in the Kay area was already thought to be caused by sorcery, it stood to follow, some thought, that Anita could not have *sida*.

Perhaps equally important to the initial "not-sent" verdict was the course of Anita's illness. Unlike Manno, she did not have any of the dermatologic manifestations of AIDS. Further, as Manno began his final decline, Anita was recovering her strength. When Manno died, Anita was hard at work in Mirebalais. To judge from the total absence of reference to Anita in AIDS-related interviews taking place in the summer and fall of 1987, it was widely assumed that she was in fact not ill with the new disorder. That Manno, too, had initially shown striking response to antituberculous medications—or some other concurrent intervention—seemed not to be relevant to this widely shared assessment. Some felt that it was *move san,* and not tuberculosis, that had "put her in bed," and observed that Anita had been successfully treated for the disorder.

In October, six months after the initiation of the antituberculous regimen, Anita declined precipitously. Her employer in Mirebalais sent her back to Do Kay. Anita had bitter words for the woman, stating that "they just use you up and when they're finished with you, they throw you in the garbage." She also felt that she had made an error, returning to "the same kind of work that got me sick in the first place. It's this kind of work that makes you weak, leaves you susceptible to all sorts of illnesses." Another villager, an elderly cousin of Mme. Pasquet, was present when Anita offered this assessment of her condition. The older woman sighed and observed: *chache lavi, detri lavi*.

Anita was sick and back in Mme. Pasquet's house during the last days of November 1987, and Mme. Pasquet's son observed that it was a shame that Anita would not be able to vote for the first time in her life. She had registered, as had the majority of young adults in Kay and surrounding villages. But none of them would have the chance to cast a ballot. November 29, 1987 may well have been a clear, bright Sunday, but many termed it *Dimanche Noir*. By ten o'clock that morning, at least thirty-four voters had been massacred by army-protected Duvalierists in Port-au-Prince alone. The elections were cancelled. "Everything's falling apart," said Mme. Pasquet, "everything. It looks as if Haiti will never change."

Anita had followed these developments with an interest that did not seem to wane as she became sicker. By early December, Anita could no longer walk to the clinic, a few hundred paces from her door. She weighed less than ninety pounds, and suffered with intermittent diarrhea. Convinced that she was indeed taking her medications, we were concerned about AIDS, especially when she recounted the story of Vincent and his illness. Her deterioration clearly shook her—and her father's—faith in the clinic, and they began spending significant sums on herbal treatments. "I had already sold a small piece of land in order to buy treatments," complained Luc. "I was spending left and right, with no results." As the treatment for tuberculosis was entirely free of charge, it was clear that Luc was spending his resources in the folk sector. He later informed me that he consulted an *amatè*, but soon abandoned that tack, as Luc seemed to agree that his daughter was an unlikely victim of sorcery. And yet the nature of her disorder had not been satisfactorily defined, whether by divination, laboratory exam, or any other means. Toward the end of 1987, Père Alexis asked the Saint-André physicians—a second had been hired—why they were dragging their feet. Luc declared himself poised to sell his last bit of land in order to "buy more nourishing food for the child." It was indeed imperative that the underlying cause of Anita's poor response to treatment be found. Blood for the requisite serologic test was drawn and dispatched to Port-au-Prince.

During one of his regular trips to the capital, Père Alexis went by the National Laboratory to see Dr. Boyer, who was becoming accustomed to visitors from Kay. She gave the bad news to the priest, and he met with Anita's physicians later that evening. "The test was positive," he said drily. Mme. Alexis said nothing, but later wondered, "What will become of Haiti if the disease is striking so many young people?" It was also at this time that Anita began receiving "prayer visits" from members of a Protestant church about forty-five minutes north of Do Kay. Anita, who kept a small Bible under her pillow, appreciated these sessions. She informed me that she was planning to pray much more regularly: "Only God can heal big sicknesses. Doctors can help, but only God can cure."

Only Luc and Mme. Pasquet were apprised of the test results. In 1983, Mme. Pasquet had been among those who had suggested that *sida* was a disorder spread by "coughing." It affected homosexual men, she said. She had also termed *sida* a "city sickness," and nothing about her goddaughter's illness led her to revise that association. Yet her other ideas about the syndrome had changed dramatically. When the question was posed on the same day that she was told that her charge had *sida*, Mme. Pasquet offered the following response: "I'm very sad to hear this news, because I know that *sida* is an infectious disease that has no cure. You get it from the blood of an infected person, or by going to bed with an infected person. . . . That's how you get *sida*." For this reason, she said, she had nothing to fear in caring for Anita. Further, she was adamant that Anita not be told of her diagnosis— "That will only make her suffer more"—and skeptical about the value of the AIDS clinic in Port-au-Prince:

Why should we [take her there]? She will not recover from this disease. She will have to endure the bumpy ride all the way to the city; she will have to endure the heat and humiliation of the clinic. She will not find a cool place to lie down. What she might find is a pill or injection to make her feel more comfortable for a short time. I can do better than that.

And that is what Mme. Pasquet proceeded to do. She attempted to sit Anita up every day, and encouraged her to drink a broth that was promised to "make her better." The godmother kept her as clean as possible, consecrating the family's two sheets to her goddaughter. She gave Anita her pillow, and stuffed a sack with rags for herself. The only thing she requested from the clinic staff was "a beautiful, soft wool blanket that will not irritate the child's skin."

Taking care of her goddaughter became a full-time occupation for Mme. Pasquet. Having weathered the dam, having raised, with her husband, ten children, she was known in Do Kay for her strength and her serenity. In one of several thoughtful interviews accorded us, Mme. Pasquet insisted that

for some people, a decent death is as important as a decent life. . . . The child has had a hard life; her life has always been difficult. It's important that she be washed of bitterness and regret before she dies. . . . I know many who died bitter people. The water made them bitter, and they died that way.

Although Mme. Pasquet can be credited with helping to counter these sentiments in Anita, the young woman did not accept her sentence without fear. In January, she said to me, "I heard I'm going to die. . . . Some people outside were talking and I heard them. I don't know who it was, but they were saying that I have an untreatable illness." Anita chose not to name this illness, but allowed that it was,

the same one that had taken Vincent. . . . I would say that as it was I who was turning him and moving him, perhaps it was the sick person's heat was too much for me. If they had taken him to the hospital, I'd know what illness he had; but it was to the *bokòr*'s house they took him.[8]

Mme. Christophe, a neighbor, was one of the first to suggest that there might be more than one way to "catch *sida.*" One could be the victim of expedited *sida,* or one could contract it "naturally," through sex or a transfusion. Although it seemed clear that there was no movement to take Anita to a *houngan,* I later went to see Tonton Mèmè, in order to ask him what he thought of Anita's history. Mèmè needed little prompting to speak about the disorder. "This form of *sida* is more difficult to treat," observed Mèmè in a tone suggesting that he had been treating it for years. "If it were a sent sickness, a man-made sickness (*maladi nèg*), why, in this case, it's the soul that is everything—as soon as it's removed, the person may be cured easily." The soul, in this context, is the same as the *mo,* the expedited dead. As it did not seem to be a sent sickness, however, Mèmè shook his head: "The child will not escape," he predicted.

When asked, "Will you be able to find a cure for *sida*?" Tonton Mèmè replied, "Yes, I think so, because if *sida* is a sickness that can be sent to someone, then I'll be able to treat it. And as soon as I do succeed, I'll send word to you." He also opined that "it will be *lafrik* itself that will treat it," adding that the rough *eskòt petro* would be the appropriate "guards" for such an unforgiving illness. Tonton Mèmè also explained that one could protect oneself against the illness. "With the help of Baron Samedi," Mèmè could prepare a drink, a *gad*:

This drink would protect you in the event that someone attempted to send [*sida*] to you. There will come a time, and it will straddle you like a person drunk on rum. You could meet one thousand people [who wished to harm you], and they would be powerless against you. The *gad* protects you against man-made illness (*maladi nèg*).

In her final month, Anita was very philosophic. She seemed to know of her diagnosis. Although she never mentioned the word *sida*, she did speak in January 1988 of the resignation appropriate to "diseases from which you cannot escape." She stated, again, that she was "dying from the sickness that took Vincent," although she was confident that she had not been the victim of witchcraft: "I simply caught it from him." Several people later confirmed this story. As Mme. Sonson put it, "We don't know whether or not they sent a *sida* death to [Vincent], but we know that she did not have a death sent to her. She had it in her blood, she caught it from him." People were talking about Anita's illness in a different way than they had discussed Manno's *sida*. Many of those interviewed in the month preceding Anita's death seemed frightened, and spoke as if personally vulnerable to the new illness. There seem to have been several reasons for this shift: one was certainly that a second case a few months after Manno's death made it difficult to construe his sickness as a freak event. Another was that, while Manno had been an outsider, Anita was *moun Kay*. A third was the banal way in which she was understood to have contracted the illness. While it might seem that one could more easily be the victim of sorcery, my informants suggested that there were "many ways to avoid sent sickness, but everyone has a family." In other words, Anita had done nothing other than begin a consensual union. She had done it precipitously and under very adverse conditions, but that was not her fault. As so many commented, "She's done nothing wrong."

Anita did not ask to be taken to a hospital, nor did her slow decline occasion any request for further diagnostic tests. What she most wanted was a radio—"for the news and the music"—and a blanket. It was during late January that Anita announced, as I sat on the edge of her bed, that "the hour has come for me to be sacrificed." She was clutching her well-thumbed Bible. She continued with what seemed to be a transposition of several lines from Saint Paul's second letter to Timothy:

The hour has come for me to be sacrificed. I have fought the good fight, I have kept faith. Now it is my job to endure suffering, and to do my job as a servant of God. Amen.[9]

By the beginning of February, Anita was afflicted with pitting edema of the lower legs; one side of her face was also swollen. She stopped eating, and asked only for another blanket, repeating "I'm so cold." On February 7, Anita sat up, and asked her godmother "for some soup and a radio"—she wanted to hear about the "events" in the capital: "They're going to inaugurate the new president tomorrow," she said sarcastically, "the one chosen in the recent *selections*." (The army-run elections held the previous month were massively boycotted, in the Kay region and elsewhere in the country.[10])

Anita's improvement was ephemeral, for the following day she began a decline that was to be her last. She was lucid, however, on several occasions, and in our last exchange recounted a dream that reflected, perhaps, some of the tensions dominant in her illness. A spirit, a *baka*, came to her and declared that she could be cured:

He came with a cup of *kleren* [raw rum], a fistful of fig leaves [*fey figi*], and seven tetracycline pills. I tried to refuse the leaves, as I heard my godmother saying "No, they're cursed by God." They made me chew the leaves and drink the *kleren*. When I did so, it turned to blood in my mouth.

Anita did not explain the significance of her dream, but it was regarded as ominous by her godmother.[11] She died shortly before dawn on St. Valentine's Day. Never sure of her own age, she had recently guessed that she might be twenty-one years old.

Anita's last rites and funeral spoke to other tensions pervading contemporary rural Haiti. By mid-morning, Luc had tied a light blue sash around his midriff.[12] When I arrived, Mme. Pasquet and her sister were weeping, as were all the children. The men, wet-eyed and silent, sat in front of the house under the newly erected *tonèl*, a gazebo fashioned of branches. By mid-afternoon, Anita had been clad in a light blue dress. Her coffin was stained reddish, and trimmed in silver tin. Also in silver were the painted words: "Reste empaix dans le paradis seleste amen." The coffin was tiny: "It only takes six boards," goes the saying, and Anita had been greatly reduced by her illness. Because there was a small plastic window in the coffin, one could see that they had placed her on top of the new blanket, which was the same color as her last outfit.

The Protestants from the neighboring church arrived, and their pastor read from the Book of Ezekiel, chapter 37. He had brought a chorus with him, and several songs followed the scriptures. The pastor then told the story of a young boy, the twelve-year-old son of a prominent *houngan,* who was ill with a fever. The boy's illness "was not simple." In spite of all the father's ministrations, the child expired, and was buried. Distraught, the *houngan* went to the cemetery at 6 P.M. and "raised the child himself." He then took him to Hinch to Pastor Daniel, a well-known evangelical Christian. When the others, the *moun djab* ("devil's people"), came at 8 P.M., they found the grave empty, and were thus thwarted in their efforts to zombify the boy. "Thrice the Pastor Daniel lay his body upon that of the dead child, saying, 'Get up, I say, and join the living.'" The child stirred. But in a uniquely Haitian twist, the moral of the story was not like that of Lazarus, or that of the child raised by Elijah. Once the child was "saved" from zombification, he was free to die a natural death. He was immediately buried again. The story served as an admonition to those concerned: do not believe that any harm will come to Anita. She is safe from zombification or any other supernatural meddlings. The story was not intended to weaken anyone's belief in the *possibility* of such matters: no one doubted, at least not fundamentally, that such things could happen.

Subsequent exchanges revealed that although those present shared, however uneasily, the vocabulary and fears of rural Haitian culture, their differing religious affiliations led to very different practices. The clash was between local tradition and a propriety of more recent vintage, reflected in a conflict between those who wished to "shake the coffin," and those who thought it offensive. The reason given for this practice, termed *dodomeya,* is most often that if the casket is pitched and shaken en route to the cemetery any *baka* ("evil spirits") or *malfektè* (evildoers) are thrown off the path. "I don't know your customs here," announced the pastor somewhat haughtily, "but we don't do *dodomeya* in our church." With that the entourage, about seventy-five strong, milled into the road. The bell up in the church tolled. A neighbor could be heard wailing up by her house.

Luc and Mme. Pasquet stayed behind. They were both hoarse, unable to speak. Luc, a man who even by local standards lived in abject poverty, spent 275 gourdes ($55) on the coffin, and an undisclosed amount on coffee, colas, and bread for the wake. Mme. Sonson later observed that Luc "ruined himself [financially] in order to expiate his guilt over having allowed the girl to go to the city and be exposed to this illness." Her husband—Luc's brother—replied sharply: "Well, it wasn't really his fault. Your son lives in the city too, and he wouldn't be there if we hadn't lost our land!"[13]

A clear trend in discussions of *sida* was the growing consensus about the new disorder. By the end of the spring, it was widely accepted that Anita had been the village's second victim of *sida*. Most agreed that she had also had tuberculosis, and three of the twenty adults polled stated that Anita had succumbed to tuberculosis, but did not have AIDS. Few mentioned *move san*. Indeed, there was a distinct decline, during the months following Manno's death, in the significance of the "blood paradigm" to discourse about *sida*. What had once been a disorder of "spoiled" or "dirty" blood, and spread by transfusions, was becoming more strongly associated with tuberculosis, a disorder well known in rural Haiti.

Although the full complement of etiological possibilities was not invoked in Anita's final days, as was the case with Manno, theories invoking various degrees of human agency did surface. By the end of her illness, distinctions between causal mechanisms operating in Manno's and Anita's illnesses became sharper. These distinctions had a great influence on a rapidly evolving collective representation of *sida*. In the eyes of a majority of those interviewed in early 1988, Manno's *sida* was sent to him by a jealous rival, or a group of them. Anita had contracted *sida* through sexual contact with a person having the syndrome. She had not been the victim of sorcery. Indeed, this would be a very unlikely fate for Anita Joseph. She, like her father, was luckless. She, even more than her father, was a victim, as was repeated many times: Anita had lost her mother, run away at fourteen, and been forced into a sexual union by poverty. She was a child without choices and she had to make a living: *chache lavi, detri lavi*. Several people, including Anita's uncle Sonson, added that they were all the victims of the dam at Peligre.

9

Dieudonné

Everything you say, I have heard before.
I understand it all; I know as much as you do.
I'm not your inferior.
But my dispute is with God, not you;
I want to argue my case with him.

Job 13:1–3

Job is not a patient man, at least not in the usual sense of the
word. He is rather a rebellious believer. . . . Job the rebel is
a witness to peace and to the hunger and thirst for justice
(those who live thus will one day be called "blessed"); he
is more than simply patient, he is a peace-loving man, a
peacemaker.

Gutierrez (1987:14)

Dieudonné Gracia was born sometime in 1963, on the top of a hill in Do Kay. He came into the world without dragging his placenta after him, recalls his mother, signaling at the outset the independence of spirit that marked his entire life. His father, Boss Yonèl, was fond of saying that his third son had "Dessalines's blood in his veins," a reference to the father of Haitian independence. That Dieudonné was quick-witted, if unruly, is clear from his school records: "Disruptive in class" is the sole remark next to one term's harvest of good grades. He received his *certificat d'études primaires* from École

Saint-André when it was still housed under a thatched roof, and was then sent by his father to Thomonde, a large town about forty minutes down the road leading north, to continue his schooling. He had not even completed one year when his father found himself unable to pay the bills. The boy had the misfortune to need cash the very year that Haiti's pigs were destroyed. Although Boss Yonèl was a busy carpenter, he had six other children; Dieudonné returned to Do Kay.

He began to work with his father, who was then working on the new school with Père Jacques. But Do Kay was "too small a place for Dieudonné," as his mother noted. "He wanted to be somewhere where there were roads and cars, somewhere where the streets make corners." Sometime during 1983, Dieudonné left for Port-au-Prince. Through a relative from Do Kay, he had found a position as the "yard boy" for a wealthy family. He spent the next two years opening gates, fetching heavy things from the cars, and tending flowers in the cool heights of one of the city's ostentatious suburbs.

While in the city, Dieudonné's close friends were in large part people whose origins were also in the area around Kay. One had arrived decades ago, when the valley was first flooded, but the others had slowly worked their way to Port-au-Prince as local options became exhausted. The time of their arrival, the place of their lodging, the nature of their work—these were all factors influenced by kinship, whether consanguineous or ritual.[1] Some, like Mme. Sonson's son, worked in factories; most worked as servants in middle- or upper-class households; a few were unemployed, and depended on the generosity of other urban kin. One young woman, who never returned to Kay but was said to have sent money to her mother, had "fallen into prostitution." She was rumored to have died in 1987.[2]

Dieudonné was invited to become a "boy" by his cousin's godmother, who worked as a maid for a wealthy Haitian family. The head of the household was a "businessman," but Dieudonné was not sure what his business was. The young man was paid $20 per month for working virtually around-the-clock.[3] Boss Yonèl recounts that his son was "well situated" in Port-au-Prince, although he did not manage to send home any money. It was enough that Dieudonné was "responsible for himself." Dieudonné returned to Kay, according to Yonèl, when he was fired by the family for whom he worked. This transpired because the young man had fallen ill "and was no longer any use to them."

Mme. Sonson, who often traveled to the city to see her own son, had heard a different story. She explained that Dieudonné became engaged in a power struggle with another young servant in the same household. In December 1988, Mme. Sonson—who in 1984 knew nothing of *sida* and in 1986 denied that it could be "sent"—detailed with confidence the means by which Dieudonné had been felled:

He got in a fight with another kid over who was going to be in charge of the yard. He sent an illness on the kid, an insanity death (*mò foli*). The boy became crazy, and his parents went through the steps to see who had sent the illness. They then displaced a person who had died from *sida,* they raised a *mò sida* from the cemetery, and sent it on Dieudonné.

She added that it was widely known that only a *mò bosal*—a person who had died without being baptized—could be sent to cause sickness.[4] Dieudonné's cousin, Tilibèt Gracia, a community health worker, had yet another story:

The person with whom he was fighting was another [female] cousin of mine. It's true that she became crazy, but it's not true that she went to a *houngan* for treatment. It was to l'Église de Dieu that they went with her. She got better, but only after being treated for *move san,* as well. Thus it was not a *mò sida* [that caused Dieudonné's sickness], or if it was, it came from another quarter. Perhaps he was fighting with another person: *le mal existe.* But my cousin is not someone who could send something on Dieudonné; she's a relative of his. She's a fatherless child.

Dieudonné knew himself to be the victim of maleficence. He accused someone, gender unspecified, of giving him a *makandal*:

I might know what happened. It might be a person. Perhaps it was a person who's left me in this state. People in Port-au-Prince know how to make *makandal,* too—they're Haitians just like everybody else. If it was a person, the person was not silly, and knew what a guy without a weapon had to do. If it was a person, then it was a *makandal,* and it had to come from jealousy.

Makandal is a term for poison or sorcery bundle. It bears the name of a famous escaped slave who terrorized the white population of mid-eighteenth-century Saint-Domingue.[5] Although the term is not used as commonly as some of the other terms for poison, it has endured for over two hundred years, and points rather directly to the source of many contemporary Haitian understandings of good and evil.

Dieudonné, in any case, became ill, and the family for whom he worked "told me to go back to my own country." Just as there remains disagreement in Do Kay as to who was responsible for Dieudonné's illness, there is also a lack of consensus on the nature and timing of this first episode, and whether, in fact, it was even related to his final illness. Dieudonné and his parents recall that he became quite ill in the last months of 1985. Yonèl remembers diarrhea and a cough; Dieudonné insisted that it started with a fever and "mental weakness." Père Jacques recalled that the young man fell ill "with debilitating diarrhea" shortly after reaching Port-au-Prince, which he estimated to be "sometime in 1984." Tilibèt believed that Dieudonné's illness in Port-au-Prince may have had nothing to do with his subsequent case of *sida*.

Mme. Sonson was among those who felt that Dieudonné's story made sense only as a whole: the city sickness was the first episode of an illness that ended three years later. She visited Dieudonné in Port-au-Prince after he had fallen ill, and recalled "he had a fever, with chills, but nothing else." He told her then that the mother of his rival had observed that *sa yon moun fè, se li li wè*; an English equivalent might be, "As ye sow, so shall ye reap." In recounting the story some two months after Dieudonné passed away, Mme. Sonson seemed more moved by this logic of retribution than by the fatal illness of her young covillager. She was as offended by Dieudonné's aggressive magic, with its less-than-fatal result, as by the *contre-coup* that she believed responsible for his death. When questioned about this, Mme. Sonson merely repeated *sa yon moun fè, se li li wè*. She deplored sorcery of all sorts, she said, but she deplored offensive magic more than its reply. Her views are widely shared in rural Haiti. Noting the "deadly character of magic, whether offensive or defensive," Hurbon adds that

one is forbidden, the other permitted. De Heusch maintains that for the Azande described by Evans-Pritchard, [magic] is part of the ethico-juridical system. This hypothesis also holds for voodoo, in which one finds destructive magic (such as sorcery) that is held to be legitimate. The *oungan*, seer and exorcist, is supposed to reestablish justice by working to detect and punish the ensorcellor, and, in any case, by "sending him back the evil." (Hurbon 1987a:262–263)

Dieudonné returned to Do Kay late in 1985. Boss Yonèl took him to see Tonton Mèmè, who reportedly "lifted the dead person" (*leve mò a*), and the young man was nursed back to health by his mother. The term *sida* was not evoked. Records in the Clinique Saint-André show that Dieudonné visited the clinic several times during the next two years, usually with complaints of recurrent diarrhea, loss of appetite, and weight loss. Throughout 1986, he presented with recurrent skin

infections in the perianal and genital areas, and antibiotics did not seem
to help. During one of these visits, it seems that Dr. Pierre considered
the diagnosis of AIDS, but Dieudonné began to put on weight, and
this lead was not pursued at that time.

Dieudonné was given a clean bill of health by his covillagers, it
seems, for his name was not mentioned in a single interview about *sida*
or tuberculosis until the last months of 1987. During the spring of
1986, Dieudonné had, by all appearances, fully recovered his health. I
first met him in the summer of 1986, when he and several other young
men barricaded the road leading through Kay: They were protesting
the arrest of several union leaders, they said, and also the dissolution
by the military of the civilian electoral council. The roadblock was one
of the first manifestations in Do Kay of any involvement in national
politics, and Dieudonné and Jean-Jacques Fardin were its principal architects. In subsequent conversations, Dieudonné painted himself as
someone who had spent some of his last months in Port-au-Prince
meeting with a group of "young nationalists." He had been invited
into the group by Jean-Jacques, whose father was the only "well-off"
person in Do Kay. Jean-Jacques had gone to Port-au-Prince to attend
high school, and knew Dieudonné as a bright and energetic person
given to "saying what he thinks." Dieudonné recalled these meetings
with nostalgia:

We used to meet on Saturday afternoons. I couldn't let the people [who employed him] know what I was doing. We talked about everything that wasn't
talked about then. The worst thing about getting sick when I did was that I
wasn't there for the 7th of February [1986, when Duvalier was deposed].

In the months following the roadblock, I saw little of Dieudonné.
He joined his father, working not with Père Jacques, but on many of
the houses being refurbished in the village.[6] He also began to work as
a day laborer for ODBFA, the most recent incarnation of the organization meant to protect the Peligre Reservoir from further erosion. For
the better part of a year, he worked with crews terracing the already
denuded hillsides of the area around Kay.

It was during this time that Dieudonné began to court an "old girl-
friend" (*ansyen menaj*) from a rural area near the town of Thomonde.
They had met years ago, as Boss Yonèl had once worked a small plot
of land in that region. When she became pregnant, Dieudonné asked
her to come and live with his parents in Do Kay. He promised to build

a house on the hill, next to that of his parents, and raise a family there. He started work on the dwelling, and finished the frame before the baby, a girl, was born. But in the late summer of 1987, the young woman fell ill with a fever. Some noted that it was the recurrence of a previous febrile illness that had resembled tuberculosis. She became delirious, and then stuporous. She died a few months after the birth of her baby.

It was not clear what had caused this tragedy. "She ate something she shouldn't have eaten" was a common assessment; others blamed the fever, qualified by many as "suspect."[7] The young woman's father was furious. He did not care for Dieudonné, who had not built a house for his daughter and *then* married. He cared little more for Boss Yonèl. The day after his daughter's death, he stormed into Kay and collected her body. It was widely rumored, after Dieudonné's sickness seemed irreversible, that he had promised to "make him go where his daughter had gone."[8]

Dieudonné was sick within a month, and for some, it was the beginning of his illness. Although in 1986 and early 1987 he had visited the clinic for recurrent diarrhea and weight loss, his cousin Tilibèt was confident that his previous afflictions were unrelated to the mortal sickness that debuted in August of 1987:

His gums began to hurt him, to bleed easily. He was coughing blood, and he had diarrhea that went on and on, and fever and vomiting. This was when he was first ill, when he was working in Savanette [a neighboring village and an ODBFA site]. It was on the way home from Savanette; he got to Christian's [also a community health worker] house, and he thought it was a cold. [Christian] gave him cold medications, and I took care of him when he came home. He got better.

Dieudonné did seem to improve, which may explain why his illness was not readily attributed to *sida*. The question was bound to resurface, however, as Manno's death and Anita's final decline had moved the new disorder center stage. By the close of 1987, *sida* was a frequent topic of conversation, and some began to ask if Dieudonné, still plagued by diarrhea and by then very thin, might not have the new "sent sickness." Others were then of the opinion that "it was [someone] in the ODBFA crew that sent [sickness] on him." But there was no consensus about the etiology of Dieudonné's affliction, unless it was that his illness was "not simple." By early 1988, few mentioned as a possibility a "simple" or "natural" illness. At least two members of Dieudonné's large extended family felt that his illness was the result of poison, an invisible "powder" laid in his path. Another termed the poison a *makandal*. It was not clear whether or not these episodes were thought to be a recurrence of his previous problems, or the onset of another illness. The majority seemed to agree with Mme. Sonson, who believed that the problem was the same that had begun years ago in Port-au-Prince.

Dieudonné had improved, but he was not cured. He spent the first two months of 1988 going from healer to healer. "The stronger he became," recalled Mme. Lamandier later that year, "the more he walked." Dieudonné was also plagued by a terrible itching, and in January sought medical care at the clinic. Even then, he preferred to discuss Haitian politics.[9] In March, he reported once more to the clinic: "Lack of appetite, loss of weight, chronic diarrhea" commented Dr. Romain in his notes. "HIV?" Père Jacques sent for Boss Yonèl "in order to ask him why he was spending what little money he had on fruitless diversions when a proper medical evaluation might be definitive." Both the priest and his wife suspected that Dieudonné might have what Mme. Alexis termed *le mal du siècle,* "the sickness of the century." Père Jacques predicted another cycle of sorcery accusations and counterattacks.

Anita's death prompted Dieudonné to speak of *sida,* but not in relation to his own illness, which he termed "weakness" (*feblès*). "*Sida* can be sent, as with Manno," he observed in late February. "But it can also be caught like tuberculosis. That is how Anita fell ill." It was then that he also wondered "whether *sida* might not have been sent to Haiti by the United States. That's why they were so quick to say that Haitians gave [the world] *sida*." When asked why the United States would wish such a pestilence on Haitians, Dieudonné had a ready answer: "They say there are too many Haitians over there now. They needed us to work for them, but now there are too many over there."

It was not until later in the spring of 1988, however, that Dieudonné and I began talking more candidly about his illness. When referring to his own condition, which continued to deteriorate, Dieudonné spoke only of weakness and "poor blood." Yet it was at about that time that he began once again to cough. Tilibèt noted that it was in early March that he began to complain of shortness of breath (*retoufman*). The records of Clinique Saint-André show that Dieudonné declined rapidly during the summer of 1988. Although he had been free of symptoms during the late spring, Dieudonné was again coughing and short of breath by late July. Again he came to the clinic. In June 1988, examination of his sputum revealed the bacillus that causes tuberculosis. Boss

Yonèl was reluctant to believe that his son could have tuberculosis, and took him to a clinic in Mirebalais: "My father wanted to be sure that's what I have," said Dieudonné, avoiding the word. "Sometimes they say that you have that, but you're really sick with something else." When asked what else, he shrugged and replied, "A cold."[10]

Tilibèt was asked to administer Dieudonné's daily shots of streptomycin, one of three antituberculous drugs that he was prescribed:

I gave him all the injections, but he didn't get much better. Then he went to [a community hospital in the town of] Pignon, and they said he had severe anemia, and prescribed more injections. Then he got much better, and even started to work again. He recovered very quickly.

By early August, Dieudonné began working on the little house next to his parents. He spoke of trying to recover his daughter, who had been taken by her mother's people. With the help of Boss Yonèl, he completed the walls and covered the roof with tin. Then he again fell ill. As Tilibèt recalls,

He had diarrhea again, and this time open sores like Manno's. He was coughing, even though he was still taking his [antituberculous] medications. It was then that people began to say he had *sida*.

Indeed, few of the villagers with whom I spoke mentioned any possibility other than the new sickness. The appearance of dermatologic lesions seemed to clinch the popular diagnosis of *sida* by leading villagers to think of Manno's illness.[11] Further, collective concern about *sida*, which seemed to subside after Anita's death, began mounting again during Dieudonné's final weeks. There seemed to be a profusion of radio programs declaring AIDS to be a "national scourge." The new consensus on Dieudonné's affliction stimulated palpable anxiety in Do Kay. "We need to know who is sending *mo sida* on Kay people," said Mme. Étienne. "Are we all susceptible?"

This anxiety was soon eclipsed by more pressing concerns. The violence in the capital had reached its zenith in the first weeks of September, when Saint-Jean Bosco, a Catholic church well known as the core of the progressive *ti legliz* movement, was brutally attacked by a group of armed men—in the midst of a crowded Sunday service. The church was then burned; over a dozen worshippers perished. The culprits, it was immediately and universally believed, were the *makout* "attachés" of the longtime Duvalierist mayor of Port-au-Prince. Soldiers stood by passively as these men ripped through the crowd. These suspicions were soon confirmed, as Haiti's self-proclaimed president—General Henri Namphy—appeared on national television with the crime's perpetrators. He was congratulating them for their patriotism.[12]

The people of Do Kay were horrified by the carnage at Saint-Jean-Bosco. So, it seemed, were a majority of Haitians, including some soldiers from the rank and file. On September 17, General Namphy was deposed by an internal coup. The following day was a Sunday, and during the intercessional prayer, one of the young teachers from École Saint-André implored God to rid Haiti of "the curse of bloody rulers" (*madichon gouvelman sanginè yo*):

> Father in heaven, you listened when the people of Israel were held in slavery. Say a word to us Haitians as we struggle here now. Say a word about those who foul your altars with the blood of the innocent. Deliver us from the curse of bloody rulers, from all brutality. Their hands are covered with the blood of those who were just doing what you said to do in Isaiah, chapter 1: Seek justice. Protect the oppressed, those who carry heavy sacks. Defend widows and street children. O, Father in heaven, only you can help us to find the solution to Haiti's problems, now and forever.[13]

In Kay, the coup was initially held to be the "deliverance" from the regime of the bloody and now universally detested command of General Namphy. Even Mme. Dieugrand, whose personal theology was quite distant from that of adherents of the *ti legliz* movement, was sure that the coup "was the direct hand of the Good Lord, sweeping away the scoundrels who dirty his temple." Dieudonné may have been short of breath, but he had a great deal to say about the recent coup. Speaking of the men who had paid their *attachés* to attack the worshippers of Saint-Jean Bosco, he predicted that "a new Haiti won't have room for people like that. They're the ones who want to shut everyone up, and if they can't shut them up, they disappear them."

My discussions with Dieudonné continued to focus on national-level political disturbances. The word *sida* never figured in exchanges about his own illness. He did not hear, or ignored, the widely circulated rumors that had him dying of *sida*; at least, we did not speak of them. He had tuberculosis, he said, a disorder that seemed, before the advent of *sida*, to be the worst of sicknesses.[14] When asked why his tuberculosis seemed refractory to treatment, Dieudonné responded with a proverb: *Maladi pa tonbe sou pyebwa, se sou nèg li tonbe.* The literal translation is, "Illness doesn't strike trees, it strikes humans." The proverb is meant to underline the inevitable association between illness and the human condition.

Shortly thereafter, however, Dieudonné hinted that his problem was a sent sickness. He did not wish to tell me that he was dealing with a sent *sida,* but he did state that "somebody, somebody who knows, told me that, if I wasn't a born-again Christian, to go for it" (*si-m pat nan levanjil pou-m degaje-m*). Dieudonné revealed this with an air of dejection. His family, however, was not ready to surrender. During the last week of September 1988, Boss Yonèl again took his son to see Tonton Mèmè. I discovered this upon going to see Dieudonné after having been absent from Do Kay for several weeks. Gaunt and gasping, he was entirely bedridden. But he told me that he would not be able to see me the following day, as had been planned; he had "a meeting." Asked if he would be seeing Tonton Mèmè at this meeting, he smiled and nodded. He acceded to my request to accompany them. At last, I thought, the old *houngan* would have a chance to try his hand at treating *sida*. But first he would have to diagnose it.

I had not interviewed Tonton Mèmè for several months. In our last exchange, in early June, he had explained that "*sida* is both natural and supernatural, because they know how to send it, and you can also catch it from a person who already has *sida*." There was no mention of his prior uncertainty of the illness, or even of its novelty. He had very formed ideas about prophylaxis against *sida*:

The *gad* is there to protect you against any kind of sickness that a person would send on you. But in such matters, one must proceed carefully: if you go overboard, you make someone crazy, and it's not worth anything to you. And also, you must not undertake this [protective rite] unless you intend to follow carefully every step, as disobedience will leave you more vulnerable to whatever they wish to send on you.

He had already protected a number of clients in precisely this fashion. The *gad* would be useless, he said, in the event that someone had already been exposed to the illness. He acknowledged then that he had not yet treated someone already ill with *sida*. Unless he had treated persons with *sida* in the four months following our last interview, Dieudonné would be his first attempt.

Dieudonné was laid on a plank of wood and carried to Mèmè's compound the following evening, September 26, 1988. There were only a dozen or so persons present: half of them related to Yonèl, and half related to Mèmè. Tonton Mèmè's wife prepared for him a drink of raw rum, spices, grape cola, and sweet, concentrated milk. He sent one of his sons off to fetch water to sprinkle on the floor of the small *houmfor*.

When I went in, two of his sons were at their drums: the smaller *ti baka* and the large *manman*. Mèmè sat in a chair by the door, and I could scarcely discern Dieudonné, who was lying in a dark recess. The portrait of a saint, in the garb of a bishop, was suspended over the sick man. The small room was impossibly crowded.

The objects on the altar were more or less the same ones I had seen on earlier visits, but there were also three pitchers (*govi*) draped with blue cloth. The altar was lit with a small kerosene lamp, and I could see that the plastic baby dolls were of the sort used as toys in the United States. There were still bottles corked with corn cobs, and adorned with black thread or hair. Two cigarettes lay near Mèmè's left side, as did a new lighter, a deck of cards, and a seashell wrapped in twine. The round yellow box contained powder and a puff; the tin box was fashioned from Budweiser beer cans. The Blessed Virgin stood to the right of a pile of rags from which emerged, spookily, the plastic duck's head. The walls were still papered with pages of *Paris Match,* but there were now many political tracts and voter's registration guides on the walls. The ceiling was hung with red and blue banners, and a faded bit of patterned cloth.

Tonton Mèmè lit a long, irregular candle, and affixed it to a jug of water at his feet. He stared into the candle, and began praying—bits of French prayers ("In the name of the Father, the Son, the Holy Spirit . . . "), the arcane *langaj* of voodoo, and Creole. Mèmè's sons began drumming, but stopped abruptly as he took the rattle in his left hand, a small bell in his right, and began shaking them vigorously near his ears. After a few minutes, Mèmè's upper body began to twitch rhythmically. It looked as if he had silent hiccups. Then Mèt Kafou took over the old man's body, greeting us with a thin voice, high-pitched and self-righteous. Each of those present, beginning with Mèmè's sons, stooped over the sitting *lwa,* and kissed him on both cheeks.

Staring into the candle, Mèt Kafou began singing in the same falsetto. Among the many verses were those relating directly to Dieudonné's illness:

> They sent on you
> Bibilo bibi
> They sent on you
> Bibilo bibi
> It's a man who did this
> A man from the city
> It's a city man

Mèt Kafou asked many questions, but often did not wait for, or inter-rupted, the answers. He would break into shrill song, and almost everyone present knew when to respond with drums and antiphons. Some present were startled by the sudden cracking of a whip, a *fwèt kach* that had been hidden near one of the drums. At one point Mèt Kafou went over to Dieudonné and waved his hands over the sick man's head and chest, singing all the while. In a softer, but quite audi-ble, voice, Kafou asked, "Who sent this *sida* death on you? It came from the city! It was sent by a man!"

I had been mistaken in thinking that this would be a healing cere-mony. All those present prayed for the return of Dieudonné's health, and Mèt Kafou blew a fine spray of his sweet drink over Dieudonné, but there were no other interventions—no *manje lwa* had been offered. It had been a diagnostic session, and a divination.

As Mèt Kafou had openly diagnosed Dieudonné's disorder as *sida*, I was able, the following day, to ask questions in a much more direct fashion. Without mentioning *sida*, Dieudonné questioned Kafou's diagnosis: "It might be that, but it might be something else. In any case, I know it was sent on me, and I know who did it." The sick man also mentioned a "new medicine for that disorder," one "recently dis-covered in New York," and wondered whether or not it could be ac-quired in Port-au-Prince.[15] Informed that effective antiviral agents were not available in Haiti, Dieudonné sighed, "I probably don't need them anyway." Yonèl also questioned the diagnosis, but with a tone that betrayed a lack of certainty.[16] Dieudonné and his family took Mèmè's divination to be a confirmation of their suspicion that it had been the young man in Port-au-Prince, and not Dieudonne's "father-in-law," who had sent the illness.

It was the day after the divination that Dieudonné observed that "*sida* is a jealousy sickness." When asked to explain more fully what he intended by his observation, he replied,

What I see is that poor people catch it more easily. They say the rich get *sida*; I don't see that. But what I do see is that one poor person sends it to another poor person. It's like the army: brothers shooting brothers. The little soldier (*ti solda*) is really one of us, one of the people. But he is made to do the bidding of the State, and so shoots his own brother when they yell "Fire!" Perhaps they are at last coming to understand this.

Dieudonné's optimism was based on the recent *coup d'état*, which was then perceived as having been led by a group of *ti solda*. It was the guarded optimism of one who had lived the preceding two years intensely, and also of one who believed himself to be the victim of sorcery. With considerable heat, Dieudonné continued his analysis of *sida* as sent sickness. "It's something new to weaken the people. It's a sickness we send on one another. *Sida* goes down, it doesn't go back up. . . . It's something to put people to sleep, like 'Long live the Haitian nation, forever united!' What happened at Saint-Jean Bosco, that's the real struggle, not all these arguments, not all these hexes." [17] He concluded our conversation with a deep sigh and the prediction that "Haiti will never change as long as poor people keep sending sickness on other poor people."

Dieudonné felt somewhat stronger after Mèmè's divination, but did little other than listen to the radio. And so he heard, as did many others, a journalist describe Do Kay as "a place ravaged by *sida*." This assessment, preferred by the Mirebalais correspondent of Radio Soleil, was widely regarded as a provocation, and was the chief topic of conversation in the days preceding Dieudonné's death. [18] When the residents of Do Kay noted defensively that "only two or three Kay people have died from *sida*," they were already including Dieudonné.

Dieudonné died in the second week of October. His mother later told me that she had been warned in advance: "A woman I know came to the clinic. . . . She was sitting with me and said, 'Oh! Look how death is near you!' So I knew the week before." Dieudonné was quietly buried in the same makeshift cemetery where Anita had been interred. [19]

Although one dissenting opinion had it that "tuberculosis killed him because it circulated too long in his blood," most agreed with Mme. Charité, who explained the relation between tuberculosis and sent *sida*:

Tuberculosis and *sida* resemble each other greatly. They say that "TB is *sida*'s little brother," because you can see them together. But if it's a sent *sida*, then it's really [*sida*] that leaves you weak and susceptible to TB. You can treat it, but you'll die nonetheless. *Sida* is TB's older brother, and it's not easy to find treatment for it.

A few years earlier, *sida* had been caught in a completely different web of associations. It had already been strongly associated with blood disorders, but had also been linked to pneumonia, homosexuality, blood transfusion, and life in the city. By the time of Dieudonné's death, the new disorder could be termed "TB's big brother" without causing disagreement. Tilibèt, for example, readily explained what was intended by the analogy, adding that "tuberculosis is like *sida* only more deadly and colder (*pi fatal e pi frèt*)."[20] Although many interviewed in the last days of 1988 and in early 1989 spoke of differences between the two disorders, it was clear that, in the eyes of many, the two disorders were intimately associated.

One of the chief similarities between *sida* and tuberculosis was the possibility of a sent death. Most were of the opinion that Dieudonné's illness had been sent by the rival domestic of long ago, or by his family. When I commented that this seemed a rather long interval between offense and retribution, Absalom Kola smiled and offered a proverb, *Bay kou, bliye; pote mak, sonje*: "He who strikes forgets; he who bears the scar remembers." Mme. Charité, who was unrelated to Dieudonné, felt that his *mò sida* had been sent by his "father-in-law." A minority opinion was also offered by Ti Zout, one of the first villagers to attend high school, and one of the original founders of Projè Veye Sante. He favored an infectious-disease model of *sida*:

Dieudonné was working in Port-au-Prince, and then he became the *plase*[21] of a girl from Thomonde, who had also spent a great deal of time working in Port-au-Prince. The girl fell ill, and was laid low with several kinds of sicknesses, such as diarrhea, scabies (*gratèl*). She even had tuberculosis. After that, she died. In my opinion, it was a bad illness this girl had, and he caught it too, because she had already had several husbands.

There seemed to have been little speculation as to why Tonton Mèmè's intervention had produced no results. *Sida* was already known as a deadly killer, and the sent dead were always notoriously difficult to pry from the living. "It's not just any sickness, this *sida*," said Tonton Mèmè when interviewed two months after Dieudonné's death. "It has to be caught early, and you have to have a great deal of knowledge to treat it."

Boss Yonèl went to significant trouble to discover the culprit. Did he then attempt to avenge his son's death? The ethnographic literature would lead one to expect such reprisals: "When the parents of someone deceased suspect poisoning," writes Métraux (1972:273), "they spare neither money nor trouble to discover the culprit and hit back." At this writing, however, it seems that Yonèl has refrained from any counterattack. Such is the opinion of Tonton Mèmè, the only *houngan* with whom Yonèl has regular contact. Mme. Sonson agrees:

Yonèl knows that they sent the sickness on [Dieudonné] because he tried to get someone out of the way. He shouldn't have done that. You can't keep send-

·ing on everyone who sends on you because you sent on them. That doesn't make sense!

Sent sickness does follow a certain logic, and it is this moral calculus that prevents every act of *maji* from initiating a never-ending spiral of attack and counterattack. We will return to the "sense" made by sorcery in a subsequent chapter. For Dieudonné, *sida* most made sense as a "jealousy sickness," a sickness emblematic of a nation of poor people distracted from "the real struggle" by the hurts they inflict on one another.

10

"A Place Ravaged by AIDS"

The suffering of mortally ill individuals can never be reduced to "cultural models" of suffering. Accordingly, we have closely examined the experience of the first three villagers to fall ill with *sida* in Do Kay. Because Manno, Anita, and Dieudonné lived in the relative intimacy of a small village, the responses of their covillagers shaped their experience, and the voices of many people from Do Kay are heard in the stories recounted in the previous three chapters. There is much, however, that these accounts do not capture. Through the misfortune of Manno and Anita and Dieudonné, *sida* became a *collective* concern. After Manno's death, the lack of interest in *sida* registered in previous years gave away to an enduring fascination and fear; innumerable stories were told, some publicly, some semiprivately—all indicative of what was felt to be at stake. By the time Dieudonné was mortally stricken, everyone in Do Kay had a stake in understanding this new and lethal sickness.

The specter of serious illness is ever-present in rural Haiti; life expectancy is short. It is not surprising, then, that the people of Kay and surrounding villages talk a great deal about these illnesses, and also about the minor complaints that are experienced regularly. It was therefore striking to note that in 1983 *sida* was not mentioned during many hours of open-ended interviewing; nor was the syndrome discussed in more casual talk. Between May 1983 and April 1984, any conversation I may have had about *sida* was prompted by my questioning. When one villager was asked if his friends were reluctant to speak about *sida,* he responded, "Why should that be? There is no one who says we can't talk about *sida.* But it is nothing we have ever seen here. It's a city sickness (*maladi lavil*)." It was difficult to discern any fear of speaking about *sida*; the syndrome did not seem to be considered "taboo" or embarrassing. It was, simply, irrelevant in the already beleaguered lives of the rural poor.

Most people had heard of *sida,* however, and several felt that they could list key features of the syndrome. Although there was some disagreement about what those characteristics might be, the following assessment, from a thirty-six-year-old market woman, was not atypical of the descriptions elicited in 1984:

Sida is a sickness they have in Port-au-Prince and in the United States. It gives you a diarrhea that starts very slowly, but never stops until you're completely dry. There's no water left in your body. . . . *Sida* is a sickness that you see in men who sleep with other men.

Although two persons suggested that "*sida* is the same thing as tuberculosis," most of those questioned mentioned three attributes: its novelty, its relation to diarrhea, and its association with homosexuality. Most of the villagers who offered such a description had heard of AIDS on the radio, or during trips to the capital.

If villagers were aware of but uninterested in *sida* by 1984, interest in the illness was almost universal less than three years later. Moreover, ideas about the disorder and its origin had changed drastically, as had understandings of etiology, course, and presentation of the malady. The case of Manno Surpris in particular influenced the views of area residents, and contributed substantially to the collective representation that was slowly emerging. All concerned agreed that the schoolteacher was the first resident of Do Kay to fall ill with *sida.* It was after Manno's death that the new disorder became part of the villagers' regular discourse. *Sida,* the new affliction that in 1984 had inspired little interest and no passion in Do Kay, had become by the close of 1987 a staple of "semiprivate" discussion. Why was it, several villagers queried, that Kay alone of the villages in the area had people sick with *sida*? If the disorder was indeed novel, as most seemed to believe, why should it strike Kay first? Some cautioned that the mysterious deaths of two persons from nearby villages may not have been due to tuberculosis after all: perhaps they died, unwittingly, from *sida*? Other questions were asked in more hushed tones: Were others, such as Dieudonné and Celhomme, ill with the disorder? Was it really caused by a "simple microbe," or was *someone* at the bottom of it all?

Rumors flew. Acéphie was said to have contracted the disorder by sharing clothes with Germaine, a kinswoman from another village on the plateau. A *bokòr* in Vieux Fonds—not Tonton Mèmè—was reported to have signed a contract with a North American manufacturing firm. The *bokòr* was to "load tear-gas grenades with *zonbi sida*." Demonstrators who found themselves in a cloud of this tear gas would later fall ill with a bona fide case of *sida*. One person with tuberculosis was cautioned not to cross any major paths, stand in a crossroads, or walk under a chicken roost, lest his malady "degenerate into *sida*."[1] Also striking was the new sense of personal fear that attended Anita's sickness. "She's one of us, she's family (*moun lakay*)," said many. If Anita could fall ill, so could anyone in Do Kay.

During the same period, village representatives of community medicine continued a series of parallel activities. At the January 1988 meeting of the village health committee organized by Père Alexis, there was discussion of initiating a much-needed antituberculosis project, one that would also embrace the task of education related to HIV. The community health workers of Projè Veye Sante held a second conference on AIDS, with the chief lecture prepared by Saul Joseph, and launched a program to make free disposable needles available.[2] But these attempts at activism seemed mired in a widely shared resignation, which cast the new disorder as a ruthless killer against which "doctors' medication" could afford little comfort. The dispirited physicians seemed to feel, just then, that any assertions to the contrary were hollow ones, that there was really nothing they could do.

There was, in fact, a similar weary skepticism about all forms of activism. The November massacre of voters had taken its toll, many commented. The people had tried, they had paid dearly, and they had failed. As more than one peasant informed me: "I'm not into politics anymore; I'm in my garden."[3] One Haitian journalist put it well: "The hope of actually living evaporated, the habit of surviving was soon back in place. The people were demobilized. The ideology of the daily bread again spread to the majority of the population, who lost faith and confidence" (Desinor 1988:172). Gone or eclipsed was the feverish energy of the preceding two years. Lost, too, was any widespread enthusiasm for civic activities, including public-health initiatives. Community meetings no longer drew large crowds, and those who did come seemed reluctant to speak their minds. People spoke of "the climate of in-security," a buzzword that seemed to be only weakly related to the incidence of violent crimes and assassination. There was much reference, at the close of 1987, to the "absence of Christmas," a holiday almost universally celebrated in Haiti, regardless of religious affiliation. The highlight of the celebration is midnight mass on Christmas Eve. Citing the climate of insecurity, a number of Catholic priests urged their colleagues to refuse to celebrate midnight mass. Père Alexis was among those who cancelled, for the first time in three decades, this most significant of liturgies.[4] One radio announcer referred movingly to "the Christmas of destruction, decay, and despair." The carol most often heard in the Kay area was titled "Nowel an Ayiti," one stanza of which was as follows:

Big shots go to the city
To stock up on supplies
They fill up their houses
To celebrate Christmas
The poor try to ease the pain
Of making fasts that they don't want
They're praying to the Lord
For manna to rain down
What are they going to eat?
Is Christmas not for them as well?
Those who can't pay rent?
Those who sleep in shifts?
Sadness fills their hearts
They're living without hope
And they find no one
To reach out and give a hand
That's Christmas in Haiti

In Kay, an increased concern with *sida* fit all too well into the almost apocalyptic winter of 1987–1988. Manno was dead and Anita was dying. The fearsome turn of national events—the election-day massacre—was related in several ways to continued hard times for "the people." The advent of *sida* was simply one of the many manifestations of these trials. Another would be the predicted return of the "big *tonton makout*," those that had been forced into exile after February 1986. Several persons whispered that some of the cruelest of the *makout*, even those rumored dead, were bringing back new weapons. One twenty-three-year-old *lycée* student from Do Kay informed me that Albert "Ti Boule" Pierre, one of the Duvaliers' most notorious strongmen, was returning from South America with "newly acquired knowledge." Ti Zout continued:

They say he went [to South America] to study the science of bacteriology. He learned how to create microbes, and then traveled to [North] America to study germ warfare. . . . They can now put microbes into the water of troublesome places. They can disappear all the militant young men and at the same time attract more [international] aid in order to stop the epidemic.

Anita's death, in mid-February, coincided with an obvious dampening of discussion of the disorder. What had once seemed a sort of struggle for preeminence between politics and *sida*—with the former eclipsing the latter whenever "the thing was hot"—was now revealed to be a more symbiotic relationship. When the muzzle was off, it was off for everything; when it was applied with new force, those with the most to lose simply spoke less. The disorder was discussed less and less as villagers stopped discussing national politics.[5] Père Alexis acridly assessed rural Haitians' growing silence: "They've been excluded from politics for a couple of centuries now. They know that no one in power really wants their opinions on things. They know they're not invited to the party." The apocalyptic mood persisted throughout the "zombi spring," as more than one of the villagers put it, but it was increasingly mute.

The silence proved transient. During the summer of 1988, public and private discussion again focused on national events. Another "hot" summer had followed the zombi spring. Haiti was again experiencing a wave of officially sanctioned repression, which attained new heights during the early fall. Rural Haitians saw themselves as passive spectators gazing at an absurd and increasingly brutal spectacle: another *coup d'état*, the bloody exactions of the urban death squads, and the more subtle but unremitting violence of a collapsing economy. "The climate of insecurity" was invoked as a free-standing explanatory response to many queries. Collective concern about *sida* began mounting again well before the death of Dieudonné.

In September 1988, Haitians at home and abroad were shocked by the massacre at Saint-Jean Bosco. This event seemed to have a special resonance in rural Haiti. "It's incredible," said Mme. Sonson in an interview two weeks after the carnage. "Just when you imagine it can't get any worse for the Haitian people, look what happens to them." These atrocities were followed by another *coup d'état*, this one applauded, however briefly, by many rural Haitians: expressing revulsion for the Sunday killings, a group of noncommissioned officers initiated the coup that brought yet another Duvalierist to power. The attachés who had carried out the grisly Saint-Jean Bosco attack found rude justice in the streets of Port-au-Prince.

Many people in Kay immediately commented that the muzzle was again off; some were not sure. A third and far less intense wave of publicly expressed concern over *sida* was nonetheless registered soon after the bloody events in Saint-Jean Bosco, when Dieudonné's illness was revealed, shortly before his death, to be another case of "sent *sida*." In the collective readings of Manno's and Anita's illnesses, popular opinion had been informed by medical or other specialist (for example, *houngan*) assessment. But Dieudonné's illness was widely thought to be *sida* well before there was medical or ritual confirmation. The people of Kay now recognized *sida,* and had much to say about its causes, its course, and possible interventions. Many of those interviewed in the summer and fall of 1988 were confident about their knowledge of *sida,* and felt that "the thing is now clear." Indeed, the rapid change in referents, the wildly discrepant understandings of the same illnesses, and professed ignorance of the disorder were becoming things of the past. A collective representation was emerging, as would become clear in the more "public" events of the fall.

For a brief stretch of autumn—the last weeks of September and the first weeks of October—the muzzle was indeed off again. *Sida,* like many other controversial issues, was the topic of much discussion. Its zenith seemed to coincide with the description, by the Mirebalais correspondent of Radio Soleil, of Kay as "a place ravaged by *sida*." In the course of a routine report from the area around his hometown, the journalist noted that "Kay is a place where there is much *sida,* and people in the area should be aware of this." Père Jacques was troubled by the report, and predicted that it would have an adverse effect on the clinic: "People will be reluctant to come to the clinic if they believe the village is inhabited by people who harbor the virus."

The priest's prediction came true, if only briefly. A substantial decrease in traffic was registered, which Dr. Roumain did not hesitate to attribute to the radio report. Yet business was again booming within two weeks.[6] The chief damage, it seems, was to the *lycée* students from the Kay area, as an interview with Saul suggests:

It led to many problems in school because when they announced the news on the radio, everyone heard it. Many students said that they weren't going to sit next to children from Kay in order to avoid catching *sida*. Everyone knows, they said, that Kay has been ruined by that sickness.

In the intensely competitive atmosphere of the regional *lycée,* such discrimination may have been the functional equivalent of sorcery accusations. The "children from Kay"—which meant those who had graduated from École Saint-André, regardless of village of origin—called a meeting. They decided to "form a committee to meet with Père Jacques, in order to ask for his advice." Their plan was to request, through Alexis, a meeting with the journalist who had posted the note, in order to ask him why he had done so.[7] They further attributed to the journalist rather unsavory motives. As Ti François, in his last year at the *lycée,* would have it, "Several people from Mirebalais have died from *sida,* but that wasn't deemed newsworthy. That's why we feel that the announcement was in order to slander the [Kay] region." Fanfan Guerrier, the son of Anita's godmother, also suggested that local jealousy contributed to the rapid dissemination of the "news." "Not everyone is happy that Père Alexis has put so much into Kay," he said in late September. "Not everyone is happy that there is such a nice clinic in the middle of the weeds, while the town [of Mirebalais] doesn't have a good one."

The students never met with Père Alexis, perhaps because they were in the midst of the academic year's first round of exams. But Père Alexis and members of his parish council seemed to have independently reached a similar conclusion: "We thought it was because the clinic had such a good reputation—everyone was singing its praises. Well, you know that that is going to make some people jealous, and that's why they slandered the area." The priest suggested that Clinique Saint-André, "hidden in the middle of the weeds," was widely known to offer better services than those available in the "big town" of Mirebalais.

Many of the villagers were disturbed less by the threat to the clinic than that to commerce. Because even the poorest of Haitian peasants depend on what is termed "public transportation," the bad publicity was widely perceived as demanding some response. The priest did in fact summon the correspondent, who subsequently recalled that "Père Alexis told us that the [news] bulletin was bad. He said that the people of Kay protested, and that we should correct the error. We did so no more than a few days later." This rectification led, he insisted, to an immediate end to the truck drivers' refusal to stop in Do Kay.[8] The journalist insisted that he meant only that "the people of Kay should avoid sexual contact with these people, not handshaking and that sort of thing. It was their own poor understanding (*movèz konsepsyon*) that led [the truck drivers] to refuse to pick up people from Kay." Others involved insisted that the effects were much more enduring. For two months, according to Saul, it was difficult for him and for other residents of Do Kay to find public transportation. There was agreement among all parties, however, that the truck drivers and the native Mirebalais students had "behaved poorly."

Although a confused welter of emotions—the fear of sorcery and sorcery accusations, the anger of conspiracy theories, and the prejudice and fear reflected in the refusal of truck drivers to stop in a place branded as AIDS-ridden—persisted in Do Kay, the dissension that had marked the previous years of the epidemic was giving way to agreement and clarity. Several of the villagers indicated that *sida* was now "understood" in the Kay area. "It was once like this with tuberculosis," observed Mme. Charité. "People were very afraid of it, and would even hide it. But the proverb says, 'Hidden sickness has no treatment' (*Maladi kache pa gen remèd*). *Sida* is like tuberculosis before there was a treatment."

Many had come to see the new disorder as not only similar but intimately related to that familiar scourge, tuberculosis. One person classed *sida* as "the worst form of tuberculosis." Mme. Lamandier referred to tuberculosis as "*sida*'s little brother. These two sicknesses look alike. They have almost the same symptoms. And they crush the [sick] person in the same manner." She nonetheless made major distinctions between the two disorders:

The person with TB (*tebe*) has more of a chance of recovery than does the person with *sida*. The person with TB, if he or she is cared for closely at a clinic, follows all the clinic's instructions, will live. But the person with *sida* has, from the moment he or she catches it, a greater chance of dying than of living.

The universal awareness of the new disorder's virulence, coupled with the current, though transient, freedom of expression, led to unprecedented public discussion of *sida*. The prime example of *sida*'s place in public discourse was the "testimonial" by Acéphie Laurent, who had been diagnosed with active pulmonary tuberculosis in February 1988. The testimonial was offered in church, in late October, less than two weeks after Dieudonné's death. Before the final hymn and blessing, Maître Gerard announced that "Sister Acéphie" had "a matter of importance that she wished to bring before the congregation." Acéphie arose and walked to front of the church. She inclined her head before the altar, went to the podium, and began to speak. Below is an edited version of what she had to say:

My brothers and sisters, greetings. I'd like to stand before you and give testimonial. It all started with a pain below my heart.[9] It took away my appetite, and I grew thin. Then I began to eat again, but still I stayed thin. I was so thin that they said I had *sida*. But I knew I didn't have it. The doctor said my sputum was not good (*kracha-m pat bon*). Truly, I was sick, but that was no reason for people to criticize me, to say I had a bad disease. I live in my mother's house; I'm in the care of my parents. I don't go looking for trouble, and here they go and say that that's what I have. I was so upset by this that I fell ill with *move san*. . . . But God lifted me up, helped me to stand. Now I'm in His Church to thank Him. To thank Him for the courage to withstand the criticism heaped upon me by everyone. Only Tilibèt [the community health worker], who gave me [streptomycin] injections, did not criticize me. She came to visit me every day. But they even called her aside to discourage her from coming to see me. . . . Some people said I should call those who slandered me before a judge. But I'll leave them to God's judgment.

There were a few "Amens" and a feeling of communal sympathy, but little other response to her outpouring. "Everyone in church was rather somber," Saul later assessed. "They had nothing to say when she said, 'Instead of slandering me, why don't you help me to pray that nothing like that ever happens?'" I later asked Acéphie who was slandering her, and she replied, "The people" (*pèp la*). In any case, she stated that her strategy was a successful one: "When they saw that [the rumor that she had *sida*] wasn't true, every one felt comfortable around me."

Acéphie's declaration did indeed trigger a more collective response to *sida*.[10] A meeting of the community council was called to discuss "problems facing our area." The reunion was scheduled, it seemed, to coincide with Père Jacques's absence. As Dieugrand, a council member, later confided, "If Père were there, people might not say critical things about the clinic." To the question, "Why was it that Kay alone of the villages in the area had people sick with *sida*?" some people had answered, "Because the clinic draws them." It was true that Clinique Saint-André received and treated its share of *moun sida*, but probably no more than any other large center. The notion that it treated an inordinately large number of persons with AIDS probably stemmed from the clinic's aggressive public-education campaign.

In any case, it seems that no "critical things about the clinic" were mentioned during the late-October meeting. This may have been due to Boss Yonèl, Dieudonné's father. The same man who had so vigorously denied the existence of *sida* and its role in his son's death was now speaking as an advocate for those with the disorder. Boss Yonèl reminded those present of the need for *tèt ansanm,* cooperation. Saul, who recorded the meeting on tape, recalled that "he stood there quite confidently, and seemed to make *sida* the main point of the meeting." "It is our duty," Yonèl said, "to serve the ill. This is true no matter what the illness. This is true even for *sida*." No one offered a counterargument.[11]

The meeting marked one of the first times that *sida* had been mentioned in a public gathering not convened by Père Jacques or by the leaders of Projè Veye Sante. But the Kay area was clearly a region where a great deal was known and said of the new disorder. By the spring of 1989, scarcely more than two years after its arrival, the inhabitants of Do Kay seemed to have come to terms with *sida*. In the first months of 1989, there seemed to be very little publicly evinced anxiety, and certainly nothing that would qualify as hysteria. "I know they say that there is *sida* in Kay," said Mme. Charité in February, "but I don't yet see it." In the same month, Mme. Fardin went so far as to express hope that an effective treatment for *sida* might soon be found. "There's still no treatment. Some time ago, it was said that a treatment would come from New York in six years. The six years are not up yet."

Less is said of the disorder, although it is clearly something that is greatly feared. So are many other misfortunes. *Sida*-the-infectious-disease and *sida*-caused-by-magic are two new slings and arrows to add to the deplorable fortunes of the Kay peasants. That this might be so is suggested by the ethnographic literature predating *sida*. Research conducted decades ago led Métraux (1972:269) to observe that "in everyday life the threat of charms, sorcery and spells makes [magic] but one more care to be listed with drought and the price of coffee and bananas. Magic is at least an evil against which man is not entirely powerless." Hurbon (1987a:260) offers a similar insight when he notes of sorcery bundles that "*wanga* are part of the daily struggle in a world already littered with traps."

When interpreted in the light of these observations, the lessons of the previous chapters should be brought to bear on our understanding of the oft-mentioned "resignation" of the rural poor. We have seen the extent to which the families of Manno, Anita, and Dieudonné went in order to care for them. If this be resignation, it is a decidedly energetic type, a sort of "opportunistic resignation."[12] When rural Haitians are

offered the chance to change their lot, they take it. But their circumstances demand a certain realism.[13] Mme. Sonson, when she was
confronted with the question of resignation, put it as follows: "It's not
that we don't care. It's just that we're sick all the time."

It seems fair to suggest that the people of Kay have maintained a
certain resilience in their travail. Though badly battered by the loss of
their land and their subsequent poverty, they have nonetheless managed
to maintain a humane discourse about suffering. The advent of *sida* did
not change this. At no point did the family members of the ill refuse
to care for their kin, as has been the case in the United States and elsewhere. Saul had a ready response to this comparison:

A family will never deny the existence of one of their own because of a sickness.
We are frightened of the illness because the Americans say that it came from
us, and also because everyone knows there's no hope. But that's no excuse for
turning your back on family. Haitians are already a people of poverty (*yon pèp
la misè*); the poor have to have the patience to struggle with their people's
sicknesses.

PART THREE

The Exotic and the Mundane: HIV in Haiti

> *On one level it has become a commonplace to say that we all inhabit "one world." There are ecological connections: New York suffers from the Hong Kong flu; the grapevines of Europe are destroyed by American plant lice. There are demographic connections: Jamaicans migrate to London; Chinese migrate to Singapore. There are economic connections: a shutdown of oil wells on the Persian Gulf halts generating plants in Ohio; a balance of payments unfavorable to the United States drains American dollars into bank accounts in Frankfurt or Yokahama; Italians produce Fiat automobiles in the Soviet Union; Japanese build a hydroelectric system in Ceylon. There are political connections: wars begun in Europe unleash reverberations around the globe; American troops intervene on the rim of Asia; Finns guard the border between Israel and Egypt.*
>
> Wolf (1982:3)

Although the human immunodeficiency virus cannot be shown to have been present in Haiti before the close of the 1970s, the country is now among those most gravely affected by HIV. As of March 20, 1990, Haiti had reported 2,331 cases of AIDS to the Pan-American Health Organization, making Haiti one of the world's twenty most affected nations. And although no large random surveys have been conducted, several epidemiologic studies of asymptomatic city dwellers reveal HIV seroprevalence rates of between 5 percent and 9 percent. Some Haitian researchers have gone so far as to suggest that HIV-related disorders have recently become the leading cause of death among adults between twenty and forty-nine years of age.

The following chapters will review the epidemiology of AIDS and HIV in Haiti. How did HIV cause such a devastating epidemic in such a short amount of time? What is known about HIV transmission in Haiti? Does it still remain a "mystery"? That such questions are critical is underscored by a February 1990 U.S. Food and Drug Administration (FDA) ruling, which banned all Haitians from donating blood. In response to this ruling, thousands of Haitians brought Miami traffic to a standstill as they shouted "Racists!" in front of FDA headquarters there. The demonstrations culminated in a mammoth rally in New York City. So many marchers—50,000 according to the police, more than twice that according to organizers—crossed the Brooklyn Bridge that it was closed to traffic for the day.

What, exactly, had prompted the recent FDA ruling? The March 14, 1990, edition of the *New York Times* explained that the decision was based on what was known about HIV transmission in Haiti:

The Centers for Disease Control have stopped publicly specifying that Haitians are at risk for contracting AIDS, but the agency's statistics still carry a category of "pattern II countries," where heterosexual transmission is the primary mode of infection. And these are defined by the World Health Organization as Haiti and sub-Saharan Africa.

In overviews of the world epidemiology of HIV/AIDS, it is often suggested that three general types of epidemiological "patterns" currently exist. Pattern I, to use the terminology of the World Health Organization Global Program on AIDS, is seen in North America and Europe. It is characterized by a preponderance of cases among gay and bisexual men, with variable attack rates among intravenous drug users. Haiti (and sometimes the entire Caribbean) is characterized along with much of Africa as reflecting Pattern II. To cite a recent review:

Pattern II is seen in the Caribbean and in large areas of sub-Saharan Africa, and differs [from Pattern I] in that heterosexual intercourse has been the dominant mode of HIV transmission from the start. Blood transfusion, the reuse of contaminated needles, and intravenous drug use contribute to a variable degree, but homosexuality generally plays a minor role in this pattern. (Osborn 1989:126)

Pattern III is used to describe areas of low incidence of AIDS.

This section, which reviews what is known about HIV transmission in Haiti, will suggest that the World Health Organization (WHO) terminology obscures more than it illuminates, especially in regard to Haiti and much of the Caribbean. In fact, many early assumptions about the Haitian epidemic, and its role in the larger epidemic to the north, have been cast in doubt by careful epidemiological research. Moreover, the course of the American pandemic, including the epidemic in Haiti, has been determined to no small extent by economic and political structures long in place.

11

A Chronology of the AIDS/HIV Epidemic in Haiti

Most chroniclers of the AIDS pandemic agree that awareness of the new syndrome began in 1980 in California. Several physicians in Los Angeles observed that *Pneumocystis carinii,* a harmless parasite to those with intact immune defenses, had caused pneumonia (P.C.P.) in several young men without recognized states of immunodeficiency. The only epidemiological clue linking the cases was the sexual preference of the men. By June of 1981, the U.S. Centers for Disease Control (CDC), monitoring the distribution of drugs used to treat P.C.P., reported that "in the period from October 1980 to May 1981, five young men, all active homosexuals, were treated for biopsy-confirmed P.C.P. at three different hospitals in Los Angeles." By the end of the summer, 108 cases of Kaposi's sarcoma and unexplained opportunistic infections had been reported to the CDC. The vast majority of cases were from California and New York. Of those afflicted, 107 were men; over 90 percent of these men stated that they were gay and sexually active.

Alerted to the possibility of an epidemic, North American public health specialists reviewed available documentation and observed that unexpected clusterings of Kaposi's sarcoma and opportunistic infections had begun early in 1977. Haitian physicians began to see similarly puzzling cases of immunosuppression shortly thereafter. The first Haitian case of Kaposi's sarcoma was detected in June 1979, when dermatologist Bernard Liautaud diagnosed the disorder in a twenty-eight-year-old woman from a city in western Haiti. She had been referred to the university hospital for worsening lower-extremity edema and had presented with nodular and papular lesions over her face, trunk, and extremities. Neither demographic variables nor clinical presentation fit the standard description of patients with the sarcoma: before the AIDS pandemic, Kaposi's had been described as a rare and slow-growing malignancy seen largely in elderly men of Eastern European and Mediterranean descent. The tumor behaved quite differently in Dr. Liautaud's patient, in whom it was aggressive and fatal. When he confirmed, later that year, the presence of the cancer in a young Haitian man, Liautaud posed the following question: Was Kaposi's of long-standing and unappreciated importance in Haiti, or was the cancer new to the country? A survey of colleagues led him to conclude that Kaposi's sarcoma was virtually unknown in Haiti. Liautaud and his coworkers reported their findings to an international medical conference held in Haiti in April 1982 (Liautaud et al. 1983).

The fact that concurrent "outbreaks" of Kaposi's had been reported in California and New York lent credence to the idea that the tumor might be related in some way to an epidemic triggered by an infectious agent, as did the increased incidence of unexplained opportunistic infections.[1] Several such infections, first noted in February 1980, were also presented in the 1982 conference held in Port-au-Prince. These suggestions of immunosuppression were strikingly similar to those recently termed AIDS in the North American medical literature. The conviction that something new and significant was afoot led to the formation in May 1982 of the Haitian Study Group on Kaposi's Sarcoma and Opportunistic Infections (GHESKIO). The study group comprised thirteen physicians and scientists who would eventually treat hundreds with AIDS while conducting important clinical and epidemiological research.

In May 1983, the Association Médicale Haitienne (AMH) devoted their annual conference to the subject of AIDS. Research presented there left little doubt that in urban Haiti, at least, a new state of immunodeficiency was striking increasing numbers of young adults, especially men. In the Haitian medical community, few doubted that the patients were ill with AIDS as recently defined by the CDC. There were, by the time of the AMH conference, twenty cases of Kaposi's sarcoma and more than sixty otherwise unexplained opportunistic infections (see table 2). Using CDC criteria, Haitian researchers diagnosed a total of sixty-one cases of AIDS between June 1979 and October 1982.

Table 2 *AIDS Cases Diagnosed by the Haitian Study Group on Kaposi's Sarcoma and Opportunistic Infections (GHESKIO)*

Year	Kaposi's Sarcoma	Opportunistic Infection
1979	2	0
1980	2	5
1981	7	9
1982	5	35
1/83–5/83	4	12

SOURCE: Pape et al. (1983)

Despite the obvious parallel—the suggestion in both Haiti and the United States of a new, acquired, and epidemic immunosuppression—there were important disparities between the two epidemics. When compared to cases in the United States, a smaller proportion of Haitians with AIDS had P.C.P., the most common opportunistic infection in North Americans with AIDS. Although the Haitian patients did have mycobacterial infections, they were almost exclusively tuberculosis; *M. avium-intracellulare,* an infection common in North Americans with AIDS, was rare in Haiti. Oroesophageal candidiasis was extremely common in Haitians with AIDS, so much so that it was suggested as an early marker for the syndrome (Guérin et al. 1984: 260). There were also disparities in length of survival after diagnosis: while mean survival after diagnosis was usually greater than a year in the United States, survival was less than six months in the majority of Haitian patients, and none survived more than twenty-four months. Despite these differences, most researchers were confident that the Haitian and North American epidemics were caused by the same organism.

The research presented in 1983 offered important epidemiologic clues to Haiti's "role" in the larger pandemic. Although the Haitian researchers had initially concluded that "no segment of Haitian society appears to be free of opportunistic infections or Kaposi's sarcoma" (Pape et al. 1983:949), AIDS did not strike randomly. Pape and co-workers found that 74 percent of all men with opportunistic infections lived in greater Port-au-Prince, home to approximately 20 percent of all Haitians. Curiously, 33 percent of all AIDS patients lived in a single suburb, Carrefour. This finding was underscored because several of the patients interviewed by Pape and other researchers reported that they had been remunerated for sex:

The prevalence rate of men with opportunistic infections in Carrefour was significantly higher than that of men in Port-au-Prince (p<0.001 by the chi-square test). This is of interest since Carrefour, a suburb of Port-au-Prince, is recognized as the principal center of male and female prostitution in Haiti. (Pape et al. 1983:948)

These investigations also revealed that only 13 percent of the remaining men with opportunistic infections were from elsewhere in the country. An equal number had been living outside Haiti: two patients lived in New York; one in Miami; one in Belgium; and one in the Bahamas. Five of twenty-one men interviewed by one of the GHESKIO clinicians stated that they were bisexual, as did two patients referred by other Haitian physicians.[2] Of these seven men, all had lived in Carrefour (four) or the United States (three). Three had had sexual contact with North American men in both Haiti and in the United States, and two others had had sexual contact with Haitian men known to have opportunistic infections.[3] Furthermore, fully half of the allegedly heterosexual men had either lived or traveled outside of Haiti. Research presented at the 1983 meetings made it clear that none of the Haitians ill with the new syndrome had ever been to Africa.[4] All denied sexual contact with persons from that continent; most, in fact, had never met an African. But 10 to 15 percent of these patients had traveled to North America or Europe in the five years preceding the onset of their illness, and several more admitted to sexual contact with tourists (Guérin et al. 1984; Johnson and Pape 1989). Other important demographic data offered by the GHESKIO team were high prevalence (71 percent) of venereal disease and histories of blood transfusion (20 percent) in these patients.

Also in 1983, members of the GHESKIO team surveyed the twenty-one dermatologists and pathologists known to be practicing in Haiti, and asked them to provide information about their experience diagnosing and treating Kaposi's sarcoma. Over one thousand biopsy specimens from the Hôpital Albert Schweitzer were also reviewed. The survey revealed that only one case of the disease had been diagnosed in Haiti in 1972, and it had afflicted a man in his sixties. The course of his illness was not known, but it had not aroused suspicions of immunodeficiency. GHESKIO concluded, as had Liautaud, that the new cases of Kaposi's represented an epidemic of recent onset.

In summary, those who attended the AMH conference could draw several important conclusions based on the data presented at these meetings: Haitians with AIDS were then largely men, though there were increasing numbers of women reporting to the GHESKIO clinic;

there was an epicenter of the Haitian epidemic in the city of Carrefour, a center of prostitution bordering the south side of Port-au-Prince; a large percentage of the early cases had been linked to homosexual contact, some of it with North Americans; the rate of transfusion-associated transmission was higher in Haiti than in the United States; although the opportunistic infections were often different from those seen in North Americans with AIDS, the Haitian epidemic was manifestly related to that in the United States; the microbial agent that led to AIDS was probably new to Haiti, as no one could report cases predating the much larger North American epidemic.

Subsequent research, based on the development of assays for antibodies to the newly discovered HIV, also suggested that the virus was new to Haiti. Blood samples drawn from adults during the course of a 1977–1979 outbreak of dengue fever were later tested for antibodies to HIV. Using ELISA (whole virus) and radioimmunoprecipitation assay (RIPA) for antibody to the p24 and gp120 antigens, it was revealed that none of 191 sera tested had antibodies to HIV (Johnson and Pape 1989).[5] The sole suggestion that AIDS existed in Haiti prior to 1979, the time at which Dr. Liautaud noted the first two cases of Kaposi's sarcoma, were the autopsy records of a previously healthy twenty-year-old man who had died in 1978, two weeks after the sudden onset of generalized seizures. Post-mortem studies at the Hôpital Albert Schweitzer revealed cerebral toxoplasmosis, an opportunistic infection common in persons with AIDS. "These data and studies from Africa," conclude Johnson and Pape (1989:67), "are consistent with the hypothesis that HIV most likely originated in that continent, came to the United States and Europe, and subsequently was introduced into Haiti by either tourists or returning Haitians."

The research conducted in the first years of the Haitian epidemic also spoke to many of the speculations of North American researchers. Was AIDS caused by "an epidemic Haitian virus," as had been suggested? Had overworked or undertrained Haitian physicians merely overlooked the disease, as others seemed to imply?[6] Was AIDS caused by an African virus brought to the United States by Haitians?[7] Was AIDS caused by an organism endemic among isolated, superstitious peasants who transmitted the organism through some bizarre voodoo practice? While some of the Haitian researchers felt that these questions had been answered by their research, which had been published in refereed, international journals, their contributions did little to dampen the apparently self-sustaining "exotic theories" that continued to influence popular opinion in the United States and elsewhere.

12

HIV in Haiti: The Dimensions of the Problem

How far has HIV spread in Haiti? Given the natural history of HIV infection, this question is best answered not by the epidemiology of AIDS, but through the study of HIV seroprevalence in asymptomatic populations. Researchers in Haiti have studied seroprevalence of HIV using both ELISA and RIPA (p24, gp120). During 1986 and 1987, sera from several cohorts of healthy adults were analyzed for antibodies to HIV (see table 3). In a group of individuals working in hotels catering to tourists, HIV seroprevalence was 12 percent. Among urban factory workers, 5 percent were found to have antibodies to HIV. In both series, *rates were comparable for men and women,* which suggested to many observers that the high attack rate in Haitian men would slowly give way to a pattern like that seen in parts of Central Africa, where men and women are equally affected. The highest rates observed were in female Haitian prostitutes (53 percent), underlining for some their role in the transmission of HIV. Few observed that high rates of seroprevalence among prostitutes might simply reflect "occupational risk"—an increased likelihood of coming into contact with a seropositive man—which proved nothing about their role in propagating the virus.

In a group of 502 mothers of children hospitalized with diarrhea and in a group of 190 urban adults with a comparable socioeconomic background, the seroprevalence rates were 12 percent and 13 percent, respectively. All 57 health workers involved in the care of AIDS patients were seronegative, corroborating data suggesting that HIV is not easily

Table 3 *HIV Seroprevalence Among Healthy Adults in Haiti*
(1986–1987)

Category	N	Mean Age (Years)	% HIV (+)
Urban Haiti (Port-au-Prince)			
Hotel Workers	25	45	12.0
Factory Workers	84	30	5.0
Pregnant Women (1986)	1,240	29	8.4
Mothers of Sick Infants	502	29	12.0
Other Adults:			
High SES	54	35	0.0
Low SES	190	33	13.0
Medical Workers	57	40	0.0
Total	2,152	37	9.0
Rural Haiti			
Mothers of Sick Infants	97	25	3.0
Pregnant Women	117	27	3.0
Blood Donors	245	32	4.0
Other Adults (rural village)	191	29	1.0
Total	650	30	3.0

SOURCE: Pape and Johnson (1988b)

spread by nonsexual contact. Overall, GHESKIO researchers found that approximately 9 percent of 912 healthy urban adults (medical workers, college graduates, factory or hotel workers, mothers of sick infants, and other adults) were seropositive for HIV.

A group of researchers based in Cité Soleil, a slum on the northern fringes of Port-au-Prince, reported that 8.4 percent of 1,240 healthy women receiving prenatal care in 1986 were seropositive for HIV (Halsey et al. 1987). In 1987, 9.9 percent of 2,009 "sexually active women" in Cité Soleil were HIV-positive; in 1989, 10.5 percent of 1,074 such women were found to have been exposed to HIV (Brutus 1989b; seropositivity in Cité Soleil was confirmed by Western blot). In Gonaives, the third largest Haitian city, 9 percent of 1,795 patients reporting to a clinic that serves a predominantly low-income clientele were found to be seropositive in 1988 (Brutus 1989a).

Other investigations confirmed the impression of high rates of seroprevalence among people living in or near the capital. Pape and co-workers also tested sera collected for other diagnostic tests and found that of 1,037 adults phlebotomized during the first six months of 1986 by three commercial laboratories in Port-au-Prince, 8 percent were seropositive for HIV antibodies (Johnson and Pape 1989). The health status of these persons is not known, but since none of the three laboratories performed HIV serology at the time of phlebotomy, the sera had not been collected to diagnose HIV infection. These samples represented about 10 percent of the total number of persons bled by the three laboratories during that period.

In compiling all available data from seroprevalence studies of healthy urban adults, one is led to conclude that a substantial fraction of urban Haitians have been exposed to HIV. In contrast, the seroprevalence rate concurrently averaged 3 percent in rural areas. The seroprevalence rate in 97 mothers of children hospitalized in the university hospital with dehydration was 3 percent; 4 percent of 245 unscreened rural blood donors had antibodies to HIV. In an area even more distant from urban centers, 1 percent of 191 adults who came for immunizations were seropositive.

What of seroprevalence among children? The GHESKIO team studied three groups of children: offspring of a parent with AIDS; children hospitalized in Port-au-Prince with diarrheal disease; and healthy, age-matched controls from the same neighborhoods as the hospitalized children. Their findings, summarized in table 4, suggest that pediatric infection with HIV is perinatal: rates are highest in the children of parents with AIDS, especially those less than one year old, when maternal antibodies may give "false" positive antibody tests. Further, the children of a seropositive father and a seronegative mother were all seronegative, also strongly suggesting vertical transmission. Disturbingly, the rates of seropositivity were identical for the children of parents with AIDS and the children hospitalized with diarrhea: 6.5 percent in both groups, and three times greater than in controls. This suggests that, in Port-au-Prince at least, pediatric infection with HIV may be leading to significant morbidity (for example, diarrheal disease) even before pediatric AIDS may be diagnosed. The relative contribution of HIV versus that of other pathogens is difficult to assess in Haiti, where infant death due to diarrheal disease has long been commonplace.

In summary, large numbers of Haitians have been exposed to HIV. The speed of spread has been great indeed: sera stored between 1977 and 1979 were found to be free of HIV. Since then, the only areas without a single seropositive adult have been small cohorts of rural Haitians. The exception has been a group of health care workers and adults from relatively privileged backgrounds, which has led some observ-

Table 4 *Prevalence of HIV Antibody in Haitian Children*

Age	Children of AIDS Parents		Children Hospitalized with Diarrhea		Controls	
	N	HIV+ (%)	N	HIV+ (%)	N	HIV+ (%)
<1	96	28	260	8	119	3
1–4	252	3	52	2	41	2
4–10	218	2	5	0	7	0
>10	43	0	0	–	0	–
Total	609	6.5	317	6.5	167	2

SOURCE: Pape and Johnson (1988a)

ers to question the conclusion, advanced early in the epidemic, that Haitians from all economic backgrounds were equally vulnerable to AIDS. As Johnson and Pape (1989:70) have recently concluded, "Collectively, these data indicate that HIV infection is widespread and more prevalent in urban areas and in lower socioeconomic groups." It is precisely this group—poor city dwellers—who were most at risk during the early years of the epidemic. They remain more vulnerable than their wealthy counterparts to HIV infection and to virtually every other infectious disease known in Haiti.

13

Haiti and the "Accepted Risk Factors"

In Haiti, the epidemiological questions posed were the same as those in other areas facing the AIDS pandemic: Who is at risk for acquiring HIV infection? How is the virus transmitted? Specifically, what behaviors or preexisting conditions might be associated with seropositivity or HIV disease? What was the extent of infection in groups engaging in high-risk behaviors? A good deal of evidence suggests that answers to these questions have changed over the years. Initial research conducted among Haitian-Americans with AIDS identified none of the "accepted risk factors"—that is, homosexuality, bisexuality, IV drug use, a history of transfusion, or hemophilia—in the vast majority of Haitians with AIDS. In Haiti, however, certain risk factors often were identified, although the factors deemed important have changed over the years.

Spurred on in large part by calls for careful research that would answer questions raised at the 1983 AMH conference, the GHESKIO investigators began to gather much more information from each new patient in an effort to identify activities or events that may have exposed that patient to HIV. Unfortunately, questions pertaining to sexual history were not standardized, and little effort was made to gather ethnographic data that might complement information garnered in the clinic. Dr. Pape developed a standardized questionnaire, which he and the GHESKIO physicians administered beginning in July 1983. They discovered that, in the majority of cases presenting at this time, "accepted risk factors" could be identified. Data on the first thirty-four patients so evaluated were presented at a Washington conference the following summer (see table 5).

The most striking revelation, considering reports about Haitians with AIDS in the United States, was that fully 50 percent of the men interviewed had a history of sexual relations with men. None of them, however, was exclusively homosexual:

The fact that all the male AIDS patients who have had sex with men are bisexual would also provide greater opportunity for heterosexual transmission of AIDS in Haiti. This also may contribute to the finding that 21 percent of our Haitian AIDS patients are women, as compared with only 7 percent in the United States (Pape et al. 1986:7).

Pape and his team further showed that fully half the women in the study had received a blood transfusion in the five years prior to onset of symptoms, and also observed that Haitian women are more likely to receive blood—often in the course of childbirth—than are Haitian men.

Did these data, which clearly demonstrated "accepted risk factors" in a majority of those studied, suggest that transmission in Haiti was through the same mechanisms as those elucidated in the United States? To determine the significance of presumed risk factors, a case-control study was initiated at the same time. The research design was ambitious:

Each of the most recent 36 AIDS patients was asked to provide three "healthy" persons to serve as controls. The controls included a sibling of the same sex closest in age to the patient, a friend of the same sex who shared social activities, and a current or recent sexual partner. (Pape et al. 1986)

Despite the audacity of this request, Pape's patients complied by recruiting twenty siblings, twenty friends, and twenty sexual partners. Interestingly, all the patients provided "current or recent sexual partners" of the opposite sex, including the men who had histories of homosexual contact. Among the risk factors studied were transfusion, the use of parenteral medications, and frequency of "heterosexual promiscuity" (arbitrarily defined as greater than twelve different partners during the six months preceding onset of their illness).

Early in the epidemic, it was noted that another potential mode of transmission of HIV is through the use of contaminated needles. In Haiti, intramuscular injections may be given by either medical personnel or, in areas without access to medical facilities, by those known to be *pikiris,* "injectionists." Disposable needles and syringes, not readily available in Haiti, are frequently reused without sterilization. Pape and

Table 5 *Risk Factors in 34 Patients*

	Males (n = 26)	Females (n = 8)
Bisexual	13 (50%)	0
Blood transfusion	3 (11%)	4 (50%)
IV drug abuse	1 (4%)	0
Spouse with AIDS	0	1 (12%)
None apparent	9 (35%)	3 (38%)

SOURCE: Pape et al. (1986)

colleagues found that, during the five-year period before the onset of AIDS symptoms, parenteral medications were received by 83 percent of male and 88 percent of female AIDS patients (Pape et al. 1985). Although the figure is by itself suggestive, injections were also reported by greater than 67 percent of controls (seronegative siblings and friends), suggesting that other factors were involved in HIV transmission.

With homosexual contact already a documented risk factor, it was hypothesized that one of the additional factors may be the number of opposite-sex partners. The female siblings and friends had a mean of one sex partner per year during the five years preceding the study and an HIV seroprevalence rate of 9 percent. Male siblings and friends, in contrast, had six or seven opposite sex partners annually and a seroprevalence of 22 percent. Although the numbers are small and the sample not random, these figures corroborate the initial impressions of those studying the epidemic: urban Haitian men were noted to have significantly more sexual partners than did urban women, suggesting a greater role for men in the spread of HIV. The predominantly male role would be further amplified if the viral agent were more easily transmitted from male to female.

An analogous mode of transmission has been described for HTLV–1, a retrovirus related to HIV, for which female-to-male transmission is thought to occur rarely, if at all (see Kajiyama et al. 1986, and Murphy et al. 1989). There are other reasons to believe that HIV is more efficiently transmitted from men to women. Some are intuitive: HIV is concentrated in seminal fluid, but often difficult to isolate in vaginal secretions. In comparing male ejaculate to vaginal secretions, it is important to note that inoculum size is of course different by several orders of magnitude. Data from the United States also suggest that HIV is inefficiently transmitted from women to men: in two studies of women whose date of transfusion-associated HIV infection could be ascertained, from 0 to 7 percent of their spouses or regular sexual partners showed evidence of HIV infection (Peterman et al. 1988).[1]

Based on the case-control study initiated in 1983, the GHESKIO team initially concluded that "accepted risk factors" were present in approximately two-thirds of Haitians diagnosed with AIDS. This figure was compared to those published in reports from the United States, where only 6 percent of Haitian-Americans with AIDS "were bisexual" and only 1 percent used intravenous drugs. As Pape et al. (1986:6) later observed, "The disparity in the data from the United States and Haiti may be attributable, in part, to a greater willingness of Haitians to provide reliable responses to personal questions in their native country and language."

The patterns that emerged in the first case-control cohort were soon shown to be shifting. Indeed, the Haitian epidemic was changing. Most striking was the changing incidence of opportunistic infections versus Kaposi's sarcoma in Haitians with AIDS. The percentage of AIDS patients with Kaposi's decreased from 15 percent of cases occurring before and in 1984 to 5 percent in cases between 1986 and 1988 (table 6).

In addition to changing clinical features, there were important shifts in sex distribution of persons with AIDS. An overwhelming majority of the early patients had been men, but the proportion of women among the GHESKIO patients was increasing with each passing year (see table 7).

Not only were sex differences in the incidence of AIDS diminishing, but "accepted risk factors" were denied by more and more patients. Such risk factors were found in only 20 percent of the first Haitian cohort (before 1983) because, it was hypothesized, a standardized approach to these questions had not been applied. In a second cohort (1983–84), risk factors could be identified in a majority of patients. Of the men, 50 percent had histories of sexual contact with both men and women. In contrast, only 11 percent of the 170 male and female AIDS patients who presented in or after 1986 reported either bisexuality, blood transfusions, or IV drug abuse.

The changing significance of these risk factors was suggested by the case-control study, in which a total of 384 persons with AIDS, of whom 278 were male and 106 were female, had been evaluated, as were 174 of their heterosexual sex partners, and 224 of their siblings and friends (table 8). Among the sex-matched siblings, none of whom had

Table 6 *AIDS Cases Diagnosed by the Haitian Study Group on Kaposi's Sarcoma and Opportunistic Infections (GHESKIO)*

Year	Kaposi's Sarcoma	Opportunistic Infection	Total
1979	2	0	2
1980	2	5	7
1981	7	9	16
1982	5	35	40
1983	8	53	61
1984	11	103	114
1985	8	136	144
1986	10	160	170
1987	8	159	167
Total	61	660	721

SOURCES: Pape et al. (1983, 1985); Johnson and Pape (1989)

Table 7 *Sex Distribution of Patients with AIDS in Haiti*

Years	N	Percent Female
1979–1982	10/65	15%
1983–1985	86/319	27
1986–1988	144/458	31

SOURCE: Marie-Marcelle Deschamps, personal communication

been transfused and all of whom denied bisexuality, 17 percent were seropositive. Sex differences in this group were not striking: 19 percent of the brothers were seropositive, as were 14 percent of the sisters. Among 108 of the patients' sex-matched friends, it was discovered that, while none of the women screened were seropositive, fully 26 percent of the men were. All but 5 percent of the male friends screened denied homosexuality or bisexuality; all of those who had same-sex sexual relations were seropositive. Blood transfusion seemed to be less important as a mode of transmission as the epidemic progressed: 2 percent of male and 3 percent of female respondents had received transfusion during the preceding five years, and none of them was seropositive.

Finally, 55 percent of 174 regular sexual partners or spouses of AIDS patients had antibodies to HIV: 61 percent of male partners and 54 percent of female partners. Only 3 percent and 6 percent of the male and female partners, respectively, had received a transfusion, and

Table 8 *Risk Factors in 559 Haitian AIDS Patients*

	1983	1984	1985	1986	1987	All
N	38	104	132	185	100	559
Bisexuality	50%	27%	8%	4%	1%	13%
Transfusion	23	12	8	7	10	10
IVDA	1	1	1	0	1	1
Heterosexual	5	6	14	16	15	13
Undetermined	21	54	69	73	73	64

SOURCE: Pape and Johnson (1988a:37)

neither bisexuality nor IV drug use was reported by either group. HIV infection among the regular sexual partners of Haitians with AIDS underlined the disturbing suggestion that AIDS was becoming "just another" sexually transmitted disease, yet there were still no data to suggest efficient female-to-male transmission of the virus.

In summary, then, there has been a marked decrease in the relative number of Haitians with AIDS reporting a history of transfusion or same-sex contact.[2] Among patients who have recently visited the GHESKIO clinic, there has been a marked increase in the proportion having a spouse or regular sexual partner with AIDS, having a history of prostitution, or denying all the "accepted risk factors." When data from all three "phases" of the epidemic are considered together, it appears that, at the outset of the epidemic, "accepted risk factors" could be identified for only 20 percent of Haitians with AIDS. A couple of years later, risk factors were identified in a majority of Haitians with AIDS, but by 1986 the number of patients with such risk factors began to decrease. The shape of this curve, which suggests a rise and fall of the importance of bisexual contact, is in all probability an artifact of research design. It is far more likely that preliminary low rates of detection of bisexual contact (and perhaps transfusion) were due to the stigma attached to homosexuality and to the nonstandardized approaches in collecting these data.[3]

A more probable curve would be one that reveals a high prevalence, among the first Haitians with AIDS, of "accepted risk factors," that is, the "North American/European" risk factors identified by the CDC. Of all of these factors, bisexual activity was by far the most significant in Haiti. With the passage of time, however, it has become increasingly clear that HIV is heterosexually transmitted, especially from men to women. By 1988, heterosexual transmission was presumed in 16 percent of patients who were female prostitutes or in those who had a spouse with AIDS; it is a probable source of infection in the patients denying all other "accepted risk factors." By 1986, these patients represented more than 70 percent of Haitian AIDS cases (see table 8). Additional evidence for heterosexual transmission of HIV is the finding that more than half of 139 Haitian prostitutes in the Port-au-Prince area were seropositive: the rate of seropositivity among sex workers increased from 49 percent in 1985 to 66 percent in 1986 (Pape and Johnson 1988a:36).

The data from Haiti do not offer strong support for *efficient* female-to-male transmission, although it is clearly not trivial: if bisexuality is decreasingly common and yet HIV seropositivity continues to increase among heterosexual men, women are necessarily a source as well as a "sink" for infection. The conclusions that may be drawn from these studies are important: HIV is heterosexually transmitted, but it is much more efficiently transmitted from male to female than vice versa.[4] At this writing, heterosexual transmission is thought to account for the majority of Haitian AIDS cases, and cases associated with perinatal transmission are increasing at a rate greater than that of the epidemic in general. In Haiti, AIDS is afflicting increasing numbers of women—especially poor women.

14

AIDS in the Caribbean:
The "West Atlantic Pandemic"

The history of the Haitian AIDS epidemic is a brief and devastating one. Less than two decades ago, HIV may not have been present in the country. Now, complications of HIV infection are among the leading causes of death in urban Haiti. How are other Caribbean islands affected? Is Haiti, as some believe it to be, an AIDS-ridden pocket in an otherwise low-prevalence region?[1] Answering these questions is no mean task, as Pape and Johnson (1988a:32) suggest:

First, in many countries there is no registry system for AIDS and it was only in 1984 that most nations started reporting cases to [the Pan American Health Organization]. Secondly, the widely used CDC case definition for AIDS is inappropriate for defining tropical AIDS and requires sophisticated laboratory support that is not readily available in most countries. In our experience in Haiti, the new CDC case definition for AIDS (CDC 1987), which relies more on HIV testing and clinical presentation, should increase the actual number of reported cases by at least 30 per cent.

Ironically, given the extreme poverty of Haiti, Haitians with AIDS stand a better chance of an adequate workup than do the citizens of several other Caribbean nations. Although Haiti has the weakest health infrastructure in the region, it has had the largest number of cases, the greatest amount of international scrutiny as "the source of AIDS," and has sustained the most substantial economic blows relative to GNP. Perhaps in part as a result of these negative forces, many Haitian physicians and researchers have been involved in the professional response to the epidemic. Haitians publish more HIV-related studies than do

141

researchers in other Caribbean countries, and the GHESKIO-run national laboratories are experienced in diagnosing AIDS and other forms of HIV infection.

Given these limitations, what do we know about the chief characteristics of the Caribbean pandemic? All of what are termed "the Caribbean basin countries" have reported AIDS cases to the Pan American Health Organization (PAHO). Among the islands, Haiti, the Dominican Republic, Trinidad and Tobago, and the Bahamas account for 82 percent of all cases reported to PAHO between the recognized onset of the epidemic and September 1987. Haiti had reported the largest number of cases in the Caribbean region, which appears to lend credence to the widely shared belief that citizens of that nation are somehow uniquely susceptible to AIDS. When the number of cases is standardized to reflect per capita caseload, however, the uniqueness of Haiti disappears: the attack rate in Haiti is actually lower than that in several other countries in the region (Lange and Jaffe 1987:1410).

During the twelve months preceding September 1987, the number of reported Caribbean cases doubled, with the largest rates of increase in Barbados, Jamaica, Martinique, Guadeloupe, French Guiana, the U.S. Virgin Islands, and Grenada. The epidemic in the Dominican Republic continues to grow: although no cases were reported in 1983, a total of 62 were reported in the subsequent two years. During 1986, the number of Dominican cases more than doubled, and as of the end of 1989, 856 cases had been reported to PAHO.

What is the nature of HIV transmission in these countries? As noted, many public health specialists speak of the entire Caribbean basin as demonstrating "Pattern II," which differs from Pattern I "in that heterosexual intercourse has been the dominant mode of HIV transmission *from the start*. . . . Homosexuality generally plays a minor role in this pattern" (Osborn 1989:126; emphasis added). The above review of the data from Haiti suggests that the WHO terminology obscures an accurate understanding of the Haitian AIDS epidemic. First, although "the start" was never accurately documented, it seems clear that same-sex relations between men played a crucial role in the Haitian epidemic; second, the WHO scheme highlights similarities between Haiti and Africa, which would be acceptable if such comparisons did not tend to draw attention away from the history of the Caribbean pandemic, which is in fact, causally speaking, much more intimately related to the North American epidemic. Third, the WHO scheme is static, whereas the Haitian epidemic is rapidly changing. Data from other Caribbean countries suggest that the WHO terminology is equally inappropriate there, and that the patterns seen in Haiti are suggestive of what has occurred in other countries in the region.

Table 9 also presents figures suggesting that homosexual contact has played an important role in other Caribbean islands. But even here finer distinctions may be drawn. "For these homosexuals," note Pape and Johnson (1988a:36) in reference to gay men in Jamaica, the Dominican Republic, and Trinidad, "sexual contact with American homosexuals rather than promiscuity per se appeared to be associated with increased risk of infection." What studies allow such a conclusion? The first case of AIDS in the West Indies was reported on Trinidad in February 1983. Since then, the number of cases has risen steadily, leaving Trinidad with one of the highest attack rates in the Americas. In an important study, Bartholemew and coworkers (1987) compare the epidemiological correlates of infection with two retroviruses: HTLV and HIV. Infection with the former virus, thought to be long endemic in the Caribbean, was significantly associated with age, African descent, number of lifetime sexual partners, and "duration of homosexuality," that is, length of time as a sexually active gay man. In sharp contrast, "age and race were not associated with HIV seropositivity. The major risk factor for HIV seropositivity was homosexual contact with a partner from a foreign country, primarily the United States. Duration of homosexuality and number of lifetime partners were not significantly associated with HIV seropositivity" (Bartholemew et al. 1987:2606). The same risk factors were documented in Colombia, also a Caribbean-basin country. In Bogota, Merino et al. (1990:333–334) observe that "significant behavioral risk factors for HIV–1 seropositivity among this sample of Colombian homosexual men included receptive anal intercourse and, for the subgroup reporting receptive roles, contact with foreign visitors."[2] The Haitian experience would suggest that Trinidad and Colombia can expect the relative significance of sexual contact with a North American gay man to decrease, as other risk factors—most notably, high numbers of partners—become preeminent.

A similar risk factor was also hypothesized for the Dominican Republic, where Haitians, long despised in the neighboring country, have come under even heavier fire as "AIDS carriers." And yet studies revealed high seroprevalence among homosexual/bisexual male prostitutes living in the tourist areas of the country—10 percent in Santiago and 19 percent in Puerto Plata. "Tourists, and not Haitians, were the most likely source of virus transmission to Dominicans, because con-

Table 9 *HIV Seroprevalence in Caribbean Homosexuals or Bisexuals*

	Jamaica			Dominican Republic			Trinidad		
	Year	*N*	*HIV (%)*	*Year*	*N*	*HIV (%)*	*Year*	*N*	*HIV (%)*
Homo/ Bisex	'86	125	10	'85	46	17	'83–84	106	40
Controls	'86	4,000	0	'85	306	2.6	'82	983	0.2

SOURCE: Pape and Johnson (1988a)

tact occurs frequently between tourists (for example, male homosexuals) and Dominicans but rarely between Haitians and Dominicans" (Koenig et al. 1987:634). Further, it seems that the epidemiology of HIV in the Dominican Republic may resemble that in Haiti to an even greater extent than did the Trinidadian epidemiology. Koenig and coworkers underline the role of economically driven prostitution among young Dominican men who consider themselves heterosexual: "Persons who engage in homosexual acts only to earn money usually consider themselves heterosexual. This situation, public health workers have indicated, is particularly prevalent in the tourist areas with young adolescents. It could explain our finding of three positive serum samples in schoolchildren from Santo Domingo" (Koenig et al. 1987:634).[3]

More recent research in the Puerta Plata area suggests that, although homosexual prostitution has diminished, another form of sexual exchange fostered by economic inequity continues to flourish. Garcia and coworkers have studied the "beach boys" who work the area's tourist hotels:

Beach boys are charming, friendly young heterosexual males who provide escort service to women tourists, most of whom are 30 years old or more. The beach boys are known locally as "Sanky Panky"—a corruption of the term "hanky panky." Because these men have contact with tourists from different countries and continents, they are often skilled, if not fluent, in English, French, German, and Italian. (Garcia 1991:2)

Although termed "brief holiday romances," the escort service typically involves "monetary compensation," and qualitative research allows Garcia (1991:2) to conclude that "beach boys have multiple sexual partners and ply their trade in an area where the prevalence of AIDS is among the highest in the country."

Epidemiologic reports from other parts of the Caribbean suggest a similar history for other growing island epidemics. Composite data from Surinam and what has been termed the "English-speaking Caribbean," which includes twenty island nations, show that while 100 percent of those diagnosed with AIDS in 1983 were homosexual or bisexual, the relative significance of same-sex contact as a risk factor for AIDS plunged to 30 percent over the next five years. Blood-transfusion–related AIDS remained low, at less than 5 percent, and pediatric AIDS continued to account for less than 10 percent of diagnosed cases. Cases among those claiming to be exclusively heterosexual and without history of transfusion or intravenous drug use have soared, from less than 10 percent before 1985 to 60 percent in 1988. The male-to-female ratio has declined each year, as more and more women fall ill with AIDS. These trends necessarily imply that the proportion of pediatric cases will also climb (Hospedales 1989).

Caribbean-wide data suggest that many of the factors that have helped to shape the Haitian epidemic have been important throughout the region. Of these factors, the most important have been economically driven and historically given: sufficient data now exist to support the assertion that economically driven male prostitution, catering to a North American clientele, played a major role in the introduction of HIV to Haiti. Why might Haiti have been particularly vulnerable to such commodification of sexuality? In a country as poor as Haiti—"the poorest country in the hemisphere"—AIDS might be thought of as an occupational hazard for workers in the tourist industry. A similar observation may be made about several other Caribbean nations.

Throughout the earlier half of this century, tourists' attitudes toward Haiti are nicely summarized by Carpenter (1930:326), whose Anglo-American guide book to the Caribbean qualifies Haiti as "a deplorable and almost unbelievable mixture of barbaric customs and African traditions." Later, in a slightly different era, Haiti's "exoticism" could be peddled as an attraction.[4] Tourism truly began in 1949, when Port-au-Prince celebrated the two hundredth anniversary of its founding with the inauguration of the "Cité de l'Exposition," a long stretch of modern buildings built on the reclaimed swampy waterfront of the capital. The country counted some 20,000 visitors that year, and slightly fewer in 1950 and 1951. During the next few years, however, approximately 250,000 tourists would spend an average of three days and $105 in Haiti—bringing in approximately 25 percent of Haiti's foreign currency (Francisque 1986:139).

There was every sign that the gains in tourism would be steady, but political instability in 1957, followed by the tyrannical rule of François

Duvalier, led North American tourists to avoid Haiti for several years.[5] This was the case even though a number of casinos located in Cuba relocated to Haiti after the overthrow of the Batista dictatorship. After he had silenced domestic opposition, Duvalier attempted to court tourists and their dollars later in the decade. In the same speech in which he welcomed U.S. Vice President Nelson Rockefeller to Haiti and promoted the country as an ideal site for U.S. assembly plants, François Duvalier suggested that "Haiti could be a great land of relaxation for the American middle class—it is close, beautiful, and politically stable" (Trouillot 1990:200).

By 1970, the annual number of visitors was close to 100,000; not counting brief layovers and "afternoon dockings," the annual tally had risen to 143,538 by 1979. Club Mediterranée opened its doors the following year (Barros 1984:750). It seemed as if tourism had arrived. Indeed, the industry, it was predicted, would soon supplant coffee and the offshore assembly plants as the capital's chief source of foreign exchange. But the effects of the "AIDS scare" were dramatic and prompt: the Haitian Bureau of Tourism estimated that tourism declined from 75,000 visitors in the winter of 1981–82 to under 10,000 the following year. In 1983–84, during the season following the risk-grouping and spate of articles in the popular press, even fewer tourists came to Haiti. Six hotels folded, and as many more declared themselves on the edge of bankruptcy. Several hotel owners were rumored to be planning a lawsuit against the CDC.[6]

Of course fluctuations in tourism and trade may be attributed to many factors, but there was little doubt in Haiti about the cause of the collapse: Haiti had been accused of "starting the AIDS epidemic." To cite Abbott (1988:255) once again: "AIDS stamped Haiti's international image as political repression and intense poverty never had." "Already suffering from an image problem, Haiti has been made an international pariah by AIDS," concluded one 1983 report. "Boycotted by tourists and investors, it has lost millions of dollars and hundreds of jobs at a time when half the work force is jobless. Even exports are being shunned by some" (Chaze 1983:41).

Tourism and poverty did bring something of lasting significance, however: institutionalized prostitution. As one physician-author put it, "This country had—as far as promiscuity was concerned—replaced Cuba" (Météllus 1987:90). And as Haiti became poorer, both men's and women's bodies became cheaper. Although there have been no quantitative studies of Haitian urban prostitution, it was clear that a substantial sector of the trade catered to tourists, and especially North Americans. Some portion of the tourist industry catered specifically to a gay clientele:

During the past five years Haiti, especially Port-au-Prince, has become a very popular holiday resort for Americans who are homosexual. There are also Haitians who are homosexual, and homosexual prostitution is becoming increasingly common. . . . For the young Haitian male between the ages of fifteen and thirty there is no likelihood of escaping the despair that abounds in Port-au-Prince. As elsewhere, those with money can purchase whatever they want. (Greco 1983:516)

Although not all gay sex was prostitution, the deepening poverty of Haiti helped to ensure that money played an inordinant role in even "voluntary" same-sex relations: "With the help of money," writes d'Adesky, "what existed as gay life in Haiti in the '60s and '70s flowed like a dream." In a report recently filed in *The Advocate,* d'Adesky writes of "hotels that catered to a gay clientele," of "discreet fucking rooms" in tourist hotels, and of slum houses that "would be emptied for a price and arrangements made." She continues by citing a North American participant in Haiti's "once-flourishing gay subculture."

"There was a gay life that was very gala and that involved various sectors of society," said AIDS activist Stephen Machon, a former resident of Haiti who saw the tail end of what some call Haiti's gay golden period. "There would be the gay guys and the working boys and the tourists, of course, and the parties would be just fabulous. Some of it took place in the streets, but a lot went on behind the courtyard walls. You could lead a very flamboyant life-style within certain limitations, and it was wonderful." (d'Adesky 1991:31)

During the AMH-sponsored conference in 1983, one Haitian-American researcher read aloud from the pages of the 1983 *Spartacus International Gay Guide,* in which Haiti was enthusiastically recommended to the gay tourist: handsome men with "a great ability to satisfy" are readily available, but "there is no free sex in Haiti, except with other gay tourists you may come across. Your partners will expect to be paid for their services but the charges are nominal." Another advertisement, which ran in *The Advocate,* assured the prospective tourist that Haiti is "a place where all your fantasies come true" (Moore and LeBaron 1986:82).

It was not long before interviews with Haitians with AIDS revealed their sexual contact with gay men from North America. In a key paper published in 1984, Guérin and coworkers from Haiti, North America, and Canada stated that "17 percent of our patients had sexual contact with [North] American tourists" (Guérin et al. 1984:256). Murray and Payne (1988:25–26) question the relevance of gay tourism in the Haitian AIDS epidemic: "Insofar as gay travel can be estimated from gay guidebooks, Haiti was one of the least-favored destinations in the Caribbean for gay travelers during the 1970s and the less-favored half of the island of Hispaniola."[7] His assessment is based only on "frequency of listing in gay guidebooks," surely a less significant indicator of the relevance of such tourism than the cluster studies which revealed direct sexual contact between Haitian men and North American gay tourists. It is important to note that the introduction of an epidemic of sexually transmitted disease need not involve some critical mass of sexual contact, but requires only that the infectious agent be introduced into a sexually active population (in this case, Haitian men). The Guérin et al. (1984) study makes this clear. Interestingly, Murray and Payne cite, an American journalist's interview with Guérin and not the research published in the *Annals of the New York Academy of Science*: "At the Haitian end of the hypothesized transmission vector, Dr. Jean-Michel Guérin of GHESKIO told [journalist Anne-Christine] d'Adesky that 'all his patients—without exception—had denied having sex with tourists.'" Yet the *Annals* article, which brought together the research of ten physicians representing research centers in Haiti, the United States, and Canada, clearly specifies which patients acknowledge sexual relations with gay tourists from North America.[8]

The existence of tourism, some of it gay, does not of course prove that such commerce was "the cause" of the Haitian AIDS epidemic, nor is it my intention to argue that it does. Such commerce does, however, throw into relief the ties between Haiti and nearby North America, ties not mentioned in early discussions of AIDS among Haitians, which often posited "isolated Haiti" as the *source* of the pandemic. In fact, a review of even the scholarly literature on Haiti would leave the impression that the country is the most "isolated" or "insular" of Caribbean countries. In an assessment resonant with the U.S. medical community's AIDS-related speculations, the author of one standard text remarks that "Haiti in 1950 was in general what it had been in 1900: a preindustrial society inhabited by ignorant, diseased peasants oblivious to the outside world" (Langley 1989:175). A more attentive study of Haiti's economy reveals that the nation has long been closely tied to the United States. In fact, Haiti plays an interesting role in what

Orlando Patterson has termed the "West Atlantic system," an economic network encompassing much of the Caribbean basin and centered in the United States:

Originally a region of diverse cultures and economies operating within the framework of several imperial systems, the West Atlantic region has emerged over the centuries as a single environment in which the dualistic United States center is asymmetrically linked to dualistic peripheral units. Unlike other peripheral systems of states—those of the Pacific, for example—the West Atlantic periphery has become more and more uniform, under the direct and immediate influence of the all-powerful center, in cultural, political and economic terms. Further, unlike other peripheral states in their relation to their centers, the West Atlantic system has a physical nexus in the metropolis at the tip of Florida. (Patterson 1987:258)

The Caribbean nations with high attack rates of AIDS are all part of the West Atlantic system. A relation between the degree of "insertion" in this network and prevalence of AIDS is suggested by the following exercise. Excluding Puerto Rico, which is not an independent country, the five Caribbean basin nations with the largest number of cases by 1986 were as follows: the Dominican Republic, the Bahamas, Trinidad/Tobago, Mexico, and Haiti. In terms of trade, which are the five countries most dependent upon the United States? Export indices offer a convenient marker of involvement in the West Atlantic system. In both 1983 and 1977, the years for which such data are available, the same five countries were most linked to the United States economically—and they are precisely those countries with the largest number of AIDS cases.[9] And the country with the most cases, Haiti, was also the country most fully dependent on U.S. exports. In all the Caribbean basin, only Puerto Rico is more economically dependent on the United States. And only Puerto Rico has reported more cases of AIDS to the Pan American Health Organization.

To understand the West Atlantic AIDS pandemic, a historical understanding of the worldwide spread of HIV is crucial. The thesis that evolving economic forces run parallel to the lineaments of the American epidemics is confirmed by comparing Haiti with a neighboring island, Cuba, the sole country in the region not enmeshed in the West Atlantic system. In Haiti, as we have seen, several epidemiological studies of asymptomatic city dwellers reveal HIV seroprevalence rates of approximately 9 percent. In 1986 in Cuba, only 0.01 percent of 1,000,000 persons tested were found to have antibodies to HIV (Liautaud, Pape, and Pamphile 1988:690). Had the pandemic begun a few decades ear-lier, the epidemiology of HIV infection in the Caribbean might well have been different. Havana, once the "tropical playground of the Americas," might have been as much an epicenter of the pandemic as Carrefour.

PART FOUR

AIDS, History, Political Economy

A number of studies have linked the history of specific disease episodes—malaria epidemics, outbreaks of typhus, or of small-pox—to wider patterns of political and economic change. Yet in limiting their time frame they have been unable to describe how these linkages have evolved over longer periods of time and how realignments in specific sets of political and economic interests have shaped the longer history of both health and health care.

Packard (1989:20)

If there are connections everywhere, why do we persist in turning dynamic, interconnected phenomena into static, disconnected things? Some of this is owing, perhaps, to the way we have learned our own history.

Wolf (1982:4)

Anthropology, Eric Wolf suggests, needs to rediscover history. In his view, anthropology needs to "transcend the customary ways of depicting Western history, and must take account of the conjoint participation of Western and non-Western people in this worldwide process" (Wolf 1982:ix). And so anthropology needed to rediscover not only the history of "victorious elites," but also the history of the "primitive" societies so often studied by anthropologists. For many centuries now, Wolf argues, these have not really been two histories at all, but one dynamic and interconnected process. In his account, "both the people who claim history as their own and the people to whom history has been denied emerge as participants in the same historical trajectory" (Wolf 1982:23). Few have appreciated the conjoint participation of the peasants of Haiti in the making of the modern world. Though traditionally portrayed as the hemisphere's most backward people, the Haitians are and have been in many respects the most modern Americans. The next four chapters attempt to show the ways in which Haiti, a product of internationalizing economies based first in Europe and later in North America, is in essence a modern entity.

I will argue here that the Haitian AIDS epidemic, and indeed the Caribbean pandemic in general, are best understood by taking the long view. It is further argued here that familiarity with the historical trajectory of the Haitian people helps us to understand contemporary Haitian responses to the advent of AIDS. Ethnography and epidemiology cannot speak to the *origins* of contemporary conditions, nor can they reveal the processes that have shaped, over time, the AIDS pandemic and social responses to it. In fact, history alone will help the ethnographer to understand why, in a small village in the central plateau, AIDS can be "sent" through sorcery or through the malevolence of the CIA, and why one hears frequent references to poisons and zombies and those spells called *makandal*.[1] The length of this study results in large part from an effort to place such "local knowledge" in the context of the larger socioeconomic and cultural systems of which rural Haiti is but a small part. In this effort, I am following not only current trends in anthropology, but the hints and even exhortations of several of my informants.

15

Many Masters: The European Domination of Haiti

Wherever the European has trod, death seems to pursue the aboriginal.

Charles Darwin (1989 [1839]:322)

In December of 1492, Christopher Columbus initiated the construction of the first European settlement in the New World. He chose a bay on the northern end of an island called *Ayiti,* "high country," by the Amerindians who lived there. The Arawakan-speaking Taino people warmly welcomed Columbus, and soon fell victims to the first chronicled genocide in the New World. Weakened by exposure to new infectious diseases, the Indians were further reduced through peonage: on each adult Taino an impossible tribute of gold was imposed. The "lovable, tractable, peaceable, gentle, decorous" Indians, as Columbus had described them, did not fare well as slaves: they sickened and died at a rate that appalled even the Europeans. Estimates of their number at the close of the fifteenth century reach as high as eight million, but the Taino and other indigenous tribes did not last long against the deadly admixture of imported infectious disease, slavery, and outright slaughter. By 1510, some 50,000 Indians remained on the island; by 1520, their number was further reduced to 15,000. Only 5,000 survivors were counted in 1530. Less than fifty years after the arrival of Columbus, the representatives of the native population could be counted in hundreds, and Moreau de Saint-Méry (1984:28) could later

153

note that "there remained not a single Indian when the French came to wrest the island from the Spanish."[1]

With the rapid disappearance of the Indians, Spanish settlers needed another source of expendable manpower with which to build forts and mine for gold. They turned toward Africa.[2] Mintz (1985:33) notes that there were already African slaves on the island before 1503. In 1504, King Ferdinand sent seventeen Africans to Hispaniola to serve as "agrarian laborers," and he promised one hundred more—for the mines—within a year. The traffic began in earnest in 1517, and Las Casas estimated that, by 1540, some 30,000 Africans had been imported to Hispaniola. The island was also the setting for an event that continues to reverberate throughout Haiti, the Caribbean, and other parts of the Americas even today: the introduction, by Columbus himself, of sugar cane to the New World.[3] The importation of Africans continued apace, and by 1568 many plantations had between one hundred fifty and two hundred slaves; some of the grander establishments boasted up to five hundred slaves (Mintz 1985:34). By the end of the century, Spanish historian Antonio de Herrera was able to observe, "There are so many Negroes in this island, as a result of the sugar factories, that the land seems an effigy or an image of Ethiopia itself" (Williams 1970:45).

But the Spanish agricultural experiments did not endure. When the Spaniards found that there was no more gold to be found on Hispaniola, the island slowly became a backwater frequented mostly by buccaneers, many of them French. Some of them settled on the northern coast, and then slowly spread southward. By the middle of the seventeenth century, the French were definitively, if illegally, installed. The slave trade was stepped up after the western third of Hispaniola was officially ceded to France by the Treaty of Ryswick in 1697. Père Labat, a Jacobin priest who visited the island in 1700, wrote that

roving, the sacking of Cartagena, the loot from the Jamaica raids, and the inland trade which has started with the mainland since the Peace of Ryswick, has filled San Domingo with gold and silver. The settlers all gamble to excess, live very well, and vie with each other in displaying their wealth. (Labat 1970:165)

The French colonialists, who called their territory "Saint-Domingue," came to be more interested in agriculture than in the quest for gold, and their method of farming required many able bodies. The slave ships traced a triangle from the European metropolises to the west coast of Africa to the Caribbean and back to Europe.[4] Their bookkeepers left chillingly precise records. One has only to compare annual "import" figures with the year-end census to see that slaves did not survive long on the plantations of Saint-Domingue. Debien (1962:50) estimates that between 1766 and 1775, the quasi totality of one sugar plantation's slaves was replaced by "new blood," most of it in newly arrived Africans. As the plantation economy reached staggering proportions, so did the demand for slave labor. Saint-Domingue had become the chief port-of-call for the slave trade. Between 1784 and 1791, the average annual import was 29,000 slaves. The territory was by then home to almost half of all slaves held in the Caribbean colonies (Klein 1986:57).

"A SECOND SODOM"

The slaves soon made the French traders and planters very wealthy, and also generated enormous revenue for France. Late in the eighteenth century, wrote Moreau de Saint-Méry, "the French part of the island of Saint-Domingue is, of all French possessions in the New World, the most significant in terms of wealth procured for its metropolis and in terms of its influence on agriculture and commerce" (1984:25).[5] From his and many other accounts, it is clear that by the mid-eighteenth century the territory of Saint-Domingue was fabulously rich. At one time or another, the territory was first in world production of coffee, rum, cotton, and indigo. On the eve of the American Revolution, Saint-Domingue, about the size of the state of Maryland, provided more revenue than all thirteen colonies. By 1789, the colony supplied three-fourths of the world's sugar:

In 1791 there were 792 sugar plantations, 2,180 of coffee, 705 of cotton, 3,097 of indigo, 69 of cocoa, and 623 raising subsistence crops. Haiti's exports to France alone that year totaled approximately $41 million. The net worth of the colony was put at $300 million. "Rich as a Creole" had become a common saying in France. (Heinl and Heinl 1978:32)

Although these figures give some idea of the pace of the slave economy at its height, they do not suggest the immense suffering that underpinned that economy. Published accounts of visitors to the territory make it clear that the planters of Saint-Domingue were notorious for their abuse of slaves. Few slaves were able to put their thoughts on paper, and so the words of the Baron de Vastey, a Haitian who had grown up a slave, are worth noting:

Have they not hung up men with heads downward, drowned them in sacks, crucified them on planks, buried them alive, crushed them in mortars? Have they not forced them to eat shit? And, after having flayed them with the lash, have they not cast them alive to be devoured by worms, or onto anthills, or lashed them to stakes in the swamp to be devoured by mosquitoes? Have they not thrown them into boiling cauldrons of cane syrup? (Heinl and Heinl 1978:26–27)

Hailing from scores of tribes, and speaking as many mutually unintelligible languages, the Africans of Saint-Domingue shared their bondage and their complicated hatred of their oppressors. It is clear from the historical records that Haitian Creole, termed by Archer (1987) a "language of survival," had taken on many of its present characteristics by the latter part of the eighteenth century. Haitian voodoo has a similar pedigree. Acknowledging that "a full explanation of the origins of this hybrid religion cannot be given," Simpson (1978:491) nonetheless asserts that "it seems likely that the Haitian *vodun* cult began to take definite form between 1750 and 1790." Although there may be a tendency to exaggerate the role of voodoo in the overthrow of slavery, there can be little doubt that many forms of resistance were organized around magico-religious themes.

Many have offered histories of voodoo, most often focusing on African contributions (for example, Herskovits 1975, H. Trouillot 1983). But voodoo, and to some extent the larger cultural systems in which it was embedded, were fundamentally the products of the plantation economy: "It is too often forgotten that voodoo, for all its African heritage, belongs to the modern world and is part of our own civilization" (Métraux 1972:365). Accordingly, voodoo has always been marked by European cosmologies. Pluchon (1987) has attempted to trace the contribution of French magic to what would later be termed the "Blacks' superstition" in Saint-Domingue and other French holdings. He demonstrates that the contribution was most significant during the seventeenth century, when most colonists were of rural French origin, and underlines similarities between the cosmologies of the masters and the slaves: "Between seventeenth-century masters and slaves, [one notes] the same magical conception of nature and the same errors of interpretation, which among the whites compounded uncertainties of faith and weaknesses of science" (Pluchon 1987:30).

The magico-religious outlook of the French contributed greatly to their fear of the slaves, to whom they attributed dark powers. French fears and African suffering, the constant threat of revolt, the ever-present whip, all lent to Saint-Domingue an ambiance of dread:

Man is never cruel and unjust with impunity: the anxiety which grows in the minds of those who abuse power often takes the form of imaginary terrors and demented obsessions. The master maltreated his slave, but feared his hatred. He treated him like a beast of burden but dreaded the occult powers which he imputed to him. And the greater the subjugation of the Black, the more he inspired fear; that ubiquitous fear which shows in the records of the period and which solidified in that obsession with poison which, throughout the eighteenth century, was the cause of so many atrocities. Perhaps certain slaves did revenge themselves on their tyrants in this way—such a thing is possible and even probable—but the fear which reigned in the plantations had its source in deeper recesses of the soul: it was the witchcraft of remote and mysterious Africa which troubled the sleep of people in "the big house." (Métraux 1972:15)

In his history of French colonial law, Moreau de Saint-Méry notes that of the eleven royal edicts issued in July 1682, three concerned "seducers," and the remaining eight, "poisoners." To judge by their legislation, eighteenth-century masters were even more skittish about black magic than their predecessors, but these laws, complained one Cap-Français doctor in 1791, "do not deter what are termed by Negroes and colored persons 'Kaperlata' from taking part . . . in certain crude, superstitious, and often annoying practices" (Pluchon 1987:19). In the last decades of the century, fear of magic and poison seemed to grip the entire white population. Another physician practicing in Cap-Français complained that all of his patients claimed they might have been poisoned. The whites, "obsessed by the black sorcery which they believed to be omnipresent, detected poison everywhere" (Pluchon 1987:34).

One of the more celebrated examples of slave resistance evokes the mood of the territory at mid-century. African-born François Macandal (sometimes, "Mackandal" or "Makandal") was by then notorious throughout the colony. After his hand was severed in a sugar mill, he became a maroon, a fugitive from the plantations, and was held responsible for the deaths by poisoning of several whites. Moreau de Saint-Méry (1984:630) asserts that Macandal "held classes" in the "execrable art" of poisoning, and that the entire colony was riddled with his agents: "In his grand scheme, he conceived the infernal project of erasing from the face of Saint-Domingue all who were not black."

According to the judge who later tried him, many of the slaves revered him: "They say that there is nothing greater on earth than the Good Lord, and after the Good Lord comes F. Macandal" (Courtain 1989: 139). With such a project—and such acclaim among the slaves—it was only a matter of time before Macandal became the authorities' most wanted fugitive.

Macandal and his accomplices were arrested on the seventeenth of January, and burned at the stake three days later. Close examination of the criminal proceedings suggests that some of the terms used in discussions of twentieth-century illness have their origins in Saint-Domingue. One of the charges against Macandal and the other men and women executed with him was the fabrication of "ouanga or poison, which are synonyms among those we have interrogated." The recipe for making these charms is recounted in the summary of the French judge, who notes that these *ouanga*, also termed *macandal*, were strapped to the thigh for protection:

It is while tying on the macandal that one expresses one's wish: to be strong in combat, to win when gambling, to be loved by the negresses, to not be beaten by one's master for *marronage* or other [infractions], to render [the master] blind to the biggest transgressions and, to use their expression, to make his heart as soft as water. (Courtain 1989:137–138)

But because these *macandals* were also sorcery bundles and implied blasphemy, pacts with the Devil, and insurrection, possession of one was decreed a capital crime.

Macandal's execution was to be public, meaning in front of the local slaves. But "as chance would have it," the stake was rotten, and Macandal's agony caused it to break. He lurched out of reach of the flames:

The negroes screamed "Macandal has escaped"; the terror was extreme; all doors were slammed shut. The regiment of Swiss guards who kept the square evacuated the execution area; the jailor Masse wanted to kill him with a thrust of the sword, while the order of the Procurer-general was to tie him to a plank and thrust him into the fire. Although Macandal's body was incinerated, many negroes believe to this day that he did not perish at the stake. (Moreau de Saint-Méry 1984:631)

The word *macandal* became synonymous with both poisons and poisoners; Moreau de Saint-Méry notes that it became for the slaves a most offensive insult. In present-day Haiti, however, Macandal is remembered as a martyr, and there is more than one "Rue Macandal" in the capital.[6]

The anecdote is singular only in its celebrity: scores of similar stories are to be found in the pages of eighteenth-century treatises and memoirs. And the accusations of poison grew more and more frequent as the century wore on. Pluchon (1987:176) writes that, with its "collective obsession with poison, its pitiless repression prompted by mere suspicion and by unshakable convictions, the North of Saint-Domingue drew itself into a hellish cycle and, attempting to snuff out crime, applied itself to torture." The cycle of repression, hysteria, and more atrocities was spinning toward its ineluctable finale: "This colony of slaves," observed the Marquis du Rouvray in 1783, "is like a city under the imminence of attack; we are treading on loaded barrels of gunpowder" (Heinl and Heinl 1978:37).

FORGING THE BLACK REPUBLIC

The Haitian Revolution has been well chronicled by its partisans, and by many scholars.[7] C.L.R. James entitled his study *The Black Jacobins* for, if Saint-Domingue might be likened to barrels of gunpowder, to borrow Du Rouvray's metaphor, the French Revolution was the spark that finally ignited them. The brittle status quo of the colony at the time of the French Revolution is sketched by Williams, who writes of five classes:

The first was the planters, the big whites. . . . They were restless under the Exclusive [trade arrangements with France]. The second was the royal officials, the representatives of the Exclusive, the symbols of the denial of the self-governing institutions. Then came the poor whites, the overseers, artisans, professional men, hating the planters above, determined to maintain the bridge that separated them from the men of colour below. The three groups of whites number 40,000. Below them came the fourth class, the mulattoes and free Negroes, numbering 28,000, possessing one-third of the real estate and one-fourth of the personal property in the colony, but denied social and political equality with the whites. Finally, there were the 452,000 slaves, many of them only recently arrived from Africa, the foundation on which the prosperity and superiority of Saint-Domingue rested. (Williams 1970:246)[8]

These demographics spelled trouble for the plantation owners. In the confusion following the events of 1789, the *grands blancs* gained control of the new Colonial Assembly by excluding their economic competitors, the mulattoes, and setting a property qualification that effectively excluded the *petits blancs*. The plantocracy, especially its strong northern faction, envisioned a self-governing Saint-Domingue, one in which their power would be unchallenged. While favoring a nominal tie with France through allegiance to the now powerless king, they rejected the authority of the National Assembly in Paris, and openly sought an end to the Exclusive. Their ambitions were resisted by the new colonial authorities, by the mulattoes, and by much of the rest of the white population, which rightly feared for its position in a more *laissez-faire* situation. The *petits blancs* sought support from others who felt their interests would be better served by remaining with France: merchants, lawyers, and others whose wealth came from their association with French trade. Briefly, their economic interests coincided with those of mulattoes. The combination was strong enough to hold in check the "Patriots," as the *grands blancs* had taken to calling themselves, and the Patriots reacted with merciless attacks on the mulattoes.

But the mulattoes were not easily silenced, and in early 1791 some of them initiated an open revolt against the status quo. While much of the mulatto clout was financial, they found political support in a French abolitionist society, *les Amis des Noirs*. But, as Williams (1970:247) tersely notes, "the issue involved was equality for the mulattoes. No one mentioned the slaves." In fact, the slaves *had* been mentioned in the debates of 1790: mulatto spokesmen made it abundantly clear that they wanted full civil rights in order to stand on equal terms with the whites—as the upholders of slavery. Though they rallied between three hundred and four hundred to their cause, the mulattoes in revolt were easily defeated by the colonial militia, and the movement's leaders were tortured and executed with the usual brutality in March of 1791. When news of the executions reached Paris and the National Assembly, popular outcry forced the reopening of the question of racial discrimination and slavery. It became clear that few of the Assemblymen could be depended upon to put into practice their loudly declared principles. Slavery was just too important financially to be abolished for mere ideology, no matter how fashionable the concepts of fraternity, liberty, and equality.

Thus far, then, the slaves had served only as pawns. Both white and mulatto factions recruited armies-in-waiting from the enslaved population. But in August 1791, the slaves took matters into their own hands. Revolts, alleged poisonings of whites by slaves, arson, and the standard battery of slave abuse led slowly to the first explosion. The insurrection of 1791 is famous in Haiti as having been precipitated by a voodoo ceremony in Bois Caiman, in the north of the colony. On the night of August 22, in a lashing tropical storm, tens of thousands of slaves set forth to wreak vengeance. Armed with picks, machetes, clubs, and fire, they razed approximately 180 sugar plantations, and perhaps 900 plantations of coffee, cotton, and indigo. At least a thousand whites lost their lives; well over ten thousand slaves were killed outright, and up to twenty-five thousand were thought to have taken to the hills.[9]

Compared with previous slave revolts, this one was remarkable in both its scale and in the degree of its organization. Although it was restricted to the northern half of the island, its symbolic message was, of course, of colonywide currency. And as a result of the merciless reprisals of the plantocracy, the numbers of rebels swelled considerably. By the end of 1791, the nascent slave army was almost one hundred thousand strong (James 1980:96). Reverberations of the revolt and the ensuing pandemonium were felt in both Europe and in the rest of the New World. The United States already had a booming business with the colony: some five hundred U.S. ships sailed to Saint-Domingue's ports each year at the time of the French Revolution. In order to protect its investments, the young republic sent $750,000 in military aid, as well as a few troops, to defend the colonists. Spain, though less interested in propping up the status quo, was also involved. But the British were by far the most embroiled in the melée. Early in 1793, upon the death of Louis XVI, war was declared between Europe's greatest powers, and Britain invaded France's Caribbean colonies.[10] The *grands blancs* welcomed the British, seeing once again the possibility of increased financial independence. But Britain's schemes were foiled by the contingencies of history and by the ingenuity of Toussaint Louverture.

Toussaint, legally a slave until the age of forty-five, is said to have introduced guerilla tactics into the slave army.[11] His organizational and military skills soon won him great acclaim and he held sway over a majority of the island's inhabitants. In April 1796, Toussaint named himself "Lieutenant Governor" of a colonial state within the French Empire. Toussaint's goal was nothing less than the restoration of economic prosperity—without slavery. His plans, however, did not involve changing the plantation basis of production. Instead, he replaced slavery with a system of contract labor enforced by a gendarmerie.[12] The Exclusive was at last overtly broken by the signing of trade agreements with Britain and the United States. The dismantling of the Exclusive did not sit well with the French, but, with a war on in Europe, France was in no position to send an expeditionary force to Saint-Domingue. Successive delegates from the metropole were expelled in 1797 and

1798. Even Napoleon, who came to power in 1799, was initially constrained to "offensives of charm towards Louverture, whom he could not yet overtly attack" (Auguste and Auguste 1985:9).

On October 23, 1801, the French offensive became less charming. Napoleon ordered that Captain-General Leclerc, his brother-in-law, lead an expeditionary force, already gathering at Brest, to Saint-Domingue. Leclerc arrived in January 1802, at the head of a formidable army of well over 20,000 men, one of the largest armadas ever to set sail for the New World. It was later to be reinforced by as many troops.[13] And the troops were not exclusively French: Auguste and Auguste (1980) refer instead to a veritable crusade, one that brought together Polish, Dutch, German, and Swiss soldiers. Leclerc attempted to follow the very precise instructions of Napoleon, whose goal was to reestablish French rule and, it was rightly suspected, slavery. Through treachery—Toussaint was captured at a parley—the architect of Haitian independence was dispatched to a prison in a remote part of France, where he died, according to Schoelcher (1982:357), a "slow death from cold and misery."[14]

After Toussaint's kidnapping, his military disciples carried on the struggle to which he had dedicated his life. Although it seemed otherwise at first, the ex-slaves and the inhospitable environment soon proved more than a match for Europe's best soldiers. Of the 28,000 regular troops initially dispatched to the colony, Leclerc was able to announce, in a letter to his brother-in-law dated 16 September 1802, that 20,000 of them were dead. Many of these had succumbed to yellow fever; the remainder, to reckless but skillfully led ex-slaves who simply feared nothing so much as the reinstitution of bondage. Leclerc's final letter to Napoleon is both desperate and telling:

Here is my opinion of this country. We must destroy all the negroes in the hills, men and women, sparing only children under twelve, destroy half of those living in the plains and leave behind not a single man of color who has worn a uniform—without this the colony will never have peace. (Auguste and Auguste 1985:236)

But it was too late: the colony was already lost to France. Two weeks later Leclerc, beseiged by the ex-slaves in Cap Français, fell ill with yellow fever. Ten days later, he was dead.

Jean-Jacques Dessalines was the symbolic successor to Toussaint. For Dessalines, considered by many to be Haiti's founding father, it had at last become clear that nothing short of total independence would do. Over a decade of violence ended almost three hundred years of bondage when the last of Napoleon's select forces were routed in November 1803. On the first of January, the island's new leaders reclaimed its Indian name.[15] The Republic of Haiti became the first independent nation in the Caribbean, or in all of Latin America, for that matter. In the hemisphere, only the United States is older. But Haiti is also the example of another first and only: there exists no other case of an enslaved people breaking its own chains and using military might to beat back a powerful colonial power.

Haiti was more than the New World's second oldest republic, more even than the first black republic of the modern world. Haiti was the first *free* nation of *free* men to arise within, and in resistance to, the emerging constellation of Western European empire. (Lowenthal 1976:656–657)

The indomitable will of the slaves and their desire for freedom was captured by Toussaint Louverture's final words as he was led to prison. Haitian schoolchildren know them by heart: "In overthrowing me, you have cut down in Saint-Domingue only the trunk of the tree of liberty. It will spring up again by the roots for they are numerous and deep."

Surveying the landscape of Haiti two hundred years after Bois Caiman leads one to a stark conclusion: equally tenacious were the rotten but deeply rooted trees of colonialism, racism, and inequality. These stumps littered the new nation in 1804, and they, unlike the rest of Haiti's trees, have proven impossible to uproot. The ruins and contradictions of colonial society, whether through prescription or reaction or deformation, have remained as the unyielding template for contemporary Haiti. For Haiti, pioneering once again, soon became the world's first "Third World" country. Neocolonialism soon proved as effective a barrier to freedom as mercantilism, and racism and grotesque inequality were virtually prescribed by the new state. As we shall see, this template has shaped the contours of the AIDS epidemic that is seen by many as merely the most recent of innumerable misfortunes that have befallen the Haitian people.

16

The Nineteenth Century:
One Hundred Years
of Solitude?

*In the face of the fact that Haiti still lives, after being boy-
cotted by all the Christian world; in the face of the fact of her
known progress within the last twenty years—in the face of
the fact that she has attached herself to the car of the world's
civilization, I will not, I cannot believe that her star is to
go out in darkness, but I will rather believe that whatever
may happen of peace or war Haiti will remain in the firma-
ment of nations and, like the star of the north, will shine on
forever.*

Frederick Douglass, "Lecture on Haiti," 1893

*The experience of Liberia and Haiti shows that the African
races are devoid of any capacity for political organization and
lack genius for government.*

U.S. Secretary of State Robert Lansing, 1918

The revolution that ended in 1804 destroyed much of the
agricultural infrastructure of Saint-Domingue.[1] Contemporary British
estimates suggest that of the more than half million blacks and mulattoes in Saint-Domingue in 1792, only 341,933 survived the revolution.
Of these, a mere 170,000 were judged to be capable of field labor
(Lacerte 1981:507). What is more, the Haitians found themselves in
a world entirely hostile to the idea of self-governing blacks.[2] Mintz

(1974b:60) puts it neatly when he suggests that the birth of Haiti was a "nightmare" for every country in which slavery endured. The new nation was completely surrounded by islands ruled by slave owners, and, for several decades, writes Campbell (1975:35), "every attempt on the part of the nonwhites of Jamaica to better their condition was considered to have been instigated by collusion with Haiti."

Similiar inspiration was attributed to the 1843 uprisings in Cuba, where a group of planters called for an end to the slave trade, not on ethical grounds, but because census results suggested that slaves outnumbered whites and freedmen. "If only nearby Haiti did not present so horrifying an example," read the proclamation, "but one that should never be disregarded so that the second edition of the same book does not come to be" (in Paquette 1988:211). One wealthy Cuban planter complained of his slaves' "stupidity and swagger," which he linked to the news from Haiti: "For the very reason that there are abolitionists, Haiti, and England in the world," he counselled, "it is necessary to correct [slaves] severely, to make them bend their backs, and to whip them, which is what truly tames them, and [the slaveholders] are quite ready to work that way" (Paquette 1988:180).[3]

The same paranoia had invaded the plantations of the southern United States. In 1793, notes Jordan (1974:147), "white refugees from Haiti came streaming into American ports, many bringing their slaves with them. That year saw the growth of a peculiar uneasiness, especially in Virginia, where many refugees had congregated." From then on, any wayward behavior among the slaves, whether collective or individual, was likely to be attributed to the example set by "that French island."

As much as they were repelled by the events on the island, America remained fascinated. The popular press regaled its readers with tales of horrible atrocities ("Who can read this and not drop a tear?"). St. Domingo assumed the character of a terrifying volcano of violence, liable to a new eruption at any moment. A single black rebellion was bad enough, but this was never-ending, a nightmare dragging on for years. Worst of all, the blacks were successful, and for the first time Americans could see what a community looked like upside down. (Jordan 1974:147)

There are indications that some Haitians did not discourage this image. Following the 1804 massacre of the French, Dessalines proclaimed, "Never again shall colonist or European set foot on this soil as master or landowner. This shall henceforward be the foundation of our constitution."[4] The new constitution, drafted by Dessalines, was meant to mark Haiti's drastic departure from the regional status quo. Haiti was officially declared an asylum for Maroons, and for any person of either African or Amerindian descent (Bryan 1984:32–33; Campbell 1975:35).

The proplantation ruling class could not afford to be too antagonistic, however, and such nationalist pronouncements were gradually toned down. Dessalines was assassinated in 1806. The new Haitian elite insisted on commodities for an international market, but the peasants—the former slaves—wished to be left alone to grow foodstuffs for themselves and for local markets. Mintz regards the formation of the Haitian peasantry as a form of resistance, one in which "an entire nation turned its back upon the system of large estates, worked by forced labor" (Mintz 1974b:61). It was an option with origins in the confused interregnum between Bois Caiman and Toussaint's constitution of 1801 (and, even earlier, in the slaves' gardens of the colony). Further, Mintz suggests, the case of Haiti is but an extreme example of a process important throughout the region:

Caribbean peasantries are "reconstituted," in that they consist in large measure of Afro-Caribbean people who took advantage of every decline, lengthy or brief, in plantation domination to settle themselves on the land, as producers of a substantial part of their own needs, and of cash commodities they might sell as individuals *to local or foreign markets*. (Mintz 1974b:61, emphasis added)

It is precisely this sort of peasantry that remains linked, through a national or foreign-born bourgeoisie, to the centers of larger economic systems. To properly understand the dynamic of these still-evolving structures, we must turn to the creaking apparatus of foreign commerce and the diplomacy that greased it.

Haiti in International Context

Producing for a world market necessitated relations with the European powers and the emerging societies of the Americas. For example, Haiti quickly sought diplomatic recognition from the sole other independent nation in the hemisphere. Such recognition was bitterly opposed by members of the U.S. Congress, especially those from slaveholding states.[5] The United States and allied European powers helped France to orchestrate a diplomatic quarantine of "the Black Republic," as the island's leaders dubbed their new country. France, after a humiliating defeat, found itself bereft of its most profitable colony; the United States wished to keep Haiti's dangerous example as far as possible from its own slaves; and even the Vatican, annoyed over the expulsion of its priests, was in no hurry to establish relations with the first New World nation to declare Catholicism its official religion.

Haiti was the outcast of the international community. Mintz (in Leyburn 1966:xxiii) argues that, in the years following the revolution, Haiti was probably less affected by external developments than any other country in the hemisphere. Logan (1968:195) writes of the erection, immediately after independence, of a "cultural Chinese Wall against white men." Lacerte blames Haiti's economic decline on the nation's "xenophobia," with the effect that "foreigners found that it was impossible to invest in Haiti, as they were doing elsewhere in Latin America, because of the barriers set up by overly restrictive legislation" (Lacerte 1981:515). That the fundamentally seditious nature of the new country would lead the imperial powers to attempt to isolate Haiti *diplomatically* makes sense. It did not necessarily follow, however, that these political maneuvers were backed up by commercial isolation. There are subtle cues, even in the work that occasioned Mintz's statement, that Haiti was always subject to foreign intervention of one stripe or another. Leyburn (1966:64n) notes, as an aside, that one early Haitian administration's "coins were so easily imitated that the country was inundated with counterfeit money. The government issued only five million dollars worth of this currency, but in 1818 twelve millions were in circulation, the surplus having been fabricated in Europe and the United States." That coins minted in the United States would so readily reach the Haitian peasantry bespeaks closer links than might readily be observed.[6]

One long-standing and disastrous link was to the nation's former metropolis. The threat of reinvasion was real, for the French kept troops in neighboring Santo Domingo until 1809. After the fall of Napoleon, France continued to refuse to recognize Haiti's statehood until the former plantation owners had been indemnified for their losses. The point was really moot as long as France was entangled in European wars. But the peace proclaimed by the 1815 Treaty of Paris meant a renewal of European harassment of the "American colonies," one of which was held to be Haiti.[7] In 1824, the French monarch Charles X pressed Haiti's President Boyer for 150 million francs and the halving of customs charges for the French trade. These conditions, accepted in 1825, led to decades of French domination of Haitian finance, and had a catastrophic effect on the new nation's delicate economy. "From a country whose expenditures and receipts were, until then, balanced," remarks Price-Mars (1953:169–170) incredulously, "the incompetence and frivolity of the men in power had made a nation burdened with debts and entangled in a web of impossible financial obligations."

The very fact of a debt to France strikes the modern observer as odd. Why might a country of former slaves feel compelled to remunerate the plantocracy for losses incurred in a war of liberation? Why would a fragile—but balanced—young economy be thus jeopardized by its leaders? The legally anomalous indemnity was a business expense. The growth of the republic was held, by the elite who saw their own survival at stake in the issue of diplomatic recognition, to be tied to continued export of subtropical commodities.[8] In his assessment of Haiti's first six decades, Auguste (1987:3) declares that the "major, essential, primordial objective, pursued in diverse ways by all our governments—from Dessalines to Geffrard—was, even when not explicitly announced, the recognition of our independence." The diligence with which Haitian diplomats pursued their goal suggests the perceived political, psychological, and—especially—economic need for recognition.

And yet it was apparent to all that the nascent peasantry had no intention of going back to the old plantation formula. Perhaps an awareness of this divergence between state and popular aspirations was in part responsible for the great ambivalence, among the first Haitian administrations, toward the plantation system. Dessalines, Haiti's first ruler and a man known for his mistrust of whites, was nonetheless committed to maintaining the channels of commerce between his country, the "neutral" European powers, and the United States. Lacerte's (1981:511) assertion that Dessalines's policy was one "of virtually sealing the country off from outside contacts between 1804 and 1806" is not supported by the historical record. Shortly after the extermination of all the French residents, Dessalines officially welcomed the commercial overtures of the English and the North Americans.[9] Haiti again began producing sugar and rum, and became an important exporter of cotton, *campèche*, cocoa, and—especially—coffee.

During the first two years of Haiti's sovereignty, the United States quickly consolidated its position as her chief trading partner. A mere four decades after its own independence had been declared, the United States boasted one of the largest merchant marines in the world. It was not long before Haitians became the very first Latin Americans to complain of Yankee imperialism. Nicholls cites a prophetic editorial that appeared in the official *Gazette* of October 1805. "Owing to its proximity, as well as to the frequent visits of its citizens to the ports of [Haiti] and to 'the pretensions to which these might give birth,' the USA [the writer] warned, might in the future be a greater threat to Haitian independence than were the countries of Europe" (Nicholls 1985:89). But it was not yet the hour of the North Americans. The United States had incurred certain obligations to France following the Louisiana Purchase, and Napoleon enjoined his North American allies to adhere to the French embargo of Haiti. After February 1806, overt U.S. trade slowed to a trickle.

It was, suddenly, the hour of the British. Shortly after the October 1806 assassination of Dessalines, his successor published, in London, a decree entitled *Adresse du Gouvernement d'Haiti au Commerce des Nations Neutres*. Henry Christophe, the anglophile autocrat who ruled the northern part of the then-divided country, "stated that all the energies of the country were being turned towards the production of goods for export" (in Nicholls 1985:91). Less than a decade after Christophe's proclamation, most of the foreign houses of commerce were British. By 1832, writes Lacerte (1981:504), "Haitian exports were valued at £1,250,000 annually of which the British share was one-half. Haiti came third, at that time, after Mexico and Peru as England's trading partner among the Latin American republics."[10]

Within a decade of Haitian independence, however, North American merchants began rebuilding their Haitian trade. By 1821, almost 45 percent of Haitian imports came from the United States; 30 percent were of British origin and 21 percent were French. Much of the nationalist rhetoric of the Haitian elite was addressed to the United States. The hypocrisy of the North Americans was revealed by their loud insistence that Britain and the other European powers recognize all the new American republics—all except Haiti, that is. "Our policy with regard to Haiti is plain," declared Senator Robert Hayne of South Carolina in 1824, a few months after President Monroe enunciated his famous doctrine: "We never can acknowledge her independence. . . . The peace and safety of a large portion of our union forbids us even to discuss [it]" (cited in Schmidt 1971:28). Some U.S. statesmen persisted in referring to the Haitians as "rebel slaves."

Haiti fared little better with the Latin American republics established later, despite Haiti's rather visionary foreign policy. In 1815, in Les

Cayes, Simon Bolivar received arms, ammunition, and food from Haiti for his expedition to South America on the condition that he free all slaves in any Spanish provinces he might liberate. Unsuccessful in his first attempt, Bolivar returned to Haiti and was then the beneficiary of more extensive aid from President Pétion. Rout (1976:177) notes that Bolivar, as president of Gran Colombia, "was partially able to fulfill his promise." But his subsequent refusal to establish diplomatic relations with Haiti, on the unsubstantiated grounds that the republic was "fomenting racial conflict," was typical of Haiti's welcome in a monolithically racist world.

The Spanish, too, made threatening, if less impressive, gestures toward Haiti. After the fall of Napoleon and the withdrawal of French troops, the Junta Central, the rickety coalition of conservatives and reformers that more or less governed the Spanish empire, announced plans to "contain" the Haitians. The dilapidated colony of Santo Domingo had been illegally ceded to the French, claimed the junta in 1810; the cancellation of several outstanding debts, the restoration of the archbishopric (the hemisphere's oldest), and the encouragement of free trade were among the reforms promised. But the machinations of the old empires were increasingly hollow; the Junta Central collapsed shortly after issuing its decree. Although an independence movement seemed to be gathering force in the eastern reaches of the island, Haitian President Boyer sought to reunite the two factions under the Haitian flag. As Logan notes, "He met no opposition: indeed—according to Hazard, writing in 1872—he was received in an enthusiastic manner, and in February of 1822 was formally acknowledged as ruler of the entire island" (Logan 1968:32).

This state of affairs prevailed until 1844, when the Dominican Republic declared its independence from Haiti. Again, a troubled interregnum followed; again, the British, French, Spanish, and North Americans vied for influence and control. The diplomatic pronouncements of these powers were consistently cast in racist terms. Although the North Americans were informed by their agents that "only the United States could save the Dominican Republic from sinking 'into a Negro province under the Haytien constitution,'" the statesmen felt that there were "not enough 'white' Dominicans to warrant recognition of the republic." The British foreign secretary had soothed his own envoy, who feared that the United States would respond to Dominican calls for annexation, with the suggestion that the United States was not likely to "choose to take into their Union, even if it were disposed to join them, a State which like Haiti contains a population chiefly composed of free Blacks" (Logan 1968:34, 36, 39–40).

More than one Haitian leader was alarmed by the calls of Dominicans for foreign, and especially North American, annexation. What, asked a number of Haitians, might come of the annexation of the better part of the island by a slaveholding nation? Referring to the indivisibility of the island declared decades ago by Toussaint, Haitian armies invaded the eastern portion of Hispaniola during the reigns of presidents Guerrier and Soulouque.[11] Haiti—or, rather, its productive class, the peasantry—paid dearly for these eastward adventures. In his summary of reasons to explain contemporary Haiti's "backwardness" when compared to the Dominican Republic, Logan (1968:196) writes of "Haiti's fear during the 1840s and 1850s that United States acquisition of the Dominican Republic would lead to the reestablishment of slavery in Haiti. This fear and the Haitian concept of the indivisibility of the island led to the futile and costly invasions of 1850 and 1855–56." Such military activities were not only failures but were also well beyond the means of a political and economic system doomed to collapse.

Crisis and Collapse

Given that both northern and southern Haiti were still selling commodities on the world market, and given the existence of conquests, battles, and international intrigue, how were several leading students of the island led to speak of a "century of isolation"? One reason may have been that early legislation, while encouraging international trade, restricted the activities of foreign merchants to stipulated port cities. Penetration into the interior was forbidden. Producers were thus often linked to the world market by intermediaries who bulked and/or processed the produce of small landholders. The result of such restrictions was a *spatial isolation* of the peasantry, not just from the "outside world," but from the other classes inside Haiti as well. To cite once again the most incisive work treating these changes: "The economic structures, the very mechanisms of extracting this surplus, made it possible to purge this peasantry without ever touching or seeing it" (Trouillot 1986:89).

The chief purgers of the peasantry were the state and the small commercial class it came to represent. Joachim (1979) and Trouillot (1986) refer to this partnership as "the Holy Alliance." Although the Alliance relied heavily on indirect taxes that masked the extent to which the peasants were gouged, the small farmers could not have been unaware of the heavy price they paid for their participation in the export economy. Despite considerable change in infrastructure and the decline of sugar, Haiti continued to produce largely the same goods as had Saint-Domingue. These were primarily subtropical commodities for export: coffee, cotton, indigo, rum, cocoa, and mahogany. A striking difference was that coffee, unlike sugar, was easily cultivated on small (under two hectares) plots.[12]

Why, then, did those owning land not simply withdraw into subsistence farming? One reason was and is that many of the items long perceived as necessary to any rural household—soap, cooking oil, charcoal, and salt, for example—could only be acquired with cash. Further, peasant families regularly needed clothing, medicines, and money for children in school. The peasants could cut their losses by refusing to devote *all* their land to produce whose price fluctuated on the world market, but they were nonetheless fully enmeshed in a market economy.

By the 1860s, the system was bursting at the seams. Dissatisfaction with the Geffrard government (1859–1867) surged among the urban poor, the small-scale merchants, the market women, the unemployed, and the progressive sector of the bourgeoisie. Much of the north of Haiti openly supported Sylvain Salnave, Geffrard's mutinous rival. In 1865, the "popular quarter" of Cap Haitien rioted, calling for an end to the Geffrard government. When the business community later turned Salnaviste, the combined force of the different factions allowed Cap Haitien to successfully stave off government forces, which had laid siege to the city. For six months, the Salnavistes held strong, and it was only by appealing to British naval power that Geffrard was able to snuff out the insurrection. Heinl and Heinl (1978:228–231) relate the bombardment of the Cap and surrounding fortifications by three of the Royal Navy's ships, one of which was destroyed in the fray. The event was a watershed: "The Geffrard government thus became the first Haitian administration openly to obtain foreign aid to remain in power" (Georges Adam 1982:34). It set a lamentable precedent.

By 1870, the preceding decade could be assessed as "ruinous." Georges Adam (1982:209) writes that "the crisis shook the nation to its very roots. By and large, the privileged classes were ruined, with the exception of the money changers and the epoch's large supply houses." The names of the surviving establishments and the products they marketed speak both to the question of isolation and to the nature of the crisis: Oliver Cutts, military supplies and victuals; Simmonds Brothers, naval munitions; White Hartmann, munitions and paper money. These details, and the entire story they inform, also reveal the increasingly important roles played by foreigners in Haitian affairs of state. Not only did expatriots bankroll and arm opposing groups, their governments directly intervened in Haitian politics.

Fighting Over the Spoils: 1870–1914

During the latter part of the nineteenth century, the decline of Haiti was apparent even to charitable observers. And observers, regardless of affiliation, were struck by the role of foreigners in the vicissitudes of the Haitian economy. It seemed to many that the destiny of the Haitian people was under the jurisdiction of foreign powers. How had this come to be, given the fiercely nationalist intentions of the founding fathers? Castor (1988b) blames the opportunism of the ruling elite, easily bought out by the *grandes puissances*.[13] As Georges Adam (1982:209) would have it, "from 1879 to 1915, the striking feature of international developments in Haiti was without contest the battle between the four imperialist powers." The last three decades of the century often seemed to have been little more than a struggle between Britain, France, Germany, and the United States for ascendancy in the Haitian economy.

Increasingly, this struggle took place in Port-au-Prince, the locus of the foreign presence in Haiti. Centralizing governments such as that of Geffrard began to sap the power of the provincial ports that had once generated the majority of all customs receipts. The export economy may have declined in absolute terms over the last quarter-century, but the products sold were the same as in colonial times. Coffee was the undisputed leader; most of it was sold to France. Haiti also continued to export cotton, cocoa, and mahogany. Janvier (1883:xx) wrote that in 1878 Haiti was engaged in "un grand commerce" with the United States, France, Britain, Germany, and Italy. Trade receipts totalled 90 million francs, of which a healthy 53 million represented exports. Ten years of peace, opined Janvier, would enable his country to triple its commerce.

Janvier's assertion was never tested, however, as peace was Haiti's scarcest commodity. He wrote in a time of relative calm, but it was to be short-lived. As the nineteenth century gave way to the twentieth, the Republic of Haiti, like many of its Latin American neighbors, came increasingly to be linked to the United States. This is not to suggest that the United States began purchasing a greater percentage of Haitian exports. Instead, *imports to* Haiti were increasingly significant to the United States. By 1851, according to Trouillot (1986:56), the United States sold more to Haiti than it did to most Latin American countries, including Mexico—this in spite of the fact that the United States still refused to recognize Haitian independence. Haitian reliance on U.S. goods grew steadily throughout the latter half of the century. "Between 1870 and 1913," records Rotberg (1971:110), "the United States increased its share of the Haitian market from 30 to about 60 per cent." The importance of the Haitian trade is revealed simply by the density of traffic between the two countries: "Well before 1900, the number of North American ships docking in our ports exceeded the number reaching all of Europe" (Trouillot 1986:57).

In the latter part of the nineteenth century and in the beginning of the twentieth, United States primacy in the Haitian marketplace was no longer seriously contested by Britain or France. Germany was its chief rival. By 1909, some two hundred Germans in Haiti controlled 80 percent of all international commerce (Rotberg 1971:112). "Haiti," complained one of its late-nineteenth-century citizens, "is in the process of becoming a colony of Hamburg" (Nicholls 1985:109). Commercial primacy was not merely established through negotiating profitable trade agreements. Warships were called in by foreign merchants who claimed, often, that debts owed them by Haitians were unpaid.

One example will illustrate. Although by no means the sole perpetrators of gunboat diplomacy, the Germans were, after their victory in the Franco-Prussian War, particularly heavy-handed in all that concerned Haiti. On the standard debt-collecting pretext, two German ships steamed into Haitian waters in June 1872. The vessels were commanded by Captain Karl F. Batsch, who bypassed established diplomatic channels by dispatching a note directly to the Haitian government. Two German commercial establishments had been damaged during recent unrest (one, it should be noted, was bombarded by a British gunboat). Batsch demanded indemnities of $15,000—by sundown. The Haitian government, temporizing, replied that one case had already been fully assessed and payment was forthcoming, but the second claim had not yet been processed. Batsch seized two Haitian vessels—the bulk of the navy—anchored nearby. The government of President Nissage Saget wavered briefly, then agreed to pay the sum. With the help of the British consul (no stranger to this sort of diplomacy), the sum was raised and dispatched to Captain Batsch.

In most respects, the "Affaire Batsch" was nothing new. But national pride, reports Turnier (1985:189), was "murdered." The history textbook used in Haitian elementary schools is a bit more explicit: "Our flag was spread over the ships' bridges and soiled in a foul manner" (FIC 1942:180). The Heinls capture the Germans' disregard for Haitians as well as the ambiance of the gunboat era by telling the whole story:

> With the special finesse Hohenzollern diplomacy reserved for lesser breeds, the German boarding parties left calling cards. When the Haitians were allowed back, they found their cherished flag spread out on the bridge of each ship, smeared with shit. It was, remarked [Haitian statesman Anténor] Firmin, the republic's first contact with the methods of German diplomacy. (Heinl and Heinl 1978:256)

Such "reclamations" were current in the German, French, British, and North American communities.[14] In 1883, Janvier estimated that a total of 80 million francs had been drained from the national coffers in just this fashion, while the French debt had drawn off no less than 120 million francs (Janvier 1883:17). Between 1879 and 1902 ("la belle époque des réclamations et des indemnités"), one conservative estimate is that $2.5 million was extorted from federal reserves in order to stave off the gunboats (Marcelin, in Joachim 1979:64).

The perpetual draining of the state treasury was of a piece with the total failure to invest in agriculture. By the end of the century, 80 percent of national revenue—most of it derived directly from peasant labor—was going to repay debts (Prince 1985:18). Soon Haiti was unable to make payments: "The foreign debt had grown to the point of exceeding the nation's capacity to repay. In 1903, it was estimated at $33,121,999. In December 1904, it was $40,891,394" (Castor 1988b:21). All this was happening in tandem with rapid population growth and the steady loss of arable land to alkalinity and erosion.

In addition to interventions by European powers, Haitian waters were violated by the United States no less than fifteen times in that "century of isolation."[15] And these violations were stepped up in the decades preceding the First World War. Castor (1988b:31) offers the following roster of foreign interventions: in 1888, U.S. Marines supported the military revolt against the Légitime government. Four years later, the German government openly supported the suppression of the movement led by Anténor Firmin. In 1912, Syrians residing in Haiti participated in an anti-Leconte government plot, during which the presidential palace was blown to bits. In January 1914, at the end of Haiti's short-lived first experiment in civilian rule, North American, British, and German forces entered Haiti to "protect their citizens." Later that year came the Affaire Peters, an English version of the Affaire Batsch, which brought a British cannon boat thundering into Haitian harbors. It left Haitian waters $125,000 heavier. In December, the U.S. Marines paid another visit, this time to claim some $500,000 from the vaults of the Banque Nationale d'Haiti. Heinl and Heinl (1978: 404–405) assert that

the United States Navy had been compelled to send warships into Haitian waters to protect the lives and property of American citizens in 1849, 1851, 1857, 1858, 1865, 1866, 1867, 1868, 1869, 1876, 1888, 1891, 1892, 1902, 1903, 1904, 1905, 1906, 1907, 1908, 1909, 1911, 1912, 1913, and, during 1914, 1915, had maintained ships there almost without interruption.

Haiti's first century was hardly one of "solitude," as some scholars have claimed. Nor is "quarantine" the appropriate analogy. Certainly, Haiti was ostracized, or diplomatically isolated. But the new republic became a useful—and used—pariah. The history of foreign involvement in Haiti was most often the predictable one of domination by the United States and European powers. The North American Occupation of 1915–1934 was not, as its apologists suggest, the sudden manifestation of a new U.S. interest in protecting the Haitians from their own corrupt rulers. It was rather the continuation of a pattern established in the nineteenth century, and in many ways the logical succession to a brand of imperialism that had already taken root throughout Latin America.

17

The United States and
the People with History

*The Occupation worsened the economic crisis by augmenting
the peasantry's forced contribution to the maintenance of
the State and of the urban parasites. It worsened the crisis
of power by centralizing the Haitian Army and disarming
[citizens in] the provinces. Of course, by putting in place the
structures of military, fiscal, and commercial centralization,
the Occupation postponed judgment day for thirty years; but
it also guaranteed that the finale would be bloody.*

Trouillot (1986:23–24)

*"Haiti means business" the brochure from the Department
of Tourism and Industry says, and indeed it does: American
business. Mean business.*

Chittester (1989:9)

*Haiti is a very important client to Florida. It is one of
our top markets. We treasure our relationship with Haiti
even though it is a poor country.*

Florida Department of Commerce,
March 1990[1]

The United States Marine Corps invaded Haiti in 1915.
To the student of Latin American history, it is hardly surprising that
penetration of foreign capital, coupled with the almost continuous invasion by U.S. warships of Haitian waters, led to an armed occupation.

As Rotberg (1971:109) remarks, "It is more surprising that the Americans waited until 1915 than that they intervened at all." In 1901, the United States sent troops into Nicaragua. In the same year, after a three-year military occupation of Cuba, the United States formalized relations of dependency with the Platt Amendment, by which Cuba became a U.S. protectorate. The island's domestic and foreign policy was thereafter almost exclusively controlled by the United States, which also claimed rights to naval bases and coal stations. The North Americans took over the customs houses of the Dominican Republic in 1905. All these countries would be militarily occupied at some point in the first two decades of the century. Colombia, Venezuela, Honduras, and, especially, Panama would also be drawn ineluctably into the "back yard" of the United States. The decades of the "Big Stick" and "Dollar Diplomacy" changed the Caribbean basin forever.[2]

As is often the case, "instability" in Haiti was the pretext for U.S. intervention. And there can be no denying that the political situation there was often anarchic. Mintz notes that "of Haiti's twenty-four chief executives between 1807 and 1915, only eight were in office for a period equal to their elected terms, and seventeen were deposed by revolution" (in Leyburn 1966:ix). In the decade preceding the occupation, Haiti was nothing if not "unstable." The causes of this instability are an altogether different issue. Although many North American and European historians seem to consider them to be largely internal, Allen, writing in *Current History* in 1930, asserted that "Haiti has been victimized time and time again by foreign merchants, foreign capitalists, and foreign governments. Had it not been for foreigners it is doubtful if a large majority of the revolutions would have occurred" (Allen 1930:125). A similar view was advanced by a commission of Americans investigating the conditions of the occupation (Balch 1927), and by a penetrating new study of Haiti's relations with "the Great Powers":

Haitian political life had degenerated quickly between 1910 and 1915. The expatriation of resources and capital by the foreign and foreign-oriented enclaves intensified this deterioration. Exploitation had been proceeding for some time, but now crises followed one another in ever more rapid succession. These were crises dictated by the structure of Haitian politics, but the structure was rapidly becoming dysfunctional as recurrent warfare sapped the nation's vital energies. By 1914, more astute members of the upper classes had begun to realize that they were killing their golden goose. (Plummer 1988:220–221)

These crises reached their apogee during the brief reign of General Vilbrun Guillaume Sam, whose jails were overflowing with political detainees. When President Sam, beleaguered by forces from the north as well as another faction based in the capital, saw that his fall was imminent, he ordered the execution of the prisoners. In the Penitencier National, 163 of 173 prisoners were summarily executed. The now-deposed president took refuge in the French embassy. A mob, which included family members of the slaughtered prisoners, formed outside the legation, stormed it, and brought President Sam to rude justice in the streets of Port-au-Prince.[3] The commander of the prison met a similar fate, the very same day.

The Marines landed near Port-au-Prince on July 28, 1915. The "Convention haitiano-américaine," promulgated later that year, granted the United States complete political and administrative control over Haiti. These arrangements were more stringent than the legal trappings of other contemporary Latin American occupations, as they granted receivership not only of customs receipts—"control of the customs houses," observed President Wilson, "constituted the essence of this whole affair"—but also of all governmental outlays. Furthermore, the Republic of Haiti could not undertake any foreign debt without the approval of the United States. The Convention was ratified by the U.S. Senate in February 1916. Other, more finely tuned documents followed, resulting in the Constitution of 1918, which Franklin D. Roosevelt claimed to have written while secretary of the navy.[4]

Of the various articles in these documents, two would have the most significant repercussions. Article X of the 1915 treaty decreed the formation of a new *gendarmerie,* this one to be trained and at the orders of the U.S. Marines. Article V of the 1918 Constitution abolished Dessalines's most famous law, which forbade foreign ownership of land. Many North American companies scouted Haiti for land for new plantations of rubber, bananas, sugar, sisal, mahogany, and other tropical produce; many of these companies were leased large tracts of land. Castor documents the concession to North American firms of 266,000 acres (see table 10).

What happened to the peasants who farmed these tracts of land? Widely discrepant responses are offered to this question. The occupying force stated that no Haitians were displaced in these transactions, several of which did not lead to the establishment of new farms or plantings. Haitian historians tell a different story. Writing in a Haitian academic journal in 1929, Georges Séjourné estimated that 50,000 peasants were dispossessed in the north alone (Castor 1988b:94).[5] Augmenting the number of the landless and unemployed was not with-

Table 10 *Land Concessions During the Occupation*

Contrat W. A. Rodenberg	125,000 acres
Haytian American Sugar Co.	24,000
Haytian Corporation Pineapple Co.	1,000
Haytian Corporation of America	15,000
Haytian American Development Co.	24,000
Haytian Agricultural Corp.	14,000
Haytian Development Corp.	2,200
Societe Commerciale Haitienne	9,000
United West Indies Corp.	16,000
Haytian Products Co.	16,000
Haytian American Co.	20,000
North Haiti Sugar Co.	400
Total	266,000

SOURCE: Castor (1988b:93)

out benefits for investors. For many, the real draw was not land, but cheap labor. "Haiti offers a marvelous opportunity for American investment," announced the New York daily *Financial America* on November 28, 1926. "The run-of-the-mill Haitian is handy, easily directed, and gives a hard day's labor for 20 cents, while in Panama the same day's work cost $3."

Peasant Resistance to the Occupation

The preceding chapters might suggest that a foreign invasion of Haiti would be resisted. It was. The existence of a commercial class with scant national loyalty might also suggest that resistance would not spring from the urban bourgeoisie. It did not. The U.S. Marines, aided by the police force of their own creation, set out to disarm a rural population that had kept its weapons from the days of the revolution. Invoking a law ratified in 1916 by the U.S. Senate, the occupying force resurrected the *corvée*—the involuntary conscription of labor crews. The round-up of several thousand men by U.S. Marines did not sit well with Haitian memories of white domination from 125 years before, and led to the "Cacos Insurrection" that soon found a latter-day Toussaint Louverture in Charlemagne Péralte. The marines responded with machine guns and even bombs, but the Cacos held the marines at bay until Péralte's assassination in November 1919. This peasant-based rebellion came to have a significant number of adherents before it was finally put down.[6]

Many Haitian lives had been lost during the "pacification period," as the marines termed their quelling of "the bandits." An in-house investigation of the rumors of "indiscriminate killings" was conducted in 1920 by Brigadier General George Barnett, former Commandant General of the Marine Corps. He concluded that 3,250 "natives" had been killed. The *New York Times* of 14 October 1920 noted that

on 2 September 1919, [General Barnett] wrote a confidential letter to Colonel John H. Russell, commanding the marine forces in Haiti, bringing to the latter's attention evidence that "practically indiscriminate killings of natives had gone on for some time," and calling for a thorough investigation. . . . "I think," General Barnett wrote to Colonel Russell, "this is the most startling thing of its kind that has ever taken place in the Marine Corps, and I don't want anything of the kind to happen again." (Prince 1985:21)

In reviewing the records over fifty years later, the Heinls note that the "best evidence, which is not very satisfactory for either side, suggests that, in putting down the Cacos, Marines and Gendarmerie sustained 98 *killed and wounded*; and from 1915 through 1920 some 2,250 Cacos were *killed*" (Heinl and Heinl 1978:462; emphasis added). The authors do not cite their sources, nor do they offer the evidence rejected. Schmidt (1971:103n), the North American authority on the occupation, suggests that 3,250 were killed in the twenty months of active resistance. According to Haitian historians, however, the cost was far more dear. After exhibiting several of the figures most commonly cited, Gaillard asks

if the total number of battle victims and casualties of repression and *consequences* of the war might not have reached, by the end of the pacification period, four or five times that—somewhere in the neighborhood of 15,000 persons. This figure is all the more impressive when it is compared to the 98 dead and wounded among the "marines" and the American and Haitian constabulary. This war, in many instances, must have resembled a massacre. (Gaillard 1983:261–262)

With peasant rebellion silenced, the occupying force went about its business. The North Americans began a process of fiscal and commercial centralization that continued the work of earlier Haitian administrations and finished off the coastal cities that had once collected the majority of the state's customs receipts. Although few of the commercial elite had protested the landing of the marines, losing control of state wealth was a heavy blow to them. The indiscriminant racism of the occupying force was also jarring to the elite, accustomed as they were to being the discriminators.[7]

What, then, is the economic verdict on the United States occupation of Haiti? Heinl and Heinl (1978:516) thought it appropriate to compare Haiti at the close of the occupation with Haiti at the close of the revolution: "In 1804 Haiti was wrecked and ravaged; in 1934, the country was modernized, solvent and thriving, with a national infrastructure passing anything in its history." No one, regardless of political persuasion, would be able to contest the assertion that postoccupation Haiti was in better shape than the smoking ruins of Saint-Domingue; and it is unlikely that the comparison occurred to anyone residing in Haiti. The question of solvency may, however, be disputed. The administration that took over in 1934 was propped up on shaky foundations: the country was heavily indebted, not to the French, but to the North Americans. It was still straddled with the 1922 loan—at $40 million, a record even for loan-happy Haiti—and both the "national" treasury and the Banque Nationale were owned by a New York bank. What is worse, the treasury was even more dependent on customs duties, on coffee especially, than before the occupation. In other words, the wealth of the state was still derived largely from the extraction of a surplus from peasant production and owed to offshore creditors.[8]

An equally damning evaluation has recently been advanced by Trouillot (1986:23–24), who argues that the American occupation "improved nothing and complicated almost everything." He suggests that the racism of the North American stewards reinforced color prejudice in Haiti, paving the way for the *noiriste* rhetoric of François Duvalier. And there were further, tragic consequences of the North American occupation. For example, the occupying force established a new frontier between Haiti and the Dominican Republic, also occupied by the United States. These arrangements granted to Haiti a swath of disputed land far from both Port-au-Prince and Santo Domingo, and some of the dispossessed peasants relocated there. In 1937, after the North Americans had left the island, Dominican dictator Rafael Trujillo, by way of redrawing the boundary, ordered the massacre of thousands of Haitians in the eastern reaches of their own country. The number of people killed during a three-day, genocidal spree has been estimated at between 10,000 and 20,000 (Castor 1988a; Hicks 1946; Price-Mars 1953).

The invasion by the marines, the quelling of peasant resistance, the rewriting of the constitution to allow foreign landholding—all point to at least one important conclusion. From the beginning of the occupation to the ascent of François Duvalier, the United States exerted enormous and unchallenged influence in Haiti. Indeed, when dividing Haitian history into periods, Hurbon (1987c:74) arrives at a tripartite schema: the period of slavery (sixteenth century–1804); the period of independence (1804–1915); and the period of American colonialization. The dates spanned by this latter epoch is given as "1915 to present."

Blood, Sweat, and Baseballs: The Haitian Economy Now

It has become a cliché in some circles to note that Haiti is the poorest country in the hemisphere, and one of the twenty-five poorest in the world. A per capita annual income of $315 in 1983 masks the fact that it hovered around $100 in the countryside. Expert opinion has been given to grim assessments and dour predictions. "From 1955 to 1975," notes Lundahl (1983:9), "Haiti's real GDP [Gross Domestic Product] increased at a yearly rate of only 1.7 percent, and at the same time, the population grew by 1.6 percent per annum. Thereafter, only marginal improvements have taken place, and these improvements do not show any signs of being of the lasting kind." Girault (1984:177) typifies the decade preceding 1984 as marked chiefly "by the slow-down of agricultural production and by a decrease in productivity. Haiti has become a net importer of sugar . . . more than 50 percent of the coffee production is consumed in Haiti." The decline of the agricultural sector, which now contributes only 32 percent of the GDP, has led to increased food importation. "With imports of approximately 240,000 tons of cereals in 1981," adds Girault (1984:179), "it is estimated that food coming from abroad represents already 23 percent of national consumption." Not surprisingly, then, Haiti has not had a positive trade balance since 1964–1965, and the gap is widening.[9] As Patterson (1987:241) notes, Haiti ranks among those circum-Caribbean countries most dependent on trade with the United States. In fact, Haiti currently acquires a larger share of its imported goods from the United States than does any other country in the region.

What *kind* of economy is prevalent in late twentieth-century Haiti? A history of agricultural *specialism* still marks the economy. Even now, the small country of Haiti ranks in the world's top twenty exporters of coffee. Some 400,000 peasants are involved in coffee production, which generated $51 million out of a total of $213 million in 1983 export earnings (Prince 1985:45). Sugar, copper, and bauxite have played significant roles in the past three decades, though they are no longer important. The same is true of sisal, for which thousands of (admittedly poor) hectares were appropriated by North American companies. Before hemp was rendered almost obsolete by nylon, Haiti was the world's third largest producer of sisal.[10]

For the past hundred years, Haitians have worked sugarcane and other harvests in a number of Caribbean countries. The migration, ostensibly seasonal, has led to the formation of important diaspora communities in Cuba, the Bahamas, and, especially, the Dominican Republic. Experts agree that "virtually no Dominican cuts cane in his own country" (Plant 1987:2). Who, then, harvests the sugar? The government of the Dominican Republic estimated in 1980 that 90 percent of the agricultural labor force on sugar plantations is Haitian. By agreement between Duvalier *père* and Rafael Trujillo, tens of thousands of Haitians are "sold" each year to the Dominican Republic. The arrangement, which netted both dictators millions of dollars, has been termed slavery by international human rights organizations.[11]

In short, the Haitian economy cannot be understood without an appreciation of its ties to other countries and of the role of migration. Insisting that Caribbean and Central American migration cannot be properly understood without reference to larger socioeconomic interactions, Patterson points out that Haiti is one of the "peripheral units" of the West Atlantic system. One of the most important processes in that system is migration.

Migration, Urbanization, and the Decline of Agriculture

The most striking recent demographic change in Haiti has been the rapid growth of Port-au-Prince. Haiti, a country of approximately six million, is generally considered to be an overwhelmingly rural nation.[12] But by 1976, 14 percent of the population lived in Port-au-Prince alone (Fass 1978:158). Although this is not impressive by Caribbean standards (more than 30 percent of Puerto Ricans now live in San Juan), the city has grown so much in the last decade that it is now estimated that up to 20 percent of Haitians residing in Haiti live in or on the outskirts of the capital, a city of more than one million that has doubled in size between 1970 and 1984.[13] And from where do these residents come? As is the case with so many "third-world" countries, internal migration has played the significant role in the growth of Port-au-Prince. Unsure of how long this trend will hold, Locher (1984:329) nonetheless states with confidence "that between 1950 and 1971 rural-urban migration accounted for 59 percent of Haitian urban growth, while natural population increase accounted for only 8 percent." Port-au-Prince has taken on many of the characteristics of a city of peasants.

And what of the peasants left behind in the increasingly inhospitable hinterlands? The visitor to rural Haiti is often struck by the aridity, the erosion, and the limitless poverty. The countryside does not even faintly resemble the one described by Christopher Columbus, who found an almost entirely forested island. Haiti seems to have been "used up." By the time *jean-claudisme,* as Duvalier *fils* termed his plan for economic growth, was firmly entrenched, the majority of Haitians had long since given up hope of attaining even a peasant standard of living.[14] Deforestation and concomitant erosion were washing thousands of acres of topsoil into the sea each year, and thousands more were being rendered useless by alkalinity.[15]

In examining Haitian urbanization, migrants to the center of the West Atlantic system must also be taken into account. As has been true for several other Caribbean nations, significant out-migration to the United States (and elsewhere in the region) has changed patterns of urban settlement.[16] It is thought that between 700,000 and 1.5 million Haitians live outside their country, the majority of them in urban North America (New York, Miami, Montreal, urban New Jersey, and Boston) or elsewhere in the Caribbean basin. If an intermediate estimate of their numbers is included in national estimates, the expatriates bring to 36 percent the proportion of Haitians living in cities.[17]

Some might object that such data are not entirely relevant to an examination of the Haitian economy. But most Haitians in North America continue to speak Creole, as do even their U.S.-born offspring; they live in Haitian communities, attend Haitian churches, listen to Haitian radio, and follow with passion developments "at home."

Students of Haitian and other Caribbean migration to the United States suggest that this is less a phenomenon of emigration than of *transnationalism*.[18] Especially telling are flows of capital: countering the long-standing capital flows out of Haiti is the money immigrants send back to relatives on the island. In 1970 alone, Haitians in the United States infused, through remittances to family members, an estimated $16.5 million into the Haitian economy—amounting to 5 percent of the Haitian GNP in that year. It was then suggested that "each employed Haitian in the United States directly or indirectly supports five family members in Haiti" (Lundahl 1983:230). Since that time, Haitian reliance on family members "over there" has only increased. In 1969, a single bank in the northwest town of Port-de-Paix, a frequent departure point, received $1,200,000 in remittances (Marshall 1979:117). Prince (1985:68) reports that remittances are now "estimated at anything from $30 million to $100 million a year."

Operation Bra-strap: Offshore Assembly in Contemporary Haiti

In addition to massive rural-to-urban migration and the continued importance of crops for exports, a new form of capitalist penetration has made even deeper incursions into a faltering agricultural economy. In the last years of François Duvalier's tenure (1957–71), Haitian assembly of U.S. goods was touted by both countries as "aid" to Haiti. The incentives offered to U.S. investors—generous tax holidays, a franchise granting tariff exemption, docile unions, a minimum wage that was but a tiny fraction of that back home—were substantial, and assured by Haiti, as Duvalier's 1969 welcome to Nelson Rockefeller suggests: "Haiti could be a vast reservoir of manpower for [North] Americans establishing reexportation industries, one closer, safer, and more convenient than Hong Kong."

Of Papa Doc's reign of terror, much has been written. As Graham Greene (1980:269) recalls in his memoirs, "Haiti really was the bad dream of the newspaper headlines." Jean-Claude Duvalier's advent is said to have marked a liberalization of Duvalierism; the newspaper headlines abroad became favorable. And yet there was no great change of heart with the passing of Papa Doc, as Trouillot has argued:

With the perspective gained from the passage of time, the two Duvalier regimes appear as two sides of the same coin. There are, of course, dissimilarities, but most of them are superficial. The greatest difference between the two regimes lay in the deepening of relations between the state and holders of capital at home and abroad, and in the increased support of the U.S. government. It was not, however, a difference in principle. On the contrary, the blueprint for the economic policies executed under Jean-Claude Duvalier . . . can be found in the speeches of François. In the late 1960s, Papa Doc . . . projected a vision of what may be described as a totalitarianism with a human face, one that rested on increased economic dependence, particularly on a subcontracting assembly industry heavily tied to the United States. (Trouillot 1990:200)

Haiti was not among those countries first favored by investors seeking conditions for optimum profit through offshore assembly. The trend was initiated in Asia, and came to Latin America in the 1960s. The businesses set up in Mexico were referred to as "export platforms" or *maquiladores*:

In 1973 there were some 448 *maquiladores* in Mexico, chiefly in electronics and the garment industry. But by this time Mexican workers had begun to organize, and companies began to look to Central America and the Caribbean for a cheaper and more docile labor force. They found what they were looking for in Haiti and El Salvador. (Chinchilla and Hamilton 1984:230; paragraphing altered)

In fact, Haiti and El Salvador are two countries that resemble each other more than the government of either would care to admit.[19] Each is poor, overcrowded, and has been ruled, until very recently, by a U.S.-backed, right-wing regime. All these factors are intimately related to the growth of reassembly plants. "Largely because of its cheap labor force, extensive government repression, and denial of even minimal labor rights," explain Burbach and Herold (1984:196), "Haiti is one of the most attractive countries for both the subcontractors and the *maquilas*." Before 1986, Haiti was well known for its "docile" workforce, a trait aggressively demanded by industrialists there.[20]

Some dispute the nature of the relationship among low wages, a repressive state, and its role in the larger West Atlantic system. Those who doubt the nature of these links should attend to the words of one of the architects of the Haitian offshore industry:

"I honestly believe," said Stanley Urban, president of the Haitian-American Chamber of Commerce and Industry, "that a dictatorship is the best form of government for these people. There are six million illiterates on that island.

Think of what the Ruskies could do there." He said, "There's more democracy for business in Haiti than for business in the United States." In Haiti labor was cheap and disciplined at a minimum daily wage of $2.64. "In other words," he exclaimed, "the whole country is virtually a free trade zone!" (Sklar 1988:115–116)

How significant is the contribution of offshore reassembly to the "Haitian" economy? Already, Haiti is the world's largest producer of baseballs, and ranks among the top three in the assembly of such diverse products as stuffed toys, dolls, and apparel, especially brassieres.[21] All told, the importance of international subcontracting is considerable: "Contributing more than half of the country's industrial exports, assembly production now earns almost one-quarter of Haiti's yearly foreign exchange receipts" (Grunwald, Delatour, and Voltaire 1984:244). By 1978, "exports" from offshore assembly operations had surpassed coffee as the number one export. Already labeled by its cheerleaders as "the most buoyant sector of the Haitian economy for the past decade," its significance in the world economy is already palpable:

At this point, let it be noted that Haiti's weight in the world offshore production system is far greater than its size (in population and income) in the world community. Of the forty-seven countries in 1980 which imported nontrivial amounts of U.S. components for assembly, Haiti ranked ninth with imports of more than $105 million. It held a similar position among developing countries in respect to value added in its assembly production which was exported to the United States. (Grunwald, Delatour, and Voltaire 1984:233)

In terms of employment, the World Bank and the United States Embassy estimate that as of 1980, there were approximately two hundred assembly plants employing 60,000 persons, a majority of whom were women. These factories were (and are) all located in the capital. "Assuming a dependency ratio of 4 to 1," add Grunwald, Delatour, and Voltaire (1984:232), "this means that assembly operations supported about one-quarter of the population of Port-au-Prince in 1980."

The assembly plants have come under heavy fire in post-Duvalier Haiti. Their critics argue that the plants exist merely to exploit cheap Haitian labor and help to perpetuate relations of dependence. What options remained for "hopeless Haiti," as the country was termed in the international aid community? Not many, answered the country's Duvalierist leaders, who in recent years cynically promoted the idea of Haiti as a diseased polity that demanded a rapid infusion of international aid. Clearly, the Duvalier governments saw a meal ticket in the international organizations. Haiti appealed to every imaginable source of aid, and especially to the U.S. Agency for International Development. The Duvaliers also turned to Canada, France, West Germany, and to the World Bank, UNICEF, UNDP, WHO, and the FAO. Hancock (1989) estimates that during the 1970s and 1980s, such aid financed two-thirds of government investment and covered fully half of Haitian import expenditures. Despite obvious evidence of massive fraud, the organizations, and especially U.S. AID, happily pumped money into the Duvalier kleptocracy:

Being so charmingly credulous, the U.S. Department of Commerce produced figures to show that no less than 63 percent of all recorded government revenue in Haiti was being "misappropriated" each year. Not long afterwards—and just before he was dismissed by Duvalier—Haiti's Finance Minister, Marc Bazin, revealed that a monthly average of $15 million was being diverted from public funds to meet "extra-budgetary expenses" that included regular deposits into the President's private Swiss bank account. Most of the "public funds" had, of course, arrived in Haiti in the form of "development assistance." (Hancock 1989:180)

But graft and thievery are only part of the story. Several studies have shown that the effects of international aid have often been highly deleterious to the local economy. For example, cereals donated under the PL 480 program have been found for sale in virtually every Haitian marketplace, thereby undercutting locally produced grains (Lappé, Collins, and Kinley 1980:97). In an important study of the effects of international aid to Haiti, DeWind and Kinley (1988) conclude that the chief effects of such aid have brought further misery to the poor (by now the vast majority of Haitians) and massive out-migration. Hancock (1989:180) examines aid to Haiti and asks, "Did the ruin of the Haitian poor occur *in spite* of foreign aid, or *because* of it?"

Port-au-Prince was also the locus of that other failed hope, tourism. For tourism brought in more than just foreign exchange; it reinforced institutionalized prostitution. Although many commentaries on prostitution in Haiti are retrospective assessments made in light of the AIDS crisis, most agree that economic desperation gave the possessors of even modest sums of money access to a sexual-services marketplace unconscionably tilted in their favor. "Fantasies came true" on payment of what was, for the fortunate outsider, "a nominal charge." What options—let alone fantasies—were left to the Haitian poor? Not many. There were few avenues of escape for those caught in the web of urban migration, unemployment greater than 60 percent, and extreme poverty.[22] Add to this combination the marked dependency of the Haitian economy as a whole on the United States, and the stage is set for what might best be termed the "West Atlantic Pandemic." For AIDS fits neatly—all too neatly, for those who like their symbolism indirect— into the misery generated in the past three centuries. Indeed, the Haitian epidemic cannot be fully understood apart from the burdensome and cumulative tragedies that preceded it.

PART FIVE

AIDS and Accusation

AIDS demonstrates how economics and politics cannot be separated from disease; indeed, these forces shape our response in powerful ways. In the years ahead we will, no doubt, learn a great deal more about AIDS and how to control it. We will also learn a great deal about the nature of our society from the manner in which we address the disease.

Brandt (1988:168)

In the next four chapters, we will turn back to the stories of Manno, Anita, and Dieudonné, and to the commentaries of the people of Kay. A number of features recorded in these accounts, including the diverse ways in which members of one community responded to a new sickness, invite further exploration. Social reponses to AIDS presented in these chapters might be classed by the dominant emotion revealed in each reaction: for example, the compassion of the families of the afflicted; the blame and anger manifest in sorcery accusations; the fear that undergirded so many responses to a new sickness. But such a typology would leave untapped an important stream of commentary, such as that found in conspiracy theories linking Kay to faraway places. In fact, one can almost discern a "geography of blame"; North American responses to AIDS reverberated throughout rural Haiti. And the accusation that AIDS had originated in Haiti triggered "aftershocks" at the far end of the fault line.

191

Of all the responses registered, accusation—the assertion that human agency had a role in the etiology of AIDS—is the dominant leitmotiv. Using an interpretive approach that draws on history and political economy—specifically, a revised world-systems theory that discerns a linked center and periphery—the following chapters will reexamine three principal forms of AIDS-related accusation: the sorcery accusations among the peasants of Kay; the AIDS-related accusations brought to bear against Haiti by North Americans, and the resulting discrimination experienced by Haitians living there; and the "conspiracy theories" that constituted a sort of Haitian reply to North American discrimination.

18

AIDS and Sorcery:
Accusation in the Village

*Good and evil are two brothers; life and death are two
brothers. All four come from God. They do not come from the
loa.*

Rural Haitian to Melville Herskovits, 1934[1]

*Human suffering is the major impetus for serving the spir-
its. . . . Understanding Vodou ritualizing in terms of the
ways in which it both comprehends suffering and amelio-
rates suffering yields greater insight than any other.*

Brown (1989a:40)

In the story told in chapter 9, it is clear that Dieudonné
Gracia attributed the central etiologic role in his illness to sorcery. And
despite the implications of his mordant critique of intraclass squab-
bling, Dieudonné designated as his aggressor a peer, another youth
from rural Haiti. Sorcery was invoked, in one way or another, as a distal
or proximal cause in each of the three *sida* deaths described previously.
What sense might be made of sorcery accusations vis-à-vis other social
responses to AIDS? What logic underlies these accusations? Into what
larger cultural system do these beliefs fit?

When posed to rural Haitians, this last query elicits quizzical stares.
That the question must be reframed is suggested by an event that occurred shortly before Manno's death. August 23, 1987, was hot and

humid by mid-morning. As it was a Sunday, many villagers were in Église Saint-André, where the lay reader Maître Gérard was leading a service. The tin roof was popping in the heat, making it difficult to hear from the back of the chapel. But we all strained to listen when Gérard announced that Brother Étienne had "two words" he wished to share.

On the previous Tuesday, reported Étienne from the lectern, someone had come to his house after he, his wife, and their children had gone to bed. A male voice called out Étienne's name three times. Étienne did not reply, and the visitor disappeared.[2] The next night, another voice called Étienne's name, again three times. This time his wife replied, "Who is it?" "It's Sonson," the voice came back. "I have something serious (*yon pawol jis*) to settle with you." Étienne, "sure that Sonson would not disturb him at such an hour," did not budge, and again the person left. The following night, Thursday, a very similar scenario ensued. This time, however, the voice responded "Rezima" when Étienne's wife asked who was calling: "It's Rezima. I have something serious to settle with you." Mme. Étienne replied that her husband was out, and there was no reply.

Early Friday morning, Mme. Étienne went to market in Domond. When she returned later that afternoon, she sat on the "porch" (really just a bit of tamped dirt covered by the eaves of the house) and fanned herself. She took off her kerchief and wiped her brow. A few minutes later, she went into the house, inadvertently leaving her kerchief on the porch. When she later could not find it, the sun had set and she was already on her sleeping mat. "Fetch me my kerchief," she said to her daughter. But the child did not want to step on the porch in the dark, and no one insisted. Everyone went to sleep. Shortly before dawn on Saturday morning, a neighbor came to the door with some money she owed Mme. Étienne. As it was almost time to go to the market in Mirebalais, Mme. Étienne went to fetch water from the fountain. When Étienne arose shortly thereafter, he found a green calabash gourd (*kalbas vèt*) in the front room. Tied to its stem was his wife's kerchief. Étienne and his family had been hexed.

This discovery, continued Étienne unconvincingly, "did not startle me too much." He did not owe anyone any money; he had not argued with anyone. He decided that, rather than go to the *bokòr* with the calabash, he wished to put the matter before the members of his church, "as it's here that I worship." He had come to see the lay reader earlier that morning. Étienne had requested a prayer meeting, but Maître Gérard had thought that a testimonial would be more appropriate.

At that point in the narrative, Maître Gérard returned to the lectern, and suggested that we "act as the true brothers and sisters of Étienne and help him to confront his problem." The lay leader concluded the mass, and announced that all those who wished could help us to "stamp out this bad thing." Well over a hundred adults filed through the doors, and traversed in disorderly procession the few hundred yards between the church and Étienne's house. Maître Gérard and three of his "acolytes"—Saul, Pierre, and Ti Zout—went into the house, a run-down, two-room shack on the north side of the clinic. The crowd began to sing familiar hymns, pray familiar prayers. Although we could not see him from the road, Gérard had lifted his voice, and seemed to be speaking in an authoritative manner. He came into the bright sunlight, dangling the calabash at the end of a black cloth. The gourd was scored with letters.

The crowd drew back in fear, and there was some nervous laughter. Maître Gérard also laughed and proclaimed, "You don't need to be afraid: it's just magic, just a little magic thing (*yon ti bagay maji*)." But the tone was forced, and everyone gave the little magic thing wide berth. Upon closer inspection, most of the marks on the calabash were elegant cursive letters: they seemed to form the words P-O-R-T-E and D-I-E-U, but it was difficult to be sure, as the letters were large, irregularly placed, and interspersed with other, more cryptic marks.

Maître Gérard crossed the road, and dashed the calabash against the hard bordering embankment. It broke open easily, and a murmur went through the congregation. Saul poured gasoline onto the gourd and the black kerchief; Ti Zout handed Étienne a box of matches. As Étienne touched a match to the kerchief, a man behind me said, "You can't burn it that easily brother," and again nervous laughter rippled through the crowd. As the flames took the kerchief and blackened the calabash, Maître Gérard had already turned back to the house. Again he went in, again the crowd sang and prayed. This time, I could see into the house, and so knew that Étienne and his wife were on their knees before Maître Gérard. The lay leader was softly reciting a prayer—a "special prayer for these kinds of circumstances," he later explained—and the couple responded with "Yes" and "Amen" at regular intervals. The three of them again emerged into the harsh sunlight, a final hymn was sung, and everyone repaired to their homes.

What is the nature of the "beliefs" so clearly shared by the majority of adults living in Do Kay? Étienne's experience serves as a useful starting point for a discussion of the AIDS-related sorcery accusation, for it cuts to the heart of the confusion surrounding Haitian "religious beliefs." The confusion stems in part from real ambiguities, from equally real ambivalences (on the part of all those concerned, including those who study voodoo), and a long list of hidden agendas.

1. *Under what aegis might we class the mutually agreed upon realities that had brought together over one hundred adult residents of this small village?*

With rare exception, ethnographers have spoken of Haitian sorcery as a phenomenon linked only to voodoo. For Métraux (1972:266), "magic is inextricably mixed up with what people are pleased to call 'the Voodoo religion.'" In a more recent review, Hurbon (1987a:264) examines sorcery accusations "in the framework of voodoo beliefs in Haiti." Indeed, the most facile answer to our question is voodoo, and it is precisely this response that is to be regarded as problematic in this chapter.

The sorcery = voodoo equation has a long history. Throughout the nineteenth century, common qualifiers of voodoo ran the gamut from "superstitious belief" to "satanic rite." Sorcery and witchcraft were held to be its very essence. Reacting sheepishly to the racism of the "outside world," many nineteenth-century Haitian intellectuals spoke of voodoo as if it were an African survival firmly on the wane. Voodoo, like Creole, had no place in the "civilized" Haiti they were trying to build (see d'Ans 1985, Hurbon 1987a). During the twentieth century, however, Haitian intellectuals, influenced in large part by anthropology, became interested in the cultural institutions of the peasantry. The opinion of the "outside world" changed little, nonetheless, as the 1933 Oxford English Dictionary's definition of voodoo would suggest: "A body of superstitious beliefs and practices, including sorcery, serpent-worship, and sacrificial rites, current among negroes and persons of negro blood in the West Indies and southern United States, and ultimately of African origin."[3]

When voodoo was outlawed during the American occupation and its practitioners persecuted, some nationalist intellectuals came to see that the task at hand was to rehabilitate voodoo. Voodoo was for them no longer superstition; nor was it satanic. It was, rather, "the folk religion" of Haiti, and it was structured by a coherent set of beliefs and doctrines. In his campaign to validate Haitian popular culture, Jean Price-Mars, an ethnologist trained in medicine, claimed that "1804 was the product of voodoo" (Schmidt 1971:23). The 1927 publication of his influential book of essays, *Ainsi Parla l'Oncle*, led to a heightened awareness of the nature and roles of religion in rural Haiti. And yet the struggle over the legitimacy of voodoo continued. The largely French Catholic clergy later joined forces with the Haitian elite and initiated the blinkered and equally unsuccessful "antisuperstition campaign."[4]

Contemporary commentary reflects these struggles, and also the contributions of the ethnographic literature. Voodoo's defenders cast sorcery as a sideshow of voodoo, and insist that its significance within the religion has been greatly amplified by Hollywood and the sensationalist press. "Voodoo is a distinct religion comprising a body of beliefs, which are themselves linked by metaphysical ideas . . . logically stemming from a secret initiation," insists Maximilien (1945:222–223). "The believer in Voodoo," writes Rigaud (1985:7), "centers his hopes and fears as strongly on it as does a follower of Christianity, Judaism, Buddhism, or Islam."

Père Jacques Alexis is no doubt among those Haitians marked by this campaign to rehabilitate voodoo. In contrast to many foreign missionaries and their Haitian adepts, Père Alexis is slow to malign voodoo as evil. He does not use terms such as *satanic* when referring to voodoo. This is not to suggest that the priest is an absolute relativist: God is, for Alexis, the way and the light. It is simply that voodoo is regarded by Père Alexis as the "historical product of a people torn from Africa." He cites approvingly the role of voodoo in the Haitian revolution, and often states that the school erected in Do Kay is "for everyone—Catholics, Protestants, and *vaudouisants*." He also believes that sorcery accusations are "magical things" and "intimately related to voodoo." Referring to Manno, the priest had remarked,

In the end, he did not have the faith that he once had. He was sure that he was the victim of magic. These sorts of beliefs are deeply rooted in Haitians. They are part of our history. While he was seeing [the internist in Port-au-Prince], he may have been to the *houngan*'s house. . . . For all you know, Manno attributed his spectacular reprive to the efficacy of another [therapeutic] system. For all you know, he stopped taking the doctor's medications early in the spring.

Here we see the double opposition of "voodoo/Christianity" and "voodoo/biomedicine." In Kay, at least, it is in the event of serious illness that many of these divisions take on their practical significance. More often, this is not an either/or decision. Although several villagers have commented that "doctors' medicines and *houngan*'s medicines don't go together," their actions often belie their words: in the event of grave illness, many rural Haitians will faithfully avail themselves of the services of both *houngan* and *doktè*. But there are many examples of prostrating febrile illness, such as syndromes caused by malaria and typhoid, that are believed by both doctors and *houngan* to demand intensive and rapid intervention. The sick person cannot be in two places at once, and the family makes a decision.[5] The case of Manno, who disappeared from the Kay area for almost one month, is emblematic of the hard choices that the people of the region must occasionally make. Recall, too, the illness of Marie as discussed in chapter 5. It is in precisely such instances, when the *houngan* wins out, that Père Alexis most loudly deplores voodoo, casting it as a trap into which fall "weak people, further weakened by fear."[6] Those living in Do Kay also regard the options as reflecting two healing systems in direct confrontation. But insofar as theologic concepts go, the beliefs of a majority of villagers are far from those of Père Alexis.

Although a rough-hewn "voodoo/Christianity" dichotomy corresponds to ethnographically real practices and beliefs, its significance to rural Haitians like those I encountered is dramatically different from that suggested by the priest. The word *vodou* itself signifies different things to different people. Based on fieldwork in southern Haiti, Lowenthal (1978:393) asserts that the word "refers simply to a type of dance often held in the Haitian countryside, which does not necessarily occur in conjunction with religious ceremonial." For the liberally educated Père Alexis, the term connotes "a system of beliefs concerning man's relation to the spirit-world, and how to get by in this world." For people from Kay and surrounding villages, the signification of the term *vodou* lies between the restrictive concept described by Lowenthal and the all-embracing definition advanced by the priest. For most of those interviewed in Do Kay, *vodou* is something one does, rather than something in which one professes faith: people are held to "do" voodoo (*yo konn fè vodou lakay yo*), and what they are doing is not simply dancing, as in the south, but propitiating the *lwa* with food. They are *moun k'ap bay lwa manje*—"people who give food to the *lwa*." In the Kay area, the offertory aspects of voodoo are mentioned as often as the aesthetic aspects of the ceremonies.

Another word often deployed in discussions of voodoo is *maji*, or "magic." The term is invoked even more frequently, however, in discussions of serious illnesses when they afflict previously healthy adults and children who "have already escaped" (*gen tan chape*) the dangerous years between birth and the beginning of school. AIDS and tuberculosis are prime examples of such illnesses, as are some acute-onset febrile states such as cerebral malaria. According to Herskovits,

A difference of the first order exists between a *traitement* to heal an illness, and magic employed to gain an end, protect from harm, or injure one another, even though the same gods be called upon to validate the healing remedies employed to effect cures as are used to actuate a *garde* or a *wanga*. (Herskovits 1975:221)

Métraux agrees that the anthropologist and the rural Haitian have two very different things in mind when each refers to "magic," but Métraux suggests that the Haitian term has an even more restricted meaning, at least for voodoo adepts: "The Voodooist regards as 'magic' any rite accomplished with evil intent" (Métraux 1972:266). He is seconded by Hurbon (1987a:262), who notes "the murderous nature of magic, whether offensive or defensive." The residents of Do Kay, regardless of religious affiliation, have a similarly restricted idea of *maji*. In the central plateau of Haiti, one elderly doctor is famous for his prowess in healing "both simple sicknesses, and those with authors." After recounting scores of his magical cures, several people expressed surprise that I would ask, "Does he not do magic?" (*Eskè li pa konn fè maji?*). One of his admirers from Kay was offended that I would think such a thing.

The indigenous term, then, is *maji*, and it corresponds best to the etic term "sorcery." In Do Kay, there are many ways of ensorcelling an enemy. In addition to the rather dramatic methods employed by Étienne's detractor, there are more subtle powders—these may be sprinkled in the yard so that one's intended victim will tread on them—and there are *pakèt*, or sorcery bundles.[7] One often hears the expressions *kout poud* ("powder hit"), *kout batri* ("battery hit"), *kout zonbi* ("zombie hit"), and *movezè* ("evil wind"). A newer method is the *kout flach*, or "flashlight hit." In order to harm someone with a flashlight beam, one must send a "dead," a *zonbi*, into the flashlight. It can then be expedited onto someone by "flashing" him or her at night. These are rural Haitian realities, and seem to have little to do with religious affiliation. In 1987, after interviewing scores of adults, I could find only two villagers who denied the possibility of the expedition of the dead as a means of causing illness. The existence of *maji*, like the existence of God, goes virtually unquestioned.[8]

My findings would be classed by Père Alexis as perfect evidence that the typical resident of Kay "is involved in both voodoo and Christianity." The villagers make finer distinctions, however, as Mme. Jolibois's observations would suggest. Even divination, she states, is not necessarily considered the province of those who make offertory to the *lwa*:

There are also *houngan* who are not involved in voodoo. If you are sick, you can have a divination (*chapit*). The *houngan* lights a candle. He speaks with the candle, speaks with the flame. If it's death, he sees black, he doesn't see red. He needs a special yellow candle, made with beeswax.

Mme. Jolibois is cited to reveal another aspect of the terminological fuzziness involved in this discussion. She is *levanjil fran*, the rural Haitian equivalent of a "born-again Christian." When she states "my father raised me with the word of Christ," she means that she has no truck with those who feed the *lwa*. Unlike the *episkopal*, who like the Roman Catholics are thought to be tolerant of voodoo, the members of Mme. Jolibois's Baptist church decry voodoo as "satanic." Her neighbors agree that Mme. Jolibois is among those who have never frequented a *houmfor*. Her social supports are largely among those who share her exclusively Protestant practices. Accordingly, while exclusive adherence or conversion to a Protestant sect may radically alter religious practice, it does not call into question a host of understandings approximated most closely by the term "rural Haitian culture." While few would insist that the *lwa* do not exist, many would agree with Mme. Jolibois that there is an enormous difference between feeding the *lwa* in such an indirect manner and participating in large ceremonies, the *raison d'être* of which is to make offerings to the *lwa*. The *lwa* exist, whether one likes it or not, and the "pure Christian" (*levanjil fran*), as locally defined, is he or she who "does not make offerings to false gods."[9]

What is the response, then, to the question, "In which category may we class the events detailed by Étienne and experienced by much of his congregation?" The category is not *vodou* as locally defined, but *maji*, which may be glossed as sorcery. Further, the larger aegis under which *maji* should be classed is not "voodoo" as used by anthropologists. For voodoo is, as Lowenthal states, "a coherent system of belief and worship," and has certain defining characteristics: "In spite of marked regional variation in almost every other regard, possession and performance are everywhere a part of Haitian religion" (Lowenthal 1978: 411).

What is left when neither possession nor performance is relevant or requisite to engagement in a process such as that which evolved on a Sunday in August? It is not that these individuals are "closet" or "lapsed" voodooists. It is rather that such understandings of *maji* are shared by most rural Haitians, and are thus a part of *rural Haitian culture,* of which the theories and practices called voodoo are but one subset.[10] On that hot Sunday, the existence of sorcery was in all likelihood not a question in anyone's mind. That the calabash existed was *prima facie* proof that Étienne had been ensorcelled, and this was as true for the most devout of the exclusively Christian as for the servants of the *lwa,* almost all of whom profess faith in a Christian God. Divergences of opinion may have been significant whether or not Maître Gérard's intervention was a sufficient reply, but there was no doubt that Étienne had been the target of the willful malice of a rival.

2. Why was Étienne the victim of malign magic?

To judge from the commentary surrounding the three villagers with *sida,* Étienne was an unlikely victim of sorcery. If unequal distribution of wealth is a chief motive for such magic, Étienne, known to be exceedingly poor, would be exempt. In his testimonial, he summarily ruled out of consideration two other usual precipitants of malign magic: "I did not owe anyone any money," he said. "I had not argued with anyone." But Étienne omitted mention of a fourth reason for ensorcelling someone: as a counterattack for aggressive magic, a "reply."

It did not take long for this mechanism to be publicly invoked to explain the green calabash in Étienne's front room. Étienne's wife had been given a pig by Mme. Alexis. When the pig died writhing on the ground, Étienne cried foul: someone had given his pig *kola,* a poison, and the writhing told him that it was "not simple." But there was no consensus, this time. Other villagers did not believe that Étienne had been the victim of magic. His pig had died of natural causes. "He should have known better," said Mme. Dieugrand. "Who would begrudge the poor man a pig?" Étienne sought the advice of an *amatè* who informed him that Rezima, Étienne's neighbor across the road, had given the pig *kola.*[11] The same *amatè* "gave it back" to Rezima, who soon lost three of his seven pigs. Mme. Sonson echoed Mme. Dieugrand:

Everyone knows that Rezima did not kill Étienne's pig. Why would he do that, with all the pigs he's got? [Étienne] was just jealous that Rezima had so many pigs, so he gave them *kola.* But now he's in over his head, poor thing, and he's frightened.

The fear is in itself diagnostic of sorcery. Étienne insists that the discovery of the calabash "did not startle me," but there was widespread sympathy for what he must have been feeling: "The sensation of being caught in an almost irreversible situation overtakes the person" (Hurbon 1987a:261). What does Étienne fear most? That he or a member of his family will next be the victims of a major illness, or a series of misfortunes. The calculus of accusation and retribution outlined in previous chapters is not irrelevant to Étienne's dilemma. He was the victim of magic, and magic is almost always used to do harm. As is clear from opinions about Dieudonné's illness, however, not all magic is thought of as unjust.[12] No one interviewed would go so far as to suggest that Étienne was getting what he deserved, but almost everyone observed that he should not have killed Rezima's pigs.

3. *What should Étienne do as an Episcopalian who is the victim of magic?*

Étienne stated that he put the matter before the members of his church, as "it's here that I worship." In so doing, he engendered the ritual interventions described above: he generated a good deal of community support, and some sympathy. Another probable step would be to divine who had placed the *wanga* in his front room, and why. I soon discovered that Étienne had also sought the services of an *amatè* skilled in divination. From the *amatè*, Étienne learned that the *wanga* had been placed by Rezima.

Knowing who had ensorcelled him, and also the reason why, should Étienne next seek to ensorcel Rezima? What steps might Étienne take to protect himself and his family? A radical option would be to escape this escalating magical war by pretending that, as a Christian, he would be protected by his faith from harm through magic. Only one person in Do Kay has undergone conversion to a radically antivoodoo Protestant sect. But even she does not deny the *existence* of magic and related practices. She merely professes assurance that she will not be its victim.

In the days following the calabash burning, several villagers were asked about the options open to Étienne. Some thought that the prudent course of action would be to seek magical protection through the use of amulets, charms, protective baths, or drinks. Many observed that Étienne should pray for God's protection. The most striking finding for me, however, was that none of those surveyed thought that Étienne should employ magic against "the person who placed the calabash" (few referred to Rezima by name). And almost no one thought that

Étienne would continue the struggle with another *contre-coup*. Although it was not possible to pinpoint the source of this mysterious consensus, it spoke of some widely held tenets regarding the "rules of the game."

4. Finally, how does maji serve as a moral barometer in a setting such as Do Kay?

As it does throughout the world, serious illness leads Haitians to ask, "Why me?" or "Why her?" In the case of grave illness in young adults, the question is posed persistently and answers emerge. These answers must make sense. That is, the answers are embedded in illness stories that render the illness meaningful. The stories must themselves be embedded in powerful explanatory frameworks if they are to prove compelling. The most important of several organizing paradigms—"the master trope"—is one that involves concepts of equality. For many Haitians, "equality" has come to mean shared poverty. Fear of magic reinforces a concern central to life in rural Haiti. Fear of magic forces questions concerning the way that villagers get along with one another, the way they share their poverty.

Events that involve *maji* fit into a number of interlocking cultural systems, of which voodoo and brands of Christianity are important but not determinant parts. In addition to the complex models that inform the experience of severe illness, other contributing frameworks include widely shared understandings of poverty and wealth, offense and retribution, good and evil.[13] Regardless of their ultimate origins—many point to West Africa, others to seventeenth-century France—contemporary understandings of *maji* took shape on the terrain of Saint-Domingue, where sorcery and poison became the slaves' best defense against their oppressors. After the revolution, these understandings endured, and great misfortune leads many latter-day Haitians to ask themselves which of their enemies are afflicting them. The lineage of these understandings is suggested by the term *makandal,* still used in Haiti to refer to poison, whether magic or toxin or both. Notably, Dieudonné Gracia remarked that his aggressor "was not silly, he knew what a guy without a weapon had to do. If it was a person [who sent the illness], then it was a *makandal,* and it had to come from jealousy."

These concerns, concepts, and fears are deeply interwoven with the realities of serious illness, and have contributed to the social construction of *sida* in Kay. The calculus of blame that emerged during Manno's illness is common in rural Haiti. When it became clear that he had been ensorcelled, Manno and his family thought immediately of his relatively good fortune at landing three paying positions in the community development project administered by Père Alexis. "Who lost out," the family soon asked, "when Manno was chosen for these jobs?" The losers were his fellow schoolteachers, who were passed over by the priest when he sought a "right-hand man" to help with the pig and water projects. Pierre, for example, was "a native of Kay, and ought to have been awarded the work before a stranger," as his aunt put it. Several interviewed also remarked that Pierre was poorer than Manno, as was Maître Fritz. Further, many suspected that Père Alexis did not care for Fritz, which led Fritz to despise Manno even more. It is for precisely this reason that Dieudonné termed *sida* a "jealousy sickness."

The obvious backdrop to sorcery in the Kay area is fierce competition in a field of great scarcity.[14] In the majority of the cases examined in previous chapters, that scarcity is material (Manno, Anita's lover, Dieudonné, Étienne), but may also be complicated by more affective considerations, as was the case with Marie (chapter 5). In the Do Kay area, sorcery accusations are also marshalled against those who advance too quickly in terms of material advantage. An often invoked proverb underlines this calculus: *Mezi lajan ou, se mezi wanga ou,* which may be translated as "the extent of your wealth is a gauge of the strength of your spells."[15] It is also important to underline that what is shared in rural Haiti is *extreme poverty,* and to hypothesize that, in settings in which there is a history of widely shared status, especially poverty, those who break out of that status are likely to be accused of sorcery, especially if they are "inside outsiders"—originally of the same class (for example, peasants) but in some way distinguishable from other members of the community. In Do Kay, Manno, the *moun vini,* was such a person. In the suburbs of Port-au-Prince, where all the rural people were *moun vini,* Dieudonné was the most recent arrival.

In a setting like Do Kay—as in contemporary Haiti generally—the most glaring anomaly is the unequal distribution of material goods, and disturbances in the social field are quite often borne of envy. In such a zero-sum setting, one person's fortune is manifestly another's ill fortune. The price of wealth for one is poverty for another. "Fear of sorcery," observes Taussig (1980:117), "is tantamount to fear of having more than others, and having more indicates failure to share. Sorcery is evil. But its roots are embedded in legitimate concerns in areas in which competition pits individualism and communalism against each other."[16]

An example of such inequity and the accusations it engenders is to be found in the case of Fardin, a livestock trader who was a water refugee. In almost uniformly poor Kay, Fardin's conspicuously nice house—four rooms, a cement floor, a spacious and well-kept courtyard—is clearly the target of no small amount of envy. Mme. Sonson, who lives across the road from Fardin and is ostensibly friendly with his wife, explained to me how he came to be "rich." He "sought the help of a *baka* [evil spirit], and the *baka* gave him money. But he had to give up his own mother! One day his date will come, and the *baka* will devour him."[17]

The tendency of rural Haitians to suspect that such pacts are at the root of the accumulation of personal wealth has been much commented on in the ethnographic literature. "The individual who begins to enrich himself in a rapid and spectacular fashion must have broken the rules of the game and gone looking for strong *pwen*; in other words, [he must have] purchased spiritual powers, bad *lwa* or *baka* in order to steal away his neighbor's vital force, or that of a member of his own family" (Hurbon 1987a:266).[18] Indeed, Métraux claims that such suspicions are unique to Haitians:

Specifically Haitian is the tendency to attribute the wealth or even simply the well-being of others to shady dealings with evil spirits. The Haitian finds it difficult to admit that anyone might become rich without having made an arrangement with a sorceror. There are always people ready to pretend they know the exact nature of the contract with a *diab* by which such and such a *grand don* was enabled to complete his fortune: to be rich is to be something of a sorceror. Naturally, all this is the eternal jealousy of the peasant, here taking the form of magical imputations. (Métraux 1972:287)

But how "specifically Haitian" are such beliefs? If Hurbon's thesis is correct, many of these are the legacy not just of Saint-Domingue, but of the inequity born of the European penetration of the New World. Similar conditions should have given rise to similar understandings—similar "structures of feeling"—of sorcery elsewhere.[19] In the Cauca Valley of Colombia, wage laborers who sport new finery or in some other way demonstrate increased income are liable to be accused, like Fardin, of making a pact with the devil. And as was the case with Fardin, it will be predicted that such men will die premature deaths because of this pact (Taussig 1980). But the correlation of magic and inequity can lead to different conclusions. Among the Chagga of Kilimanjaro, for example, "poverty may lead the community to suspect [the poor man] of malice, and consequently he or his wife may be accused of sorcery or witchcraft when misfortunes befall his more fortunate kinsmen" (Moore 1975a:137). Writing of the dynamics of accusation in Haiti, Hurbon (1987a) notes that the accused are usually "the weakest," and observes that women are most often accused.

Maji in Do Kay more often follows a somewhat different logic. In sixteen cases of more or less public sorcery accusations leveled between 1986 and 1988, eleven of the accused were men. Most frequently invoked as the ultimate cause of *maji* in Kay were "issues of inheritance, jealousy, the trampling of someone in his own space," which Hurbon (1987a:264) regards as secondary. On a third point, however, local sorcery accusations are as Hurbon describes them: involving persons who are also poor and disempowered. It was Manno's peers who were accused of sending the dead, and this pattern was to be repeated in subsequent AIDS-related accusations.

There are no hard-and-fast rules that would enable us to discern the moral logic behind all sorcery accusations. What is clear, however, is that sorcery runs up and down grades caused by perceived inequality. In her study of kuru in Papua New Guinea, Lindenbaum (1979:146) made a similar observation: "A geography of fear tracks unequal relations." *Sida*-related accusations also reflect the concerns of a "people of poverty," to use one villager's phrase, competing in a field of great scarcity. That sorcery accusations remain curiously intraclass was deeply disturbing to Dieudonné, who asked, "Why is it always the poor attacking the poor?" One answer is simply that the poor *are able* to attack their peers, or the even poorer. For, to paraphrase Dieudonné, "the guys without weapons know what they can and cannot do." The rulers of Haiti have put in place many safeguards to assure that there are no contemporary echoes—even purely symbolic ones—of 1804.

For much of the past 186 years, the foreign-supported elite has relied on village-level lackeys to implement its taxation and its repression. Most of these lackeys—rural constabulary, *macoutes,* enlisted men—are themselves from the impoverished peasant class. And so there have been few struggles openly pitting the poor against their oppressors; there have been many struggles among the poor. Some of these struggles have been magical, in the Haitian sense of the term, and have yielded nothing in the way of advancement for the rural poor. That the tragedy of these arrangements does not escape popular consciousness is suggested by the often invoked proverb: "Rotten teeth can still sink into ripe bananas." No matter how poor and disempowered one is, there will always be another who is even weaker.

19

AIDS and Racism:
Accusation in the Center

Homosexuals in New York take vacations in Haiti, and we suspect that this may be an epidemic Haitian virus that was brought back to the homosexual population in the United States.

Dr. Bruce Chabner, National Cancer
Institute, December 1, 1982

There were no AIDS in the USA until the illegal criminal Haitian dogs came.

Anonymous, sent to Haitian community agency in
Miami (postmarked May 1983)

Maybe they will kill me in Haiti. The government doesn't forget anything there. But this is worse. This is no country for black people. I will never come back, no matter what.

Affidavit of Beauvoir Pierre,
October 20, 1989, awaiting deportation
to Haiti by the U.S. INS

From the first years of the North American epidemic, when AIDS was widely termed the "gay plague," members of the gay community answered homophobia with a rich cultural response that included artfully staged demonstrations, denunciations in the straight and gay presses, and an effective movement to provide services to gay men with HIV disease. Gay cultural activism in response to AIDS has brought us novels, poetry, plays, movies and even television specials. The dimensions and ardor of this response have been much commented on in the literature on AIDS in North America, and served to focus early debate about AIDS-related discrimination on the nation's abundant homophobia. But the debate may have been too narrowly focused, as one assessment suggests: "In this country, AIDS has so far evoked less pointedly racist reactions than in Europe, including the Soviet Union, where the African origin of the disease is stressed" (Sontag 1988:62). Haitians living in the United States would vigorously contest Sontag's assertion. As early as 1981, members of the Haitian community denounced the racism inherent in the stigmatization of Haitians—*qua* Haitians—as "AIDS-carriers." They have done so loudly and in chorus. How were these voices missed by as astute an observer as Sontag? "Their voices have been unheard," one Haitian anthropologist believes, "because of their triple minority status as black, foreign, and French- and Creole-speaking" (Laguerre 1984:9).

Nor were Haitian voices heard in a debate on Haitian migration to the United States, a debate that began to intensify a decade ago. In chapter 17, the current economic and political conditions of Haiti were outlined, including the phenomenon of the massive out-migration that has also gathered steam during the past three decades.[1] Beginning in the 1960s, Haitians came to the United States both legally and clandestinely, in airplanes and in boats, for many of the same reasons that had drawn previous waves of immigrants: to escape violence and poverty, to raise families, to work. Although Haitians have sought employment outside their country throughout this century, the majority of those currently living in North America arrived during the past three decades. It was during the Duvaliers' dictatorships that state-sponsored violence was coupled with decreasing agricultural productivity and what seemed to Haitians to be irreversible immiseration. Haiti became, as many have observed, an exporter of people: professionals, intellectuals, merchants, craftsmen, and, especially, manual laborers.

These refugees were not welcomed in the United States, and many were clapped into detention by the U.S. Immigration and Naturalization Service:

Although the seventies were a time when immigrants in general came under attack, immigrants other than Haitians were not detained simply because of their nationality; Haitians, however, were rounded up and placed in federal "detention centers" that were in fact concentration camps. Haitians were por-

trayed as ragged, wretched, and pathetic and were said to be illiterate, superstitious, disease-ridden and backward peasants. They became visible scapegoats
for the failure of U.S. capitalism. (Glick-Schiller and Fouron 1990:337)

The INS argued that Haitians were "economic refugees," fleeing poverty and thus inadmissible as refugees. The flight of the Haitian people,
many Haitians countered, is as political as it is economic: it is migration
prescribed by political economy. The contemporary political-economic
conditions in Haiti make it impossible for most Haitians to live and
work in Haiti.

The "Mystery" of AIDS in Haitian-Americans

The ongoing disagreement over what constituted a "political refugee" was fanned when North American human rights advocates joined Haitians in deploring the detention as illegal and inhu-
mane. AIDS emerged at the very height of this debate:

As if to add fuel to the fire of protest over Haitian refugees, shortly after a three-
judge panel of the Court of Appeals for the Eleventh Circuit in Atlanta upheld
[Judge] Spellman's decision to release 1,800 Haitian detainees from fourteen
detention camps, the popular media were rife with reports of the spread of a
deadly new disease. (Laguerre 1984:13)

By November 1981, just a few months after what would later be
termed AIDS was first reported in the medical literature, a number of
Haitian immigrants had been seen in Florida hospitals with infections
characteristic of the syndrome.[2] Several more cases were soon reported
among Haitians living in the New York area. The U.S. Centers for
Disease Control (CDC) announced, in July 1982, that thirty-four
"Haitians residing in the United States" had been stricken with opportunistic infections (CDC 1982a). Seven of these patients were women.
In the same year, Canadian officials also learned of such infections in
a Haitian immigrant. In a study published in January 1983, Viera and
colleagues described AIDS in forty "previously well Haitians," several
of whom were recent immigrants. Pitchenik et al. (1983) reported "a
new acquired immunodeficiency state," detailing opportunistic infections in "twenty Haitian patients living in the Miami-Dade area in
Florida." The title of a similar report in the *Journal of the American Medical Association* announced "Unusual Causes of Death in Haitians Resid-

ing in Miami" (Moskowitz et al. 1983). Ten cases in Haitian-born persons were soon reported from Montreal (Ernst et al. 1983, and LeBlanc et al. 1983).

Unlike other North American patients meeting diagnostic criteria for AIDS, the Haitian immigrants denied that they had engaged in homosexual activity or intravenous drug use. Most had never had a blood transfusion. Almost all other cases of the syndrome known at the time implicated one or more of these risk factors. Although the CDC had previously released data on AIDS in heterosexuals, "the article on Haitians constituted the first complete report focusing directly on persons outside the 'homosexual' category" (Oppenheimer 1988:282). "The Haitians," notes Choi (1987:19) in a review of AIDS epidemiology, "remained the wild cards," and AIDS among Haitians was, in the words of many researchers, "a complete mystery."

Treichler (1989:34) has observed that "when one aspect of the AIDS story is declared impenetrably mysterious, reason and control must be elsewhere recuperated." Indeed, U.S. public health officials were faced with the task of tidying up the nongroupable cases. In order to accurately assess risk among Haitian immigrants, a sound knowledge of the size of this population was necessary. However, no such data were available. Instead of acknowledging its inability to make an assessment of risk, the official—and spuriously low—figure of 200,000 recent Haitian entrants was initially used as the denominator.[3] The resulting conceptual round-up officially brought *all* Haitians together in a "risk group."[4] The CDC had inferred that Haitians *per se* were in some way at risk for AIDS. On March 4, 1983, the CDC referred for the first time to four "high-risk groups," underlining similarities between the evolving AIDS epidemiological patterns and those that had been seen with hepatitis B. Soon, members of these groups were popularly termed the "Four-H Club," a shorthand reference to homosexuals, Haitians, hemophiliacs, and heroin-users.

The CDC report acknowledged that each of the four groups delineated—which were, more accurately, homosexual men with multiple sexual partners, hemophiliacs, users of intravenous drugs, and recent Haitian immigrants—probably contained many individuals who were not at risk for AIDS (CDC 1983:466). "Nonetheless," observes Oppenheimer (1988:282), "no calibration of degree-of-risk was introduced, so no distinction could be drawn. As no microbe had been isolated, risk designation was, in effect, synonymous with carrier status, even among scientists, not to speak of the news media and among the general public."[5] Thus was born the new equation, "Haitian = AIDS carrier," or, as Saint-Gérard (1984:72) put it, Haitians as "the AIDS vectors." Within weeks, the popular press seized on the CDC inference as a news item, and thus the addition of Haitians to the risk groups prompted innumerable unflattering portrayals of both Haitians and Haitian-Americans.

And there was more to come. In a calculus of blame that surprised few Haitians, the disease was said to have *come from* Haiti. Siegal and Siegal (1983:85) offer what they call "compelling" evidence of the link between Haiti and the origin of the American AIDS epidemic: three cases of transfusion-related transmission (only one of which, date unspecified, took place in Haiti), and the case of a former nun whose sole sexual contact was said to have been in Haiti, where she worked for thirty years. She died in Canada in 1981 "of a disease that her doctors retrospectively recognized as AIDS." According to the authors, these "compelling" data "suggest that the disease is quite prevalent in Haiti; that it predated AIDS in the United States; and that it may be endemic there" (Siegal and Siegal 1983:85).

During the first half of 1983, which Leibowitch (1985:69) terms "the highly imaginative period" of AIDS research, similar speculations appeared in all major medical journals and in a variety of other scholarly publications. And these exotic theories were propagated even as Haitian researchers answered them with surveys showing that Kaposi's sarcoma and opportunistic infections were new to Haiti.[6] The theories were echoed in the popular presses, both straight and gay, and the North American folk model of Haitians was quickly renovated to make room for the new qualifier, AIDS-carrier. Public perception along the eastern seaboard seemed to have added "AIDS" to the folk model that had previously relied so strongly on voodoo imagery.

An Epidemic of Discrimination

In a recent study of the U.S. response to AIDS, the spread of HIV was compared to that of polio, another virus that struck young people, triggered public panic, and received regular attention in the popular media. "Although these parallels are strong," notes the author, "one difference is crucial: there was little early sympathy for victims of AIDS because those initially at risk—homosexual men, Haitian immigrants, and drug addicts—were not in the mainstream of society. In contrast, sympathy for polio patients was extensive" (Panem 1988:15).[7] The opprobrium felt by all deemed "at-risk" was great indeed. There were important differences, however, in the nature of the scorn meted out to members of the different groups, the nature of their responses to discrimination, and the resources available to respond to the needs of these communities. Further, the logic by which the groups were defined varied radically from group to group:

The Haitian people as a whole, marked *hereditarily* by its ethno-cultural features, found itself, with regard to AIDS, in the same position as other sociocultural groups with sociologically *acquired* characteristics: homosexuals or intravenous drug users. The crime of racial discrimination with regard to the entire Haitian nation was imminent. (Leibowitch 1985:79)

The effects of these speculations upon Haiti were indeed disastrous. The burden of the new syndrome was not apparent before 1983—after all, forty AIDS cases did not add up to much against a background of tuberculosis, typhoid, malaria, malnutrition, and political repression. But the effect of AIDS-related *discrimination* would be instantly palpable. As late as the fall of 1982, notes Abbott (1988:203),

Haitians had no inkling of the havoc that would be wrought by the advent of AIDS, a problem that very shortly the world would blame on Haiti and accuse her of exporting. As punishment, her people would be officially listed as one of the "four H's" at high risk of AIDS.

The material effects of these social forces were apparent even to foreign observers, and 1983 brought Haiti only deepening crisis as the year progressed. The tourist industry was the first to fall. By 1980, tourism had become one of the country's largest sources of foreign currency, and generated employment for tens of thousands living in and around Port-au-Prince. By 1983, it had become almost nonexistent.

For many Haitians, AIDS was perceived as the proverbial last straw, and outside assessment concurred: "Nowhere in the hemisphere is poverty so harsh," blared *U.S. News and World Report* on October 31, 1983. "Now the backlash of the AIDS scare is making it worse." But the anti-Haitian backlash may have been felt as keenly in North American cities. In March 1983, the United States Public Health Service recommended that Haitian-Americans not donate blood, and school blood drives openly excluded Haitian adolescents. As veterans of calumny, Haitians living in the United States and Canada were quick to sense the prejudices that underpinned many of these responses:

The AIDS epidemic came at a time when the U.S. government policy, as evidenced by Coast Guard interdiction of Haitian vessels and by the prolonged incarceration of new Haitian arrivals in Krome and other camps, seemed to most Haitians to single them out as special targets of a racist and exclusionary attitude pervasive in this country. (Nachman and Dreyfuss 1986:33)

In New York City alone, reports from many quarters seemed to confirm Haitian charges. A schoolteacher related that "children of Haitian origin are being taunted in the school because of the connection in the scientific literature and the public media between Haitians and AIDS" (Sencer 1983:25). A physician working at a Brooklyn hospital reported that "on several occasions we have received phone calls from prospective employers of Haitians asking if it was safe to employ them" (Landesman 1983:35). In Brooklyn, walls on the margins of a predominantly Caribbean neighborhood were sprayed with "Haitians = Niggers with AIDS." By 1984, it had become clear to the newly formed AIDS Discrimination Unit of the New York City Commission on Human Rights that the effects of the risk-group classification on the local Haitian community were "devastating." One member of the unit reported that "Haitian children have been beaten up (and in at least one case, shot) in school; Haitian store owners have gone bankrupt as their businesses failed; and Haitian families have been evicted from their homes" (Sabatier 1988:47).

Stories about the tribulations of Haitians living in Canada and elsewhere in the United States soon circulated. A social-service organization in South Florida reported that, following the inclusion of Haitians on the CDC listing, it was suddenly unable to find job placements for a majority of its clients.[8] The same organization also received hate mail, which conveyed such slogans as "Hire a Haitian—Help Spread AIDS," and "There were [sic] no AIDS in the USA until the illegal criminal Haitian dogs came." One letter, postmarked July 15, 1983, had the following warning:

On Tuesday, July 19th we are mailing 6,000 of the below notices to all hotels, motels, and restaurants in South Florida. "Tourists and businesspeople are avoiding the South Florida area because of the plague of AIDS, hepatitis and TB spread by the criminal, illegal aliens of Haitian origin. If you employ a Haitian, discharge him as soon as you receive this letter. Help South Florida."

Several of these were signed "United Taxpayers Association." A Miami-based tropical medicine specialist reported "several calls a day" from anxious citizens, and reported that "people have sent Haitian house-helpers to the clinic for physical check-ups, because they're afraid of AIDS."[9] Another journalist reported that "just trying on a pair of shoes in Florida sometimes became a traumatic experience, because sales-people declined to let anyone who looked Haitian near the merchan-dise" (Shilts 1987:322).

The CDC, the FDA, and Other (Haitian) Household Acronyms

Although Haitians living in North America often dis-agreed over homeland politics, there was an initial show of unity when they were confronted with AIDS-related discrimination. One Boston cab driver, speaking in 1985, linked the apparent unanimity to the im-pact that such discrimination had on the immigrants' ability to make a living: "We are slow to anger, even when they are insulting us. But these are rumors that are keeping us from living." That these sentiments were widespread is suggested by a number of the songs popular at this time, including those which mentioned AIDS explicitly. One popular performer, Ti Manno, titled a 1984 album "SIDA." In the title cut, he decried the disorder as another means of "rich corrupt countries" to oppress poor and black people. As such, it was nothing new:

Through his music, Ti Manno, more powerfully than any of the self-identified Haitian leaders, had attacked the stigmatization of Haitians as carriers of AIDS. The stigmatization was for him *one aspect of the general rejection of Haitians by American society and the world,* a rejection that he countered with assertions of Haitian pride and a strong positive Haitian identity. (Glick-Schiller and Fouron 1990:329–330; emphasis added)

Most Haitians shared Ti Manno's interpretation of AIDS-related discrimination. The struggle to confront North American racism briefly united the fractious "diaspora."[10] And yet the consensus soon proved ephemeral. Some Haitians, especially those living in the United States "illegally," were reluctant to voice anti-American sentiments. In dias-pora communities throughout North America, Haitians were caught between their badly battered nationalist pride and the drive to survive. This double bind led to damaging attempts on the part of some to con-ceal Haitian identity. Casper (1986:201) cites a poignant example of the effects of the AIDS stigma on Haitian-Americans: "A Haitian man without AIDS states: 'People avoid shaking my hand when they know

I'm Haitian. And my wife and I won't speak Haitian at the laundromat because other people are afraid to use the same machine as us. We can pass as Jamaican.'" Syndicated columnist Ann Landers leapt to the defense of a light-skinned Haitian woman whose South American husband had taken in recent months to introducing her as French. "Haitians Did Not Bring AIDS to U.S.," ran the headline of her nationwide column. In Boston, it was more of the same. One taxi driver put it as follows:

My wife and I have lived here [in the U.S.] for fifteen years, and we speak English well, and I do O.K. driving. But the hardest time I've had in all my life, harder than Haiti, was when people would refuse to get in my cab when they discovered I was from Haiti. It got so we would pretend to be from somewhere else, which is the worst thing you can do, I think.

In the two years following the 1983 classing of Haitians as a "risk group," community activists attempted to rally Haitians around the issue. Physicians and community leaders in New York and South Florida formed coalitions in order to counter what they claimed to be a racist and specifically anti-Haitian stance. These coalitions conducted seminars, community meetings, and lobbied public health officials regarding the risk groupings.[11] They inundated the editors of medical and popular presses with letters deploring what they took to be a scientifically flawed argument made acceptable—and even popular—by racism. "The response of public health officials and AIDS researchers to Haitian protest has ranged," note Nachman and Dreyfuss (1986: 33), "from outrage to sympathetic understanding."

Among the more sympathetic institutions was the usually sluggish New York City Department of Health. Under considerable pressure from Haitian-American community leaders, the department excised "Haitian" from its official list of risk groups in the summer of 1983. The category was not easily removed, however, from the list then firmly established in the popular imagination. As one Haitian-American physician complained, "After all the wild theories of voodoo rites and genetic predisposition were aired and dispelled, and the slipshod scientific investigations were brought to light, the public perception of the problem has remained the same—that if Haitians have AIDS, it is very simply because they are Haitians" (Smith 1983:46).

Although most of their commentary has focused on North American racism, many Haitians were especially angry with public health authorities, most notably the CDC. Indeed, the name of this previously obscure branch of the public health service became a household acronym among Haitians. Mustering scientific data, notably those showing that attack rates for AIDS were lower in Haiti than in several other Caribbean islands and in most U.S. cities, the Haitian community groups insisted that the CDC abandon its classification. The CDC resisted, maintaining once again that each risk group was expressly stated to have large numbers of persons not at risk. Furthermore, the CDC had not meant to imply that persons were at risk of AIDS through mere casual contact with members of the risk group. If such fears existed, they were discriminatory; the CDC regretted such misinterpretations. The Haitians, however, were not readily placated:

The apology of the CDC missed the point. Grouping individuals may be traditional in epidemiology, both as a means of intervention and as an analytic prerequisite. The political or social consequences of such grouping are rarely examined. In this instance, even if the fear of casual transmission could be eradicated, the groups identified would still be seen as bearing a strong negative relationship to the life-sustaining blood supply. They were created, qua groups, to signify their potential status as carriers of tainted blood and as contaminators. Moreover, the analogy with the highly contagious hepatitis B virus reinforced the association of casual or vertical transmission, particularly for health-care providers. (Oppenheimer 1988:283)

The struggle between Haitian groups and the CDC continued throughout 1984. In April 1985 the CDC at last removed, without comment, the term "Haitian" as a risk-group designation. But community leaders were quick to point out that the stigma remained. In a review of the effects of the classification among Haitians in South Florida, Nachman and Dreyfuss (1986:33) reach the following conclusion:

One might at least charge the CDC with poor judgment in treating AIDS as no more than a medical issue and ignoring its social, economic, political, moral and other dimensions. By ignoring these, health officials have seriously hurt the Haitian community. A similar charge can be leveled against medical researchers and clinicians who assume that their scientific and medical priorities are shared by members of the nonmedical community.

The Haitian community of researchers is similarly resentful: "When the CDC removed Haitians from the list of risk groups, it refused to admit it made an error," commented Dr. Jean Pape (Sabatier 1988:46) in 1987. "Even now the CDC continues to stigmatize Haitians by preventing them from donating blood in the United States."

Actually, it was the U.S. Food and Drug Administration (FDA) that until recently barred Haitians from donating blood in the United States. The FDA had originally stipulated that Haitians who had reached the United States after 1977 could not donate blood. On February 5, 1990, the agency issued a ruling prohibiting *all* Haitians from donating blood. The dimensions of the imminent Haitian response to this ruling were not foreshadowed by a news story that ran less than two weeks after the ruling was made: "School Cancels Blood Drive After Haitians Are Barred."[12] If the Haitian reaction had been somewhat timid in the early years of such rulings, this time members of the diaspora community reacted with unanimity and in great numbers. The *New York Times,* in an article headlined "Now, No Haitians Can Donate Blood" and published on March 14, 1990, reported that "more than 5,000 Haitian-Americans [marched] outside an F.D.A. office in Miami last week, snarling Miami International Airport traffic. 'Racists!' the crowd chanted." In the popular press and on television, there seemed to be widespread incomprehension.[13] Why all the fuss over being prevented from donating blood?

Indeed, the fuss did not make sense to those who did not regard the FDA ruling as related to a host of other slights stretching back over the century.[14] In the Miami demonstration, there were frequent references to American racism, U.S. support for the Duvalier regime and its successor juntas, the incarceration of Haitians at Krome, and even the U.S. occupation of Haiti. Similar demonstrations soon followed in other cities on the eastern seaboard. On innumerable placards, the FDA was rebaptized the "Federal Discrimination Agency." Following a large Boston rally, in which thousands of Haitians deplored the FDA ruling, representatives of the U.S. government felt obliged to reply:

"When people donate blood they are given a list of questions on sexual activity, hemophilia, things that might lead one to be at a higher risk," explained Brad Stearns of the FDA. "Those questions don't work as well where heterosexual activity is a primary means of transmission. Haitians are not a higher risk group per se, but we don't have effective screening devices."[15]

If effective screening devices were lacking, some queried, then why was Haiti singled out? Because singling out Haiti was an "American specialty," riposted Haitian leaders, underlining the consonance between blaming Haiti and the long tradition of official American anti-Haitianism. Other Caribbean countries had higher attack rates and equally complex patterns of transmission, and yet natives of these islands were not included in the ruling. One sympathizer editorialized in the *Boston Globe*:

If the FDA were honest about geographic bans, it would have halted blood donations by all San Franciscans. In that city, the new case rate last year, according to the federal Centers for Disease Control, was ten times that of Haiti, 114.5 per 100,000. The FDA would also have banned natives of San Juan and New York City, where the respective rates were 86.8 and 69.4. . . . Most of you readers would have been banned. The city [of Boston] said its new case rate last year was 58.1 per 100,000. The CDC's rate for greater Boston is 16.0, still higher than Haiti's.[16]

The Haitian protesters, however, did not mention these regional data, preferring instead to dwell on the motivations of the North Americans: "We Haitians look at all of this as connected," one community activist was quoted as saying. "We know that for ten years now, the U.S. has been trying to eliminate us from the country, after they let Duvalier destroy ours."[17] Several of the placards expressed solidarity with inhabitants of "Africa," in reference to the banning of blood donations from those originating in "sub-Saharan Africa." In fact, the common refrain at these rallies was "Let's fight AIDS, not nationality."

Instead of losing steam after major protests in all the cities with large numbers of Haitians, the movement seemed to grow, culminating in a mammoth rally held on April 20, 1990, in New York City. So many marchers—fifty thousand according to the police, more than twice that according to organizers—crossed the Brooklyn Bridge that it was closed to traffic for the day. With the support of a broad coalition of African-Americans, including newly elected Mayor David Dinkins and the Reverend Jesse Jackson, lower Manhattan became a sea of black faces. The New York-based Haitian press ran lead stories about the demonstrations for days on end:

Such a crowd, it was remarked, had not been seen in New York since the 1968 funeral of Martin Luther King: 150,000 Haitians and non-Haitians—and even more according to some estimates— marching on April 20 to protest the FDA's discriminatory decision to exclude Haitians from the list of [potential] blood donors under the pretext that they are carriers of the AIDS virus.[18]

Taken aback by this unanticipated and unaccustomed attack, the FDA immediately formed an advisory panel to reconsider the February ruling. Within a week of the New York rally, the panel called for an end to donor bans based on nationality or geography: "We'd like to do it as quickly as possible," remarked one FDA spokesperson to the press.[19] The move, applauded by Haitians everywhere, was deplored by the *New York Times* in an April 29 editorial: "The FDA needs to think more carefully before accepting its committee's advice. Preventing discrimination is a high priority. Keeping the blood supply free of deadly disease and ensuring adequate supplies surely ranks even higher." Evidently, the leadership of the FDA agreed, for the agency did not implement its own panel's recommendation. The Haitians continued organizing. Large rallies were held in several U.S. cities, including one Washington march from the Capitol steps to the headquarters of the FDA. Finally, in December 1990, the FDA formally rescinded its ban on Haitian blood.

While the debate over the blood supply continued, one thing had become clear: AIDS-related discrimination was an issue that could mobilize diaspora Haitians like no other. Indeed, the attendance at the New York rally surpassed that expected by all concerned. "The number of protesters—college students, factory workers, and families with picnic baskets—surprised the Police Department, which had expected several thousand people."[20] "Haitians Surprised, Too" ran the headline of a subsequent article examining the phenomenon.[21] Why did these rallies draw such large crowds? Why did even those Haitians who were once frightened of publicly espousing "anti-American" positions attend these demonstrations? Why did the largest Haitian demonstrations involve AIDS-related discrimination and not, let us say, U.S. support for the military junta that had betrayed the elections of 1987? The answers to these questions were suggested by the sorts of people who attended the events: workers and students. Haitians had come to the United States to work and study, activities that had become impossible in Haiti. And AIDS-related discrimination compromised these activities more than any of the other forces that had demoralized these communities since their establishment.[22]

Racism and Exoticism in American Folk Models

If the Haitian response deserves close study, so too does the stimulus of their protests. What might explain the profusion of theories about a Haitian origin of AIDS? Why was so much attention paid to the red herring of voodoo?[23] Why were such theories so widely and uncritically accepted? What might explain their resonance among North Americans in the popular *and* scientific sectors? In a review of the response of the U.S. press to the AIDS epidemic, Albert (1986: 174–175) notes that Haitian-Americans "present preexisting characteristics of an already non-normative character. They are black, tend to be poor, are recent immigrants, and the association of Haiti with cult-religious practices fuels the current tendency to see deviance in groups at-risk for AIDS." In other words, the Haitian cases fit the already established script: the incidence of AIDS in Haitians served to *reinforce* the stigma experienced by those with AIDS. For this to be so, there must have been strong, preexisting "folk models" of Haitians.

In fact, the press drew upon readily available images of filthy squalor, voodoo, and boatloads of "disease-ridden" or "economic" refugees. Several articles even made oblique or direct references to cannibalism. Dr. Jeffrey Viera, the senior author of the 1983 paper that helped to put Haitians on the risk list, later remarked,

The original reports of AIDS among Haitian immigrants were sensationalized and misrepresented in the popular press. Some news broadcasts pictured scantily clad black natives dancing frenetically about ritual fires, while others caricatured Haitians with AIDS as illegal aliens interned in detention camps. The fact that the majority of the Haitian AIDS victims fit neither of these stereotypes was ignored. The impression left with the public in many instances was that AIDS was pervasive throughout the Haitian community. Unlike the homosexual or drug addict, the Haitian was a highly visible victim of the epidemic who could be singled out by virtue of his ethnic and cultural features. (Viera 1985:97)

Dr. Viera was joined by many other researchers in pinning the blame on the media. But the popular press was in many ways upstaged by the medical-scientific community, whose members had long been the preferred sources of the popular press when writing about AIDS. In a letter published in the February 28, 1983 edition of *New York Daily News,* Dr. Jeffrey Viera admits that, in the course of an interview he accorded a wire service, "references to voodoo were made in the context of a discussion of theoretical means of transmission of putative infectious agent among susceptible individuals." Dr. Viera also observed that "magic rituals sometimes transfer blood and secretions from person to person. Women have been known to add menstrual blood to the food and drink of partners to prevent them from 'straying'" (Viera 1987:121–122).[24] Similar theories were floated by several other prominent members of the scientific community.

Social scientists were equally quick to grant voodoo a role in disease transmission. An essay by Moore and LeBaron attempts to make "The Case for a Haitian Origin of the AIDS Epidemic." Although it appeared in 1986, and thus cannot be said to have contributed to the birth of this widely believed theory, the essay summarizes what is most important about a special brand of theory:

When understood as the systemic interrelation of underdevelopment, environmental—and consequently, physical and emotional—stress, a politically entrenched voodoo cult that thrives on the first two, and a small but distinctly offbeat tourist industry, is one in which the AIDS epidemic could well have originated. (Moore and LeBaron 1986:78)[25]

That brand of theorizing may be termed "armchair anthropology," and it fits most neatly into a symbolic network that stresses exoticism and the endemicity of disease. But as chapters 11–14 reveal, there was never any evidence that the organism causing AIDS was endemic to Haiti, nor has there ever been the slightest evidence to back the idea that voodoo practices played a role in transmission of an infectious agent. On the contrary, evidence suggests that the syndrome was new to Haiti, and that it had been brought to the island by North Americans or by Haitians returning from North America, and that sexual transmission and contaminated blood transfusions accounted for the majority of the early cases.

The epidemiology of HIV in the Caribbean might lead us to conclude that theories proposing Haiti as the source of AIDS represented the blaming of the victims. Such, at least, was the opinion of many Haitians, as the popularity of Ti Manno's composition "SIDA" suggests:

Americans have a certain flaw:
Whenever they have problems
They lay the blame
On the backs of poor people

This "American flaw" has been noted by sociologists who study the United States. In his study of the American tendency to blame victims, for example, Ryan (1971:10) recalls a tendency among the ancient Greeks to label strangers as "savages, weird and inhuman creatures." Ryan continues:

Blaming the victim depends on a very similar process of identification (carried out, to be sure, in the most kindly, philanthropic, and intellectual manner) whereby the victim of social problems is identified as strange, different—in other words, as a barbarian, a savage. Discovering savages, then, is an essential component of, and prerequisite to, Blaming the Victim, and the art of Savage Discovery is a core skill that must be acquired by all aspiring Victim Blamers. They must learn how to demonstrate that the poor, the black, the ill, the jobless, the slum tenants, are different and strange. They must learn to conduct or interpret the research that shows how "these people" think in different forms, act in different patterns, cling to different values, seek different goals, and learn different truths.

The conceptual distancing that has long marked foreign commentary on Haitians was central to popular North American discourse about AIDS and Haitians.[26] The unabashed anti-Haitianism of the nineteenth century was now more muted, but resonated with "the art of Savage Discovery" that lent such long life to exotic and Haitian-origin theories about AIDS. In the early years of the North American AIDS epidemic, the CDC and other august institutions spent an inordinate amount of time investigating feeble leads in the urban gay community and among Haitians living in the United States: "One might fairly infer," noted Oppenheimer (1988:271), "that the CDC was prematurely ready to find the etiology of the mysterious disorder in an exotic subculture."

Exoticism was only one possible form of commentary on Haiti and AIDS. There was another, more virulent strain of speculation that resonated with a symbolic web built around *race*. Racism may be overt or it may be subtle, cloaked in biologic and evolutionary parlance. Gilman (1988a:102) suggests that, for many, the associative logic ran like this:

The fact that AIDS was found among heterosexuals in Haiti could only be evidence that Haiti was the *source* of the disease. Heterosexual transmission was labeled by investigators as a more 'primitive' or 'atavistic' stage of the development of AIDS. The pattern of infection in the U.S., where the disease existed only among marginal groups (including blacks), was understood as characterizing a later phase of the disease's history.

The racism network was of course related to that turning about cultural difference, but offered a "coherence" and discursive tradition of its own. One such tradition tapped into a well-entrenched mythology of venereal disease. Fee (1988:127) recounts how syphilis came to be construed, in twentieth-century Baltimore, as a "black disease." She underlines the role of "white doctors [who] saw blacks as 'diseased, debilitated and debauched,' the victims of their own uncontrolled or uncontrollable sexual instincts and impulses."

Although the exoticism/racism semantic networks[27] are not discrete, it is possible to suggest that North American *experts* tended to rely on the former, whereas the latter was more often deployed in the popular sector. Quite frequently, however, these two symbolic systems were melded together into a comprehensive model that embraced both racist and exotic qualifiers. Apparently innocuous speculations, once introduced into the exotic/racist symbolic network, could be elevated to new heights of absurdity. For example, Sabatier (1988:45) reported that scientists "proposed that Haitians may have contracted the virus from monkeys as part of bizarre sexual practices in Haitian brothels."[28] North American scientists repeatedly speculated that AIDS might be transmitted between Haitians by voodoo rites, the ingestion of sacrificial animal blood, the eating of cats, ritualized homosexuality, and so on—a rich panoply of exotica:

Some U.S. researchers proposed that AIDS began with an outbreak of African swine fever in Haitian pigs, and that the swine virus had been passed to humans. Others suggested that a Haitian homosexual may have contracted the swine virus from eating undercooked pork, and then passed it on to homosexual partners from the United States during acts of prostitution. Another idea was that animal sacrifice and other voodoo rituals could explain the origins of human infection. (Sabatier 1988:45)

Although none of these assertions were bolstered by research, they were given air in all the nation's most prestigious medical journals.

The flow of speculation—from journalists to scientists—traveled in both directions, often through interviews accorded the popular press by the researchers themselves. But what efforts were made to conduct culturally sensitive epidemiologic studies to examine risk factors among Haitian-Americans with AIDS? Why did researchers repeatedly refer to transmission in that community as a "complete mystery"? In Miami, for example, culturally obtuse questionnaires and questioning had yielded, not surprisingly, a long list of "patient denies" for behaviors known to place individuals at risk for AIDS.[29] Leaving aside linguistic and cultural barriers, those administering questionnaires were asking for histories of a number of venereal diseases that Haitian entrants knew to be reasons for exclusion from the United States. And it was also well known that these data were to be sent to a U.S. government agency. Interagency squabbles (between, for example, the CDC and the INS) regarding patient confidentiality were of little relevance to the Haitians interviewed, several of whom were heard to comment, "*Leta se leta*": "the state is the state." At the height of debates over this research, investigators must have been concerned about front-page headlines such as "Haitian AIDS Victim Battles to Stay in U.S."[30]

It was not until later that the validity of this research was seriously challenged within the scientific community—and then only at the insistence of the stigmatized. When the investigations conducted in Miami were reexamined and the Haitian patients still living were reinterviewed, at least ten of the sixty-two men who had denied homosexual contact allowed that they had, in fact, had sexual relations with other men.[31] These revelations helped to reshape, to a small extent, the way that AIDS research was conducted among Haitians living in the United States. When Haitian-American physicians complained that exotic theories were merely reflections of North American prejudices, they also added that, although Haitians could do a better job conducting such investigations, more influential North American scientists monopolized research monies. In 1985, a bargain was struck, a coalition formed, and a multicenter investigation of risk factors was initiated. The "Collaborative Study Group of AIDS in Haitian-Americans" initiated the first and (so far) only controlled study of risk factors for AIDS among Haitians living in the United States. Compiling data from several North American research centers, the investigators reached the following conclusion: "Folklore rituals have been suggested as potential risk factors for HTLV-III/LAV transmission in Haiti. Our data do not support this hypothesis" (Collaborative Study Group of AIDS in Haitian-Americans 1987:638).

Careful study of the hypotheses emanating from the scientific sector reveals that they were not so very different, in the end, from the popular semantic network that surrounds the label "Haitian." Historical regard suggests the importance to this associative network of racism and voodoo. Even cannibalism, the most popular nineteenth-century smear, was resuscitated. Also indispensable was the geographical and cultural distancing that plays a role in rendering exotic anything that is Haitian. That these associations continue to play important roles in determining the boundaries and content of a North American semantic network about Haiti is suggested by a recent popular novel. In Sanchez's *Mile Zero,* set in Key West in the not-so-distant past, we learn that there is "some weird stuff going down in town," and that "ever since the last boatload of Haitian refugees came in it's been getting weirder" (Sanchez 1989:59–60). The "last boatload" of Haitians had perished in their efforts to escape Haiti. In one scene, a policeman appears on television, fielding questions from reporters: "There's no proof of cannibalism on this boat. I don't know where that rumor got started. These people died of exposure, starvation and drinking seawater. There will be an investigation. Yes, one survivor. No, I already told you, no signs of cannibalism have been exhibited on any bodies" (p. 24).

The one survivor is Voltaire Tincourette, a peasant who is hauled off the boat clutching an amulet. He is taken to an INS detention camp that recalls Krome. Voltaire hails from the southern mountains of Haiti: "*Paysans* up there have really been isolated, more African than Haitian," announces the book's protagonist. "Very superstitious people," he adds, in response to his interlocutor's whistled "*Grande* voodoo" (p. 43). The Africa-Haiti connection needs to be underlined, and it is done so by an omniscient narrator, who appears to be the Devil. He too is Haitian, and he offers the following warning: "Do you see the green monkey grinning in Africa, high in the tree? The green monkey has a secret he shares with me and withholds from you" (p. 252). It seems that the reader is to infer that the monkey also shared, through unspecified routes, his secret with Voltaire. He and another Haitian, Hippolyte, escape from the camp, and flee on foot until Voltaire is struck by a car and killed. His autopsy is recalled in the context of other medical examinations of the inmates:

They found some men had yaws, a flesh-rotting disease the United Nations claims had been wiped out. They found something else, a lingering pneumonia which wastes a person away. The pneumonia is linked to a virus in Africa, started by a green monkey or something, nobody knows for certain, so it doesn't have a name. Immigrant Haitians have the highest chance of developing it, except for homosexuals. The doctors had no idea how many men in camp were homosexuals, they know to a man how many were recent arrivals from Haiti. They asked permission to run tests on blood from Voltaire's body. He had the green monkey virus, they figured Hippolyte had it too. (p. 323)

These passages from a popular novel offer a classic example of the network of meanings evoked in the United States at the mention of Haiti. The story of Voltaire is a more florid version of the pseudoscientific hypotheses of Moore and LeBaron (1986) and many others. All these speculations resemble one another; they do not resemble what is known about HIV and AIDS in Haiti and among Haitian-Americans. It is precisely individuals like Voltaire Tincourette—"*Paysans* up there [who] have really been isolated"—who have not, in reality, been exposed to HIV. And yet *it is this preexisting network of meanings that has shaped to such a large degree the Haitian experience of AIDS.*[32]

The North American popular and medical presses continue to draw on and reinforce this symbolic web. One North American journalist has spoofed such attitudes in a recent study of Haitian politics. Commenting on the attitudes of her colleagues dispatched to cover the collapse of the dictatorship in 1986, Wilentz (1989:22–23) suggests the power of this symbolic network and the place of AIDS within it:

If Duvalier left it would be big news. Family in power for thirty years. Blood-thirsty dictatorship. Fall of the Tontons Macoutes. Beautiful wife flees with millions in jewels. Chaos in the streets. All this, added to the regular Haitian features, made the editors back in the world's capitals salivate: Plenty amid poverty ("Great.") Voodoo's hold on the peasantry. Voodoo's hold on the elite? ("Maybe. How do we illustrate it though? That's my problem. You see?") Voodoo and the Catholic Church. Just plain voodoo. ("Yeah, uh-huh. Good idea. Great pictures.") Deforestation. ("Can we get art? I mean, face it. Tree stumps. Do they read?") Drought? Boat People. ("Get me those bodies that washed up in Florida. Who took those pictures?") A refrigerated suite in the palace where wife and friends store their furs. ("Yeah, but has anyone ever *seen* it?") And now AIDS. The best.

The experience of Haitians living in the United States calls into question overly simplistic understandings of AIDS-related discrimination. In his study of *AIDS in the Mind of America,* Altman (1987:62, 67) relates episodes of discrimination against gay men seeking health care. He notes in passing, however, that the "experience of Haitians and drug users with AIDS is undoubtedly even worse. Unfortunately, it is extremely difficult to get any documentation of this." Perhaps better documentation would have led to increased solidarity among groups classed as at-risk, solidarity sadly lacking in the history of the American epidemic: "It has been extremely difficult for me to fully empathize with the experience of, say, drug users and Haitians," continues Altman, "and this book reflects my own position in the world as a white, middle-class gay man."[33] North American gay men were themselves heard to echo the Haitian origins theories, and also to amplify or misconstrue the role of Haitians in the U.S. epidemic.[34]

Although it is not argued that North American racism *directly* affected the epidemiology of HIV—the political economy of the region contributed much more to disease distribution—it is argued that racism helped to determine *social responses* to AIDS. In chapter 21, we will expose the roots of the phenomena examined here, and try to explain the tenacity of such images of Haitians. In the next chapter, however, we will examine the symbolic rejoinders of the scapegoats. Although most could not publish their replies in prestigious medical journals or newspapers, members of the Haitian community nonetheless conceived and circulated their own countertheories to explain both the origin and the rapid spread of AIDS. The most common of these was the assertion that the virus causing AIDS had been created willfully, in a United States military laboratory. This theory was equally popular in sub-Saharan Africa. "One of the main attractions of the theory is undoubtedly that it blames the United States for AIDS. It has appeared repeatedly in Third World newspapers, by authors who view the U.S. debate over the possible African origins of AIDS as evidence of racism and a determination to blame Africans" (Sabatier 1988:66). The next chapter shows that Haitians, the first victims of the "origins" speculations, elaborated conspiracy theories well before their African counterparts.

20

AIDS and Empire:
Accusation in the Periphery

*If we relinquish the compulsion to separate true representa-
tions of AIDS from false ones and concentrate instead on the
processes and consequences of representation and discursive
production, we can begin to sort out how particular versions
of truth are produced and sustained, and what cultural work
they do in given contexts. Such an approach illuminates
the construction of AIDS as a complex narrative and raises
questions not so much about truth as about power and
representation. To understand the ways AIDS comes to be
articulated within particular cultural contexts, the major
problem is not determining whether a given account is true
or false but identifying the underlying rules and conventions
that determine whether that account is received as true or
false, by whom, and with what material consequences.*

Treichler (1989:48)

Blame has played an important—and often destructive—
role in social responses to AIDS. The early suggestions that AIDS
originated in Haiti led to a great deal of unnecessary suffering. They
also led to a counterattack from the disempowered people who had
themselves been blamed. The counterattack was not violent, nor did it
lead to the recovery of lost jobs or housing. It did nothing to augment
the number of tourists visiting Haiti. It was, in fact, an entirely rhetorical measure: the elaboration of theories suggesting that powerful

human agency played a role in either creating HIV or in using AIDS to denigrate Haitians and other blacks. Though entirely symbolic, these rejoinders have had a significant effect on the ways in which AIDS came to be discussed in Haiti and elsewhere. This chapter attempts to make sense of the content and distribution of these accusations by juxtaposing them with information that rarely surfaces in curt dismissals of conspiracy theories.

Conspiracy theories have been a part of the AIDS scene since the advent of the syndrome. In the autumn of 1982, a radical exiled Haitian political faction circulated a flier denouncing AIDS, an acronym then freshly coined, as "an imperialist plot to destroy the Third World." The flier was easily dismissed as the paranoid propaganda of a fringe group, but it soon became clear that such thinking was much more common among Haitians than were the politics espoused by the group. In fact, many of those then speaking of the origin of the sickness spoke of the role of human agency in its creation. For example, a number of my rural Haitian informants insisted that AIDS had been created and then spread as part of a "North American plot." Others linked AIDS-related discrimination against their compatriots to "schemes to denigrate Haitians." Similar theories have also been reported by others studying the role of Haitians in the "third epidemic" (see, for example, Nachman and Dreyfuss 1986). To cite some of the comments encountered in as "isolated" a village as Do Kay:

One market woman in her mid-fifties angrily denounced AIDS as part of "the American plan to enslave Haiti. . . . The United States has a traffic in Haitian blood. Duvalier used to sell them our blood for transfusions and experiments. One of these experiments was to make a new sickness."[1]

A number of villagers linked AIDS to a plot to destroy the Cuban swine population. Mme. Fardin put it this way: "The CIA doesn't like Cuba, so they let loose a sickness among their pigs. But the sickness spread to Haiti, killed all our pigs, and then infected us. It is the sickness they call *sida*."

A voodoo priest in a neighboring village was reported to have signed a contract with a North American manufacturing firm. He was to "load tear gas grenades with *zonbi sida*." Demonstrators who found themselves in a cloud of this brand of tear gas would later fall ill with a bona fide case of *sida*.

A twenty-three-year-old *lycée* student from Do Kay whispered that Ti Boule Pierre, one of the Duvaliers' most notorious strongmen, was returning from South America with "newly acquired knowledge": "They say he went [to South America] to study the science of bacteriology. He learned how to create microbes, and then traveled to [North] America to study germ warfare. . . . They can now put microbes into the water of troublesome places. They can 'disappear' all the militant young men and at the same time attract more [international] aid in order to stop the epidemic."

More than one informant offered variations on the following theme: "Of course they say it's from Haiti: whites say all bad diseases are from Haiti."

From the first years of the pandemic, conspiracy theories were heard just as often in urban Haiti. In work attributed to the urban collective KAP, the "Coordination of Progressive Artists," the refrain of a song decrying the conditions of contemporary Haiti turns abruptly to AIDS:

> The Americans made AIDS in their laboratories.
> Faithless, lawless scoundrels,
> they made us carry the cross.
> Together with the FDA
> and a bunch of other worthless people,
> they nailed us upside down.

Following the success of the massive anti-FDA demonstration in New York, two well-known Haitian artists composed and recorded "FDA w'anraje"—"FDA, you're crazy." In the second verse are the following lines:

> It's true our country has no money
> It's true our country's full of poor people
> But you know all too well that you're the cause of this
> You're the ones who brought us drugs
> You're the ones who invented AIDS to kill off black people
> To hold onto your power, rule all nations.[2]

Investigating AIDS in Haiti for a U.S. magazine, a physician went to interview Dominican prostitutes in Carrefour. "AIDS!" responded one of them. "There is no such thing. It is a false disease invented by the American government to take advantage of the poor countries. The American president hates poor people, so now he makes up AIDS to take away the little we have" (Selzer 1987:60).[3] One young student, waiting himself for an "AIDS test," explained to a North American journalist that AIDS was part of the "American plan."

> "You get so many people to move to the city to work in your factories," he said, "and then suddenly you realize you can't give them all jobs. All those people together, without jobs and money—they're bound to stir up some sort of revolution, so you decide you're going to get rid of them. You can't do it with guns, though, because that would be inhumane. So you give them AIDS. It's part of the American Plan, people are saying. It makes sense, so I sort of believe it. People say that the CIA developed AIDS, and you know that the Americans are always saying there are too many Haitians." (Wilentz 1989:270)

Although such constructions were common in Haiti, they may have been encountered even more frequently among Haitians in the United States. It is these Haitians, more than any others, who felt the weight of AIDS-related opprobrium most directly. Some of the commentaries were strident denunciations of North American racism; others recalled the conspiracy theories heard in Haiti. A few examples illustrate the tenor of such rhetoric:

> A schoolteacher in a bilingual program for Haitians, who had lived in the United States for over a decade, made the following observation in 1985: "The Americans have always resented Haiti, ever since 1804. Being strong, they can punish us, humiliate us. The AIDS thing was a perfect tool (*bagay sida a, se te yon zouti pafè*)."

> A young janitor, working in a large Boston hospital, had been in the United States for several years when he was diagnosed with *Pneumocystis carinii* pneumonia. He had responded quickly to an intravenous solution of pentamidine; it was hoped that the aerosolized form, then an experimental protocol, would keep the lung parasite quiescent after his discharge. Soon after initiation of the novel treatment, he no longer felt short of breath; his spirits began to lift. His physician would have been startled, no doubt, to hear the following speculation, divulged at the end of a long discussion about his illness: "I'm beginning to think it was just a cold. Maybe I don't have what they say I have. Maybe it's just a cold, but they needed to get me into their experiment. They're always looking for guinea pigs for their experiments, and they especially like to try things out on Haitians."

> A group of Haitian teenagers attending Boston public schools participated in a community-based AIDS prevention project. The teens

directly engaged the issue of racism and the role it has played in the AIDS epidemics in the United States and in Haiti. At the end of a group discussion of the history of the AIDS-Haitian connection in this country, one of the teens asked whether or not the adult facilitator thought the U.S. officials "had done this to Haitians on purpose." The question was turned over to the teens; each was asked to venture his or her opinion. Without hesitation, sixteen of the teens replied "on purpose." The seventeenth was "not sure."

Such assessments resonate with another assertion, one in which human agency again plays the significant role in the genesis of suffering. This time, however, it is the causative agent itself that is held to be fabricated by U.S. military researchers. In August 1983 the progressive weekly *Haiti Progrès* ran an editorial that set the tone in at least one part of the Haitian community. Acknowledging that AIDS was a syndrome caused, ultimately, by a virus, the author warned against reductionism:

The AIDS Affair, in spite of these scientific suppositions, can not be taken as just one more disease without taking into account all the catastrophes that it could trigger. There are certain [Haitians] who put their faith in their U.S. citizenship or their status as "integrated individuals" without losing sleep over the imperialist beast. However, the case of the massacre of the Jews by the Nazis, or that of the Israeli army's assassination of the children of Beirut, or that of the lynching of blacks by the Ku Klux Klan, all of these bloody episodes show us how the dominant classes can efficiently make use of the weapon of "race" to remove from the scene a population whose blood is medically judged to be "impure."[4]

The editorial introduced a three-part essay in which Jacques Arcelin promulgated a theory: AIDS, he agreed, was caused by a "biological organism." It was infectious in nature. In contrast to emerging medical dogma, however, that biological organism was created in a laboratory in Fort Detrick, Maryland, the fruit of long years of germ-warfare research.

Of all popular commentary on AIDS, it is precisely such conspiracy theories that the mainstream press has found the most incomprehensible. Often, the print media avoid citing such accusations; at other times, they are referred to without comment. Reluctance to address such accusations was especially clear in coverage of the 1990 New York demonstration, which, as noted, brought together tens of thousands of Haitians. For example, the *New York Times* sandwiched the following paragraphs between descriptors of the marchers ("relaxed and jovial") and their effects on traffic:

Some protesters said they believed reports that AIDS had been created by the Government in laboratories and that the Government was infecting blacks on purpose. Speaker after speaker echoed that belief. . . . "We want the white folks to know that AIDS is their weapon and we're going to turn it back on them," bellowed a speaker who was not identified. "AIDS is a germ created by white folks to kill black folks."[5]

Such theories, whether "bellowed" or printed in broadsides, are not unique to Haitians. Similar allegations have come from several sub-Saharan African nations. Some have focused on the racism under-pinning the AIDS-origins theories: "Although the Haitian hypothesis collapsed," noted Chirimuuta, Harrison, and Gazi in *West Africa* in 1987, "the idea of black people as the source of AIDS was too attractive to abandon" (Clarke and Potts 1988:309). African print media have also carried dozens of versions of a rumor that terms HIV the product of the North American military establishment:

The asymmetry of the AIDS "origins" research has left a breach into which conspiracy theories can march. If the Africans often see in Western discussion of an African origin of AIDS a wish to blame the epidemic on Africa, so many Third Worlders have found attractive a counterblame theory: that AIDS was unleashed on the world by germ warfare experimentation in the U.S. Defense Department laboratory at Fort Detrick, Maryland. (Sabatier 1988:63)

African-Americans have also found such theories attractive, and they have received regular attention in the gay presses of North America and Europe.[6] But it seems that the chief purveyors of the "conspiracy theory," initially attributed to *Pravda*, have been Haitians and Africans—in other words, precisely those who have been themselves accused of introducing AIDS or HIV to the industrialized West.

Conspiracy theories pose explanatory challenges to those sympathetic to "third world" critiques of the United States. Others term such ideas "rubbish," or attribute them to Soviet stooges. Some scientists have been baffled by the conspiracy theories, protesting that they are not racists and furthermore had no intention of blaming Africans or Haitians. Luc Montagnier and Robert Gallo, credited with the discovery of HIV, responded to such accusations with bewilderment: "We deeply regret, and in fact do not understand, an interpretation of our work and opinions on the origin of HIV that finds bigotry or suggests we blame anyone."[7] Bewilderment from scientists was in many ways predictable. As Treichler has noted, conspiracy theories are embedded in a discursive tradition quite different from that in which much "conventional" AIDS discourse has been couched:

The notion that AIDS is an American invention is a recurrent element of the international AIDS story, yet one not easily incorporated within a Western positivist frame, in part, perhaps, because it is political, with discursive roots in the resistance to colonialism; the Western response, accordingly, attributes it to ignorance, state propaganda, or psychological denial. (Treichler 1989:43)

What might happen if we were to insist that such commentary is worthy of investigation? What might happen if we were to proceed as if our informants were themselves experts in a moral reading of the ills that afflict them? What follows is an attempt to extend a "hermeneutic of generosity" to the very notions dismissed as paranoid rubbish by the experts. Such an exercise leads us once again to an interpretive analysis accountable to history and political economy, the force fields from which the conspiracy theories initially arose.

1. *"Whites say all bad diseases are from Haiti."*

In the United States, popular acceptance of the scientific community's allegation that AIDS came from Haiti was rapid and complete. Equally pervasive was the notion that merely being Haitian put one at exceptionally high-risk for AIDS: "To be a Haitian and living in New York City meant that you were perceived as an AIDS 'carrier'" (Gilman 1988a:102). A similar misconception came to hold sway in South Florida, so much so that in May 1983, in Miami, "Jack Campbell, owner of the Club Baths chain of forty-two bathhouses, brushed off questions of the baths' role in the epidemic by insisting that most of Florida's AIDS cases were Haitians, and it wasn't a problem for gays. This was not accurate" (Shilts 1987:306).[8]

The preceding chapter has observed a resonance between the appearance of AIDS among Haitian-Americans and a preexisting framework in which Haitians, and especially Haitian "boat people," were conceived of as "disease-ridden." It is instructive to reexamine certain documents with an eye toward how they construe Haitians as disease-carriers. Most hate mail from the "United Taxpayers," for example, makes direct reference to *disorders other than AIDS*. To cite once again a postcard mailed to a Haitian community-based organization in Miami:

Tourists and business people are avoiding the South Florida area because of the plague of AIDS, hepatitis, and TB spread by the criminal, illegal aliens of Haitian origin. If you employ a Haitian, discharge him as soon as you receive this letter. Help South Florida.

Another postcard, mailed on the same day, declared, "Hire a Haitian—Help spread AIDS and Hepatitis."

Where did the references to hepatitis come from? To tuberculosis? In the years preceding the index cases of AIDS among Haitians, the newspapers of southern Florida carried several stories in which hepatitis, tuberculosis, and typhoid were linked to Haitians. Headlines such as "Haitian Health Crisis Hits Dade"[9] and "Typhoid Is Discovered at Haitian Camp"[10] were not uncommon. In 1979, according to the first of these articles, Florida Governor Bob Graham was asked to declare parts of northwest Miami a "special health emergency zone." The following paragraphs are from the story:

State and county health officials said yesterday that local resources are overstrained in meeting the widespread medical problems among the estimated 15,000 Haitian refugees in Dade County.

They said the refugees suffer from such communicable diseases as tuberculosis and venereal infections, as well as from malnutrition, anemia, dysentery, diarrhea, intestinal parasites, skin disorders, and complicated pregnancies.

By 1982, Haitians were popularly associated with several infectious diseases, especially tuberculosis. "First-in-nation TB Rate Linked to Haitian Influx" blared the *Miami News* of April 1, 1982. In a telephone survey of 274 Dade County residents, 74 percent of those polled felt that such diseases were "reasons for rejecting Haitians."[11] The work of anthropologist Steven Nachman is worth citing at length:

In 1981, Miami had the highest rate of tuberculosis in the country: 87 cases per 100,000, which was seven times the national average. Three hundred and forty-six cases were reported that year, of which 169, or 38 percent, were Haitian. Newspapers made much of this, and many Haitians had difficulty finding jobs because potential employers were afraid of them. Some public health officials even suggested that Haitians were resistant to ordinary tuberculosis chemotherapy, which did not help matters.

Events have shown that this public reaction was minimal in comparison to that prompted by AIDS, but at the same time it had considerable impact on the Haitian community. Leaders in that community were alarmed at the public outcry, and some regarded the issue of tuberculosis in conspiratorial terms. It was a plot to stigmatize Haitians. (Nachman n.d.:1–2)

Haitians have encountered similarly phrased hostility in Canada, where they have also been accused of importing AIDS. The advent of AIDS in the Dominican Republic, French Guiana, and the Bahamas—which have higher AIDS attack rates than does Haiti—merely augmented the already strident anti-Haitianism that has existed for decades there.[12]

The North American image of Haitians as "AIDS-carriers" usually invoked reference to the Haitians' poverty, their race, and their "foreignness." None of these attributes was mentioned to elicit sympathy. As noted in the preceding chapter, the image of exoticism played a significant role in the social construction of "the Haitian mystery." In her book, *AIDS and Its Metaphors,* Sontag (1988:48) suggests that "there is a link between imagining disease and imagining foreignness. It lies perhaps in the very concept with wrong, which is archaically identical with the non-us, the alien." The concept of race also played a role in the portrayal of Haitians as disease-ridden. The fact that Haitians are overwhelmingly of African descent and that AIDS was already known to be a sexually transmitted disease brings to mind the earlier part of the century, when white North American physicians could refer to blacks as a "notoriously syphilis-soaked race" without raising too many eyebrows (Jones 1981:27).

Few countries have been more marked by association with endemic infectious disease than Haiti. Syphilis was referred to by the Spanish as "the sickness of Hispaniola, believing it to have come from what is now Haiti when Columbus returned from his voyage to the Americas" (Sabatier 1988:42). "There is an inveterate opinion that syphilis had its European origin in Haiti," begins Holcomb (1937:13) in a study that attempts to disprove "the Haitian myth." As Lawless (n.d.) has shown in his exhaustive review of Haiti's "bad press," the entire nineteenth century was pocked with European and North American assessments of Haiti that described it as full of filthy, disease-ridden, cannibalistic savages. In an important study of Haiti's relations with the "Great Powers," Plummer devoted a significant part of her analysis to the weight of this literature of condemnation:

Haiti has long been the subject of lurid tales of voodoo rites, bizarre crimes, and capricious customs, none of which the writers of these narratives witnessed. This sensationalism originated in the early nineteenth century, but Americans and Europeans had hardly modified their disparaging tone by 1900 and continued to harp on the themes of black eccentricity and misrule. . . . Dispersed throughout this anthology are reports of cannibals who kidnapped, sacrificed, and feasted on young children. (Plummer 1988:71)

The North American visitor Samuel Hazard (1873:410) regaled his large audience with tales of Haitian garbage "left there intact to impregnate the air with the seeds of contagious disease. . . . But such is sanitary law in this enlightened (?) Republique d'Haiti." Sir Spenser St. John, the British envoy to Haiti, published a "study" of Haiti in 1884. In it he deplored widespread cannibalism, including the exhumation and ingestion of corpses, and "the intolerable stupidity of the inhabitants" (St. John 1884:5). The book became an instant best-seller.

The tone of foreign assessments of Haiti hardly improved with the passing of the century. There is nothing unusual about the tenor of Carpenter's *Lands of the Caribbean,* a travel guide popular in the 1930s:

Haiti, at the time of the American intervention, was a deplorable and almost unbelievable mixture of barbaric customs and African traditions. . . . Even in the cities, the Americans found unspeakable sanitary conditions, and diseases were prevalent all over the republic.[13] Most of the people are so superstitious that modern medical treatment has to be forced on them, and the practices of local medicine men and witch doctors combated. The religion of most of the natives is largely a survival of African superstitions and the voodooism of the Gold Coast jungles. Some travelers claim that in the most isolated regions of the republic human sacrifices are still made, and that cannibalism has not yet been entirely abolished. (Carpenter 1930:236–237)

Compare Carpenter's commentary to a recent article examining the difficulty of luring tourists to Haiti. In a 1991 report titled "If It's Tuesday, This Can't Be Haiti," an American journalist notes that cruise ship passengers who disembark in the "private tropical paradise" of "Labadee" are not even informed that they are in Haiti:

It's hard to sell Haiti as a tourist paradise when popular perceptions of the place make a visit fall into the category of "Holidays in Hell." Dire poverty, AIDS, child slavery, zombies, voodoo animal sacrifices and political violence are just some of the negative images facing tour operators. A U.S. government travel warning "strongly advises" Americans to avoid Haiti.[14]

The "Haitians = disease" carriers equation has been strongly reinforced by the AIDS pandemic, as *U.S. News and World Report*'s recent assessment of the current political unrest in Haiti would suggest:

Haiti today is distinctly unpromising soil for democracy. For one thing, there is the poverty, the worst in the hemisphere. For another, there is disease. Although statistics on the number of AIDS cases are still incomplete, one study of pregnant women in the slum of Cité Soleil found that 10 percent were carrying the virus. (Lief 1990:36)

For Haitians, then, the branding as AIDS-carriers fed into preexisting stereotypes, long deployed by foreign commentators speaking of Haiti. As throughout the nineteenth century, what was in question was corporate identity, especially their "Haitianness" and their "blackness." In light of this, it is less surprising that Haitians residing in the United States were quick to sense the difference between behaviors that put one at risk for AIDS and the designation as a "risk group"—"that neutral-sounding bureaucratic category which also revives the archaic idea of a tainted community that illness has judged" (Sontag 1988:46).

2. "The United States has a traffic in Haitian blood."

As for the "traffic in Haitian blood," there is once again more than meets the eye. There is, first of all, the splendid metaphoric connotations of a "traffic in blood," which both history and poetic license would authorize as an apt description of three centuries of Haitian history. But the accusation goes well beyond its poetic value. Precisely such a commerce was assured by the Hemo-Caribbean and Co., financed with U.S. and international capital and organized by Duvalier's cronies.[15] In his account of the fall of the Duvalier regime, Ferguson (1987:62) documents the role of *duvalieriste* Luckner Cambronne in commercial trade in Haitian blood when he noted in passing that the *makout* leader "had been implicated in a particularly unsavoury scandal which involved the selling of Haitian blood and plasma to American hospitals and laboratories (\$3 per litre was paid for the exceptionally antibody-rich blood)." It was estimated that at the height of activity some five tons of plasma were shipped each month to North American laboratories owned by Cutter Laboratories, Armour Pharmaceutical, and Dow Chemical. The plasma was sold for seven times what it cost to collect. This brisk and profitable trade earned Cambronne the epithet "Vampire of the Caribbean" (Abbott 1988:171; Prince 1985).[16]

The tale proved lurid enough to merit a few stories in the international press. Biochemist Werner A. Thrill, technical supervisor of the operation, posed the following question to *L'Express,* the French weekly: "If the Haitians don't sell their blood, what do you want them to do with it?" (Saint-Gérard 1984:111 n. 7). The scam was finally, if timidly, denounced by the local press, but it was not the exposé that led to an end to Hemo-Caribbean and Co. In his study of the discovery of HIV, Leibowitch tells the tale in full. He notes that North American hemophiliacs have for years been the beneficiaries of factor VIII, a coagulant distilled from the plasma of thousands of donors:

The blood used in North America, before 1975, came largely from Latin America and the Caribbean, *notably from Haiti*. Since the beginning of the seventies, the blood industries used donors whom they could pay cheaply. The purchasers did not lack a certain sense of opportunity: in 1973, the Nicaraguan earthquake claimed many victims and drew the sympathy, as well as the material and physical aid, of many volunteers from all parts of the Western world. Temporary camps were installed in comfortable, modern tents. In one of these, a huge one at that, a company producing the machine to "milk" plasma installed its devices by the dozen. It was to gather a huge collection of plasma for commercial use at the rate of several hundreds of liters per week. Elsewhere, we recall the rumors of scandals provoked, from 1970 to 1972, by the traffic in blood from Haiti. Bad blood, evidently, as some will have concluded, glancing at Haitian blood at the moment of AIDS. And yet, the thing is unlikely. After 1973 Haitian blood was no longer legally imported to the United States. Since the technology of massive plasmapheresis was now widespread, America would no longer have to depend on that particular blood source. After 1975, the Federal Food and Drug Administration would no longer grant its seal of approval to Haitian blood, nor to the majority of its former South American suppliers. (Leibowitch 1985:63–64; emphasis added)

Leibowitch also notes that this commerce allows us to conclude that the Haitian "donor-sellers" were not carriers of HIV before 1976. This conclusion leads to another of the "conspiracy theories," that concerning the origins of the American pandemic.

3. "The Americans gave us AIDS and then said we gave it to the world."

The observation that AIDS came to Haiti from the United States is made more frequently than any other save one: the "Americans" blamed Haiti for giving the world AIDS. Many commentators treat these statements as reflecting once again a Haitian tendency to paranoia. Others dismiss such suggestions as just plain incorrect. As the previous chapters have shown, however, there is much to be said for the theory as stated by history-conscious Haitians.

Let us look at the first half of the allegation, "Americans gave us AIDS." The epidemiology of HIV in Haiti underlines the contributions by Haitian researchers to the scientific literature on HIV. Dr. Jean Pape and his coworkers have advanced evidence to suggest that HIV was indeed introduced to Haiti by North American tourists. In 1985, however, the following paragraph appeared in a newspaper story titled

"AIDS Virus: From Monkey to Man: Disease Likely Entered America via Zaire, Haiti."

During the mid-1970s, there was a cultural exchange of about 10,000 people between Haiti and Zaire, both French-speaking countries, says NCI [National Cancer Institute] associate director Dr. Peter J. Fischinger. The virus may have crossed the Atlantic in that exchange and then moved from Haiti to New York after the island became a popular vacation spot for gay men.[17]

In addition to the usual inaccuracies (there was no cultural exchange of this scale with Zaire, ever; neither country is French-speaking), the article makes no mention of the evidence, published in refereed scientific journals by researchers from both Haiti and the United States, showing that there were no connections between Haitians with AIDS and Africa. Histories of sexual contact with North American tourists, in contrast, were offered by several of the first Haitians to fall ill with AIDS.[18]

As for the second half of the allegation, "They said we gave it to the world," the story recounted in the preceding chapters would seem to need little further scholarly buttressing. The suggestion of a Haitian origin for the organism that caused AIDS and the assertion that Haiti was "the source" of the North American epidemic were both formulated by North American physicians and disseminated widely by the North American press. This fact is widely appreciated in Haiti and by Haitians living in North America.

Paranoia or Sociological Imagination?

Similar exercises could no doubt be contrived for each of the "conspiracy theories" cited above.[19] But an even more important component of this exercise would be to reexamine the stories and words of Manno, Anita, and Dieudonné, as well as those of their covillagers, in light of the historical trends and epidemiological findings detailed in the preceding chapters. Anita, for example, insisted that she had "caught it from a man in the city." But she tended not to focus on this distal cause, preferring to speak of "the real reason" for her illness: namely, her poverty. She had a lover at a young age "because I had no mother." "When I saw how poor I was," she explained, "and how hungry, and saw that it would never get any better, I had to go to the city.

Back then I was so skinny—I was saving my life, I thought, by getting out of here." Anita was equally insistent about the cause of her family's poverty. "My parents lost their land to the water," she said, "and that is what makes us poor." If there had been no dam, insisted Anita, her mother would not have sickened and died; if her mother had been living, Anita would never have gone to the city; had she not gone to Port-au-Prince, she could not have "caught it from a man in the city."

Like Anita, Dieudonné tended to cast things in sociological terms. In so doing, he only amplified a trait widespread in Haiti. Not everyone in Haiti speaks as do many of the voices cited in these pages, but the changes of the last few years have given reign to a culturally sanctioned tendency to read the world as socially constructed. Dieudonné "wondered whether *sida* might not have been sent to Haiti by the United States. That's why they were so quick to say that Haitians gave [the world] *sida*." When asked why the United States would wish such a pestilence on Haitians, Dieudonné had a ready answer: "They say there are too many Haitians over there now. They needed us to work for them, but now there are too many over there." Here again, Dieudonné's assertions are not incompatible with data on Haitian migration to the United States and also on the type of work that Haitian entrants do there. As noted, Dieudonné also observed that "*sida* is a jealousy sickness." When asked to explain more fully what he intended by his observation, Dieudonné replied,

What I see is that poor people catch it more easily. They say the rich get *sida*; I don't see that. But what I do see is that one poor person sends it to another poor person. It's like the army: brothers shooting brothers.

Again, Dieudonné's assertions are more or less bolstered by existing epidemiological data. AIDS is indeed a disorder of poor people, and becoming more so; he had not seen a rich person with AIDS (though such cases have been reported in Haiti). The brothers-shooting-brothers simile falls short of the mark: it is more often sisters who are being "shot." Dieudonné casts *sida* as a disorder of the poor, and Anita's story reveals the mechanisms of her own impoverishment, as well as that of her covillagers. As has been noted throughout this study, both the dam and the AIDS epidemic—and a good many other misfortunes—are due in large part to Haiti's lamentable position in a network of relations that are economic as well as sexual.

The connections between sorcery accusations and conspiracy theories should be apparent. It is not that Haitians are "superstitious."

It is not that they indulge in "paranoid fantasies." On the contrary, reading these accusations with a hermeneutic of generosity leads the ethnographer to *trouvailles* such as that indicated by allegations of "a traffic in Haitian blood." The only fantasy in much of this commentary is the fantastic talent of some rural Haitians to point to the effects of impersonal or historical forces in the lives of poor Haitians. Surely this is what C. Wright Mills meant when he wrote of the "sociological imagination":

The sociological imagination enables its possessor to understand the larger historical scene in terms of its meaning for the inner life and the external career of a variety of individuals. It enables him to take into account how individuals, in the welter of their daily experience, often become falsely conscious of their social positions. (Mills 1959:5)

The sociological imagination is clearly manifest in Dieudonné; it is reflected in many incisive Haitian proverbs, and in the commentaries of many of the villagers cited here. Its origins may well lie in the slave colony of Saint-Domingue, where the "natural powers such as those of storm, drought, and disease paled before social powers such as those of the slaveholder" (Brown 1989a:67). Life on the plantations engendered a healthy respect for human agency and served as a template for latter-day understandings of causality.

Regardless of their ultimate origins, Haitian readings of AIDS and social responses to it are redolent of their readings of the world in general—a world where power and wealth and health are so unevenly distributed. To cite once again Mme. Lamandier's reply to the struggle between North American and Haitian researchers on the origin of the Caribbean pandemic: "A roach is never right in front of a chicken." With the balance of power as it is, the most Haitians can hope for is that their "conspiracy theories" will give pause to those bent on pinning the blame on Haiti.

21

Blame, Cause, Etiology, and Accusation

*What are the origins and implications of the language used
to talk about such concepts as behavior, risk, persons at risk,
modes of transmission—interpersonally and "epidemically"
(Greek for* among the people*)—agents of transmission,
health, and illness?*

*What is the nature of the bodies said to be most "at risk" for
AIDS? How are these bodies gendered? What is their
discursive history?*

*What are the differences between "dominant" and "op-
positional" accounts of this complex phenomenon?*

Treichler (1988a:232)

As long as we have known about AIDS, blame and accusation have been prominent among the social responses to the new
syndrome. These responses have been prominent enough to be labeled
by many the "third epidemic," eclipsing, at times, the epidemics of
AIDS and HIV. In the preceding three chapters, we have examined
three different types of accusation born of the AIDS pandemic: the sorcery accusations registered in a small Haitian village; the accusations
of North Americans (scientists, the press, the popular sector) blaming
Haiti for the organism causing AIDS and also for the American pandemic; the counteraccusations of Haitians as embedded in conspiracy

244

theories. Having examined the content and logic of each, we may now ask how these disparate kinds of accusation compare to one another. The purpose of this chapter is to draw on the preceding chapters—ethnographic, epidemiologic, historical, and interpretive—in order to present a critique of these responses to AIDS.

All three forms of accusation impute to human agency a significant role in the propagation of a dreaded sickness. In village Haiti, sorcery credits human beings with the capacity to "expedite" AIDS to an enemy; in North America, disease-ridden foreigners are identified and blamed for a worldwide pandemic; in Port-au-Prince or New York, conspiracy theories impute to the powerful evil motives, either the desire to weaken the ranks of outcasts (homosexuals, Haitians, intravenous drug users), or to defame black people. In each case, then, one social group attributes unsavory motives to another.

The similarities are superficial. Sorcery, AIDS-related discrimination, and conspiracy theories are in fact markedly different responses to the same sickness, and each reflects to no small extent the culture from which it springs. Compare the three in relation to their immediate effects. If we were to review a vast anthropological literature, we would see that sorcery can have negative effects on individuals and communities. A similar vein of commentary exists in the ethnographic literature on voodoo, and elite Haitians are fond of underlining the exploitative aspects of the religion. Père Jacques Alexis, tolerant of voodoo, finds sorcery difficult to caution: "It doesn't hurt anyone if you blame a microbe," he observed in 1987, "but blaming someone else for your misfortunes leads to division and hatred." And yet close examination of the ethnographic material from the Kay region demonstrates that at no point did physical harm come to any of those accused of sending sickness. The violence is entirely symbolic, an advantage underlined years ago by a leading student of Haitian sorcery:

Better cast a spell on someone than stab him. I am disposed to believe that sorcery explains the low percentage of murders committed in Haiti. A person who casts a spell on his enemy already satisfies his hatred—and avoids the kind of action which, if actually executed, would be much more serious. (Métraux 1972:271)[1]

In chapter 18, a somewhat functionalist reading of Haitian sorcery was offered, as sorcery's role in signaling infractions in the social code was underlined. Sorcery served to shore up communitarian traditions in rural Haiti, where increasing poverty was also leading to increased inequity. Anthropologists have often offered similar analyses of sorcery in other settings. In her study of kuru, which was also locally attributed to sorcery, Lindenbaum (1979:146) observed that "in the absence of alternative methods of settling disputes, sorcery may serve to regulate relations between individuals who must cooperate and also compete. . . . Sorcery seems designed not to interrupt, but to modulate the process." This modulating role, as noted, is underlined in a study of sorcery in South America: "Fear of sorcery is tantamount to fear of having more than others, and having more indicates failure to share" (Taussig 1980:117).

Regardless of how one feels about the symbolic aggression inherent in Haitian sorcery accusations, they involved no physical aggression. This has so far proven true in each of the AIDS-related sorcery cases in Do Kay. At this writing, three years have passed since Manno's wife swore to wreak revenge on her husband's aggressors. Although Alourdes Surpris left the area shortly after Manno's funeral, she has since returned. She continues to frequent the clinic, and her daughter now attends École Saint-André. To the visitor, the family courtyard seems peaceful, even though Alourdes shares it with her cousin and Maître Fritz, "the master of the affair." In an interview conducted early in 1990, Alourdes dismissed her vow to get even: "I don't believe in that sort of thing. It's not Christian to kill people, no matter what they've done."

It should be noted, as well, that sorcery is a model of *pathogenesis* widespread in rural Haiti. Indeed, Brown (1989a:38) argues that "healing is the *primary* business" of voodoo and of other religious traditions of the Afro-Caribbean area. In the area around Kay, *houngan* are consulted when several critical criteria are met. These include, usually, the strong suspicion that the illness in question has been caused by *direct* human agency, and the fear that the illness will be fatal. Ascription to a body of well-defined beliefs (for example, "voodoo") is certainly not one of these criteria, nor is regular participation in the ritual activities of a voodoo temple. As the fees of an accomplished *houngan* may be high, some care is taken to avoid triaging banal or "simple" illnesses to this sort of healer. But there are few other options when the stakes are high. The nationwide physician/population ratio is 18 physicians per 100,000 Haitians, compared to 250 physicians per 100,000 U.S. citizens. And the figures are substantially different in each of Haiti's four administrative districts. Do Kay is located in the

"Région Transversale," by far the most underserved region in the entire country.

In short, sorcery accusations, for all their flaws, are often triggered by severe sicknesses because they speak to questions of etiology, pathogenesis, and socially sanctioned therapeutic response. The same cannot be said of the other forms of accusation—AIDS-related discrimination and conspiracy theories—which are "macrosociological" models constructed to assign blame on top of etiology. Their role in explaining sickness does not include answers to the inevitable question of how AIDS comes to be embodied in the afflicted.

North American accusations, feeding on xenophobia and above all racism, do not compare favorably on any point to the sorcery of the rural Haitians. AIDS-related discrimination against Haitians has led to loss of jobs, eviction from rented housing, and violence. The suggestion that HIV originated in Haiti has the additional disadvantage of being entirely incorrect, as were all the *canards* floated about voodoo, cannibalism, monkeys, and the host of other fantasies mentioned in the preceding chapters. Conspiracy theories, in pale contrast, are revealed as the rhetorical defense of the powerless victims. Yet, conspiracy theories contain considerable amounts of truth when examined not as isolated anecdotes, but as lessons drawn from the last five hundred years of Caribbean history.

Of all these types of accusation, only one blames the victims—AIDS-related discrimination. In the United States, an invidious distinction between "innocent" and "guilty" AIDS sufferers has become entrenched. In a recent essay, the illness experience of Anita Joseph was compared to the care accorded "Robert," a gay North American man with AIDS. A native of Chicago, Robert spent his last days in a large teaching hospital in Boston. It was proposed that the striking differences in the experiences of Anita and Robert were inextricably related to the core cultural values of the societies in which each lived and died:

Robert's illness raises issues that turn about questions of autonomy and accountability. The concept of autonomous individuals who are solely responsible for their fate, including their illnesses, is a powerful cultural premise in North American society. On the positive side, this concept supports concern for individual rights and respect for individual differences and achievement. A more ominous aspect of this core cultural orientation is that it often justifies blaming the victims. The poor are viewed as unable to pull themselves up by their own bootstraps. Individual effects of powerful social forces beyond personal control are discounted. Alcoholics, those dependent on drugs, smokers who have developed emphysema, obese victims of heart attacks, chronic pain patients, even some sufferers from cancer—those who bottle up anger or who unbottle high-fat, low-fiber diets—all are seen as personally accountable for their disorders. Illness is said to be the outcome of their free choice of high-risk behaviors.

In contrast, in Haiti and in many African and Asian societies, where individual rights are often underemphasized and also frequently unprotected, and where the idea of personal accountability is less powerful than is the idea of the primacy of social relations, blaming the victim is also a less frequent response to AIDS. (Farmer and Kleinman 1989:146–147; paragraphing altered)

Who and what did get blamed by Haitians? The majority of my informants laid at least part of the blame on historical exigency, unjust social structures, and North American racism. When individuals were blamed, the accused were invariably the peers of the accusers or powerful people. More often they were powerful *classes* of people.

The moral calculus underpinning Haitian accusations would seem to be almost the obverse of that in which North American blame was embedded. In the United States, accusing fingers were pointed at poor or otherwise marginalized people: homosexual men, Haitian immigrants, intravenous drug users, and prostitutes.[2] Ryan (1971:22) has argued convincingly that blaming the victim is "central in the mainstream of contemporary American social thought, and its ideas pervade our most crucial assumptions so thoroughly that they are hardly noticed." Its chief perpetuators, he suggests, are often social scientists or others with vaguely humanitarian ideals—especially those charged with elaborating social policies in the United States. The effects of this ideology, asserts Ryan, are far-reaching:

The generic process of Blaming the Victim is applied to almost every American problem. The miserable health care of the poor is explained away on the grounds that the victim has poor motivation and lacks health information. The problems of slum housing are traced to the characteristics of tenants who are labeled as "Southern rural migrants" not yet "acculturated" to life in the big city. The "multiproblem" poor, it is claimed, suffer the psychological effects of impoverishment, the "culture of poverty," and the deviant value system of the lower classes; consequently, though unwittingly, they cause their own troubles. From such a viewpoint, the obvious fact that poverty is primarily an absence of money is easily overlooked or set aside. (Ryan 1971:5)

"Blaming the victim" as an explanatory principle has marked Haiti, and especially poor Haitians, for as long as they have existed as African-Americans. From the days of Las Casas, Africans in the New World were blamed for their own enslavement, whether as descendants of Ham, or the victims of internecine tribal aggression, or as depraved inhabitants of a dark continent: "The Negro's cultural difference commonly served as the justification for his enslavement, reinforcing the myth that he had been rescued from heathen darkness and taken to a land of spiritual light" (Davis 1975:47). At the height of the Enlightenment, chattel slavery could be ignored or even justified by leading liberal thinkers.[3]

Nineteenth-century visitors to Haiti, almost exclusively citizens of the great powers that had created or maintained plantation slavery, wrote scathing reports about the young republic. After the turn of the century, representatives of powerful nations deplored the upheaval they helped to foment and finance. Progress was impossible in a setting of constant "revolution," complained the arms merchants, bankers, and the gunboat-dispatching diplomats who wanted to shape Haiti. And yet Haiti, as Allen (1930:125) relates, was "victimized time and time again by foreign merchants, foreign capitalists, and foreign governments."

The architects of the American occupation made few attempts to mask a very common sentiment: the real source of Haiti's problems lay in the fact that black people were incapable of self-government. Witness the comments of U.S. Secretary of State Robert Lansing, who in 1918 wrote that "the experience of Liberia and Haiti shows that the African races are devoid of any capacity for political organization and lack genius for government."[4]

The American occupation of Haiti had been brutal and unabashedly racist, but fashions have since changed. Blaming the victim has been updated. Increasingly, the ideology is "cloaked in kindness and concern, and bears all the trappings and statistical furbelows of scientism; it is obscured by a perfumed haze of humanitarianism" (Ryan 1971:6). Beginning during the occupation, the United States has dispatched to Haiti various "scientific missions" composed of sundry well-paid consultants who investigate and then hold forth on Haiti's problems and, especially, Haitians' shortcomings. International organizations have followed suit, and blaming the victim again seems to be the dominant ideology. Its most recent incarnation has been the foreign-aid apparatus, which has funneled millions into the Swiss accounts of the Duvaliers and their cronies. That a solidly entrenched blame-the-victim ideology underlies much of this "development work" is suggested by strong U.S. support, for example, for a Bureau of Nutrition that finds the causes of malnutrition to lie largely in the cognitive deficiencies of poor mothers.[5] Occasionally, these deficiencies are attributed to very real injustices, but these form neither the focus of study nor the locus of intervention for the agencies. Education is their answer. Such tactics are entirely compatible with blame-the-victim philosophies:

First, identify a social problem. Second, study those affected by the problem and discover in what ways they are different from the rest of us as a consequence of deprivation and injustice. Third, define the differences as the cause of the social problem itself. Finally, of course, assign a government bureaucrat to invent a humanitarian action program to correct the differences. (Ryan 1971:8)

In its fulminant form, such as that spouted by a former director of USAID's Haiti mission, the blame-the-victim ideology locates the causes of poverty and suffering in Haiti squarely within the crania of the Haitian people: *Underdevelopment is a State of Mind* is the title of Harrison's (1985) study of Haiti and Latin America.[6] Many others working for international organizations seem to share Harrison's position: "This is a place of superlative negatives," said a Western aid official (Abbott 1988:338). "The poorest, the most illiterate, the most backward, the most superstitious." Reading Haitian history with a hermeneutic of generosity leads to a very different formula. Haiti is indeed a country of negative superlatives: it has been the most aggressively stripped and impoverished country, and its citizens have been pushed further backward than any other people in the New World.

In summary, many factors are important in an effort to understand the experience of Haitians in the United States during the early years of the AIDS epidemic. The most important of these, no doubt, are related to the dominant culture's responses to the "strange" occurrence of AIDS in Haitians. A tendency to blame victims underpins many of these responses. Yet it does not by itself fully illuminate the story recounted in chapter 19. To illustrate, take the example offered by Samuel Butler's satirical novel *Erewhon,* which relates the fortunes of a British traveler who stumbles upon a strange land. In Erewhon, the sick are punished and criminals are nursed back to health. The treatment accorded North Americans with AIDS has triggered numerous references to the country of Erewhon. The comparison fails to do justice to the Haitian immigrants' experience, however, for the treatment accorded them has never been charitable, be they sick or well. The contribution of *racism* to anti-Haitian sentiment is suggested by Butler, for it was the protagonist's "fair features" that spared him any further abuse: "If my hair was really light and my eyes blue and complexion fresh, I was to be sent up at once to the metropolis in order that the King and Queen might see me" (Butler 1970:91). North American responses to Haitians are embedded in a tendency to blame victims, endemic racism, *and* a folk theory of Haitians that depicts them as both exotic and infected—infected because exotic and exotic because infected.

In a recently published novella, Nobel laureate Saul Bellow offers great insight into the importance of each of these to the dense network of associations underpinning North American responses to AIDS in Haitians. The protagonist of *A Theft* is Clara Velde, "a corporate executive specializing in women's fashions." She is described on the book's jacket as "a genuine heroine, a woman of great depth and unsuspected capacities of wisdom and love." Her capacities of love are not so limitless, however, as to include Frederic, the "disgusting girl-fucker" who uses Clara's Austrian guest "as his cover to get into the house" and steal one of Clara's precious rings (Bellow 1989:71). Frederic is Haitian, "one of those boat people lucky enough to reach Florida a few years back" (p. 87), and Clara likes nothing about him, not even his voice— its "Frenchy slickness was offensive" (p. 84). One of her biggest mistakes had been in "letting [the Austrian woman] bring Frederic into the apartment and *infect* the whole place" (p. 71; emphasis added). The heroine's opinion of Haitians in general is poor: "These people came up from the tropical slums to outsmart New York, and with all the rules crumbling here as elsewhere, so that nobody could any longer be clear in his mind about anything, they could do it" (p. 73).

The *Bahamas Guardian* has termed Haitians "the pariahs of the Caribbean," for they have received a similar welcome from other countries.[7] The contemporary phenomena described in the previous chapters are in large part the result of a poisonous combination of a North American tendency to blame victims, a racism that has spread to every country in this hemisphere, and a surprisingly widespread and consistent "folk theory" of Haitians. The exercise of applying a historically conscious hermeneutic of generosity to Haitian "conspiracy theories" underlines the enormous differences between North American and Haitian attempts to blame, to accuse, and to understand the moral logic of this most recent affliction.

22

Conclusion: AIDS and an Anthropology of Suffering

Our consciousness has become more global and historical: to invoke another culture now is to locate it in a time and space contemporaneous with our own, and thus to see it as a part of our world, rather than a mirror or alternative to ourselves, arising from a totally alien origin.

Marcus and Fischer (1986:134)

Pigs, AIDS, immigration, support for the Duvaliers, military aid—it's hardly surprising that, with Baby Doc gone, resentment toward the United States has reached the boiling point.

Massing (1987:49)

The wicked man will disappear from the place
*   where he used to live;*
And his sons will give back
What he stole from the poor.

Job 20:9–10

Haiti's first democratically elected president took office as this book was going to press. In an entirely unexpected turn of events, the leader of the persecuted progressive church—the very priest whose church was in 1988 attacked and burned down around him as he said mass—was elected by an overwhelming majority in a field of eleven candidates. President-elect Jean-Bertrand Aristide had just published *In the Parish of the Poor,* a book about his country:

> Haiti is the parish of the poor. In Haiti, it is not enough to heal wounds, for every day another wound opens up. It is not enough to give the poor food for one day, to buy them antibiotics one day, to teach them to read a few sentences or to write a few words. Hypocrisy. The next day they will be starving again, feverish again, and they will never be able to buy the books that hold the words that might deliver them. (Aristide 1990:67)

Indeed, poverty is the central fact of life for most rural Haitians. To live in a village is to witness the struggles of the poor as they confront the deepening economic crisis that currently grips Haiti. Anthropological research conducted there is inevitably mired in a world of want, and ethnographic texts should reflect the hunger and fear and sickness that are the lot of most Haitians. But describing suffering, no matter how touchingly, is not a sufficient scholarly response to the explanatory challenges posed by the world pandemic of HIV disease. AIDS in Haiti fits neatly into a political and economic crisis, in ways that demand explication—patterns of risk and disease distribution, social responses to AIDS, and prospectives for the near future are all illuminated by a mode of analysis that links the ethnographically observed to historically given social and economic structures. Our ability to confront and prevent HIV infection in a humane and effective manner demands a holistic understanding of this new sickness.

Anthropology is uniquely equipped to investigate a new disorder, but the anthropological study of AIDS should be more than a search for "cultural meaning," that perennial object of cognitive and symbolic inquiry.[1] Haitian readings of AIDS have much more to teach us, particularly when we attend closely to the experience of the afflicted. Their commentaries, and those of their families, force us to lift our eyes from the local dramas of a small village. Indeed, many of the women and men cited in these pages seem to demand that we understand their current suffering in the light of past afflictions and current poverty. Some, such as Anita, have exposed for us the mechanisms by which they have been "put at risk" for exposure to HIV. Others have explicitly linked contemporary travails to the oppression and struggle that have long been the heritage of the Haitian poor. The net is cast wide, taking us to Port-au-Prince, to the United States, and far back in time.

An anthropology of AIDS poses important methodological and theoretical problems for medical anthropology. It is a new sickness, and it has spread rapidly across the boundaries (First World/Third World) that anthropology has helped to create and maintain. What is needed, methodologically, is a time-oriented ethnography that can

show how local events and local commentary on them can be linked to a variety of processes unfolding simultaneously on very different scales of time and place, and to note the difference between what might be called the "foreground preoccupation" of the actors or commentators on these events, and the "background conditions" informing their situation that figure much more prominently in the preoccupations of the historically minded ethnographer. (Moore 1987:731)

Moore refers to "very different scales of time and place," and in this study I have attempted to parse three different "temporalities" that may be shown to be relevant in a study of *sida*.[2] Village-level consensus on a new sickness may itself be conceived as a stream of temporality, an immediate and intimate flow involving the ethnographically observable experience of a relatively small group of individuals. In Kay, for example, the gathering consensus as described in chapter 10 was a stream winding through a series of events—the rumor of *sida*, its advent as manifested in Manno's illness (soon revealed to be tuberculosis, yet not "simple" tuberculosis), the suspicion of sorcery, and Manno's lingering death.

Processual ethnography helped bring into relief changes in what was important to the people of Do Kay. *Sida* was one important concern, but so were the growing political violence and the worsening economic crisis. What comes into focus may well be termed structure, but only if it is agreed that structures change, and at varying rates: "That such structures of relevance are contested, indeterminant, and changing (even for the ethnographer) mean that the ethnographer's descriptions are always about a local moral world that can only be known incompletely and for which the relative validity and reliability of observations must be regularly recalibrated" (Kleinman and Kleinman 1989:7). The ethnographic portions of this study were written to expose one intimate stream of temporality, and to reveal its significance in the shaping of a local moral world.

The Large-Scale in the Local

The local moral world of Do Kay was further shaken by other changes less amenable to direct ethnographic observation. The collapse of the dynastic Duvalier regime may not have led immediately to a new form of government for the Haitian people, but it did lead to important symbolic transformations that were widely felt in rural Haiti. The sudden eruption of national political issues was eventually shown to have an effect not only on the form and substance of illness narratives and on the nascent representations embedded in them but also on the *lived experience* of sickness. The salience of the political changes described in chapter 6 for understanding *sida* is subtler but no less relevant than the local events and structures. These may be termed "larger-scale" changes as they affected, in various ways, the majority of Haitians. This was as true of the residents of Do Kay as it was of the inhabitants of Port-au-Prince. It was also true, if to a lesser extent, of Haitians living in Boston, New York, Miami, and elsewhere in the diaspora.

Again, such larger trends may be elucidated through processual ethnography, but this time a village-level analysis proves inadequate to the task at hand. Certainly, reflections of these events were "ethnographically visible." Such reflections were duly noted. But there was much more to them than could ever meet the ethnographer's eye. Furthermore, the flow of these changes was experienced as far more rapid than the intimate stream described above. The impression of an increased tempo was shared by the natives of Kay, who after 1986 spoke of *evenman sou evenman,* "event after event." Changes in the way villagers spoke of their trials were the local reflection of large-scale events. When a peasant from Do Kay wondered if "perhaps these motherless *makout* might not have fashioned a microbe to do their dirty work," the relationship of his theory—and especially his ability to enunciate it in public—to the events of February 1986 was apparent. These types of commentaries, though clearly related to identifiable events (here, to rumor of a mass poisoning in Port-au-Prince), were permitted by the gradual "unmuzzling" of the Haitian poor. Some account of these events and processes should be worked into the ethnographer's rendering of setting, even if that ethnographer is a medical anthropologist studying an infectious disease.

Manifestations of international links demand no less attention. When Mme. Jolibois made reference to a cousin in New York who had lost her job "because they said she was a Haitian and an AIDS-carrier," a chord was struck between the story and persistent rumor of mistreatment of Haitians in North America. If one takes seriously some variant of world-systems theory—and Mme. Jolibois suggests we should—such rumors warrant investigation by the researcher whose fieldwork was conducted in rural Haiti. AIDS-related discrimination in New York or Miami represents distant shocks along the same fault line; in time, they will be transmitted to village Haiti, where they may trigger even larger reverberations. And of course HIV, an infectious intracellular organism, serves as the most insistent reminder that contemporary anthropology must take seriously a mode of analysis that underlines the interconnections too often elided in our discipline's past.

An attempt to gauge the effects of these national and international rumblings reveals a second stream of temporality, one related to events and trends in the lives of an entire people, and suggesting the outlines of relations between a powerful center and a peripheral client state. It is thus a "geographically broad" stream of temporality. In order to follow through on the promise of this geographically ambitious analysis, one must tap a third stream of temporality, no less broad in scope but reaching far back in time.

AIDS, History, Political Economy

When the people of Do Kay speak of *sida* as "the last thing," they are hinting that an ahistorical analysis of their current dilemmas will fail to reveal the true nature of their suffering. It is the historical gaze that brings into view earlier "things"—not only the Peligre dam and its effects on the lives of the villagers, but also the aftereffects of events that took place centuries earlier, and yet still may be shown to have sculpted the Haitian AIDS epidemic. In a study of another illness common in rural Haiti, oblique reference was made to both the geographically broad and the "historically deep" streams of temporality:

It is inexcusable to limit our horizons to the ideally circumscribed village, culture, or case history and ignore the social origins of much—if not most—illness and distress. An interpretive anthropology of affliction, attuned to the ways in which history and its calculus of economic and symbolic power impinge on the local and the personal, might yield new understandings of culturally evolved responses to illness, fear, pain, hunger, and brutality. (Farmer 1988a:80)

The present study again argues that "history and its calculus of economic and symbolic power" help to explain *why* members of a particular community came to understand illnesses such as tuberculosis and AIDS in the manner in which they did. The category of "sickness" is socially constructed, certainly, but on what foundation? Of what materials? According to whose plan, and at what pace? Historical perspectives also help to explain why Haiti, and not, say, Cuba, has been hit hard by HIV and its attendant stigma. To illustrate, let us examine these in fact indissociable strands—history and political economy—one at a time.

The historical strand is in many respects the most rewarding. In few places in the world will the ethnographer find cultural institutions that are more incomprehensible without a familiarity with three centuries of history. This is not surprising, if one pauses to reflect that the aboriginals of Haiti were, to a person, exterminated and "replaced" by kidnapped Africans. Contemporary religions of Haiti, such as voodoo or Protestantism, have well-charted histories, if one wishes to plumb the archives. The same may be said of the professional and informal ("folk") institutions providing care to the rural sick. Haitian kinship is more similar to that of eighteenth-century France than to that of West Africa, contrary to popular non-Haitian conceptions. Many of the agricultural practices have their origins in the small "slave gardens" of Saint-Domingue, or in the hidden cultivations of the Maroons. Napoleon's *Code Noir* weighs heavily on the *codes ruraux* of nineteenth-century Haitian legislation. The class structure of the entire country is derivative of the colony that preceded it. It seems, often enough, that all that impinges on life in a village like Do Kay has been born in Haiti in the discernible past.

The events of the past three hundred years are manifestly those that furnished rural Haiti with the "raw materials" for the representation of a new illness: *sida,* an illness that could be "sent" on an enemy with the help of a *bokor*; *sida,* an illness against which few *wanga* seemed efficacious; *sida,* a sickness that was not so annihilating, according to Alourdes Surpris, that a *zonbi* could not be raised from the grave after death from the new disorder; *sida,* a sickness that could force Dieudonné to ask whether or not he had been given a *makandal*—all these attributes of AIDS have their origins in the colonial epoch, and the lineage of these ideas may be studied in the historical record.

Given that historical study is a defensible and, indeed, necessary undertaking for an anthropologist, it seemed logical to turn to the methods of the historian. The insights of the *Annales* school, for example, find application in rural Haiti.[3] The quest for the above-mentioned "raw materials" of the illness representations and other social responses encountered in Kay brings the researcher back to the eighteenth century; the quest for the origins of the contemporary cultural, political and economic structures leads even further back in time. But the fruits of my own historical investigations were not entirely in keeping with the historiography of Braudel (1972) and his students, who had suggested that mere events would be rendered more meaningful by elucidating their significance in larger—and longer—trends. Instead, the events of 1986 (Duvalier's departure, first case of AIDS in Kay), 1979 (first documented case of AIDS in Haiti), and 1956 (flooding of the valley) were illuminated by other events and short-term processes: the arrival of Columbus; the European decimation of the Amerindians; the initiation of the African slave trade; the growing French domination of Saint-Domingue; the "flowering" of a colony based on slave labor; the revolution that formed Haiti; the formalization, through the American occupation, of Haiti's place in the West Atlantic system; the signing of the Export-Import Bank loan that funded the dam; the growth of tourism; and so on. The "underlying structures" seemed rather pale reflections of a series of massive upheavals. Chastened by Braudel's warning that *histoire événementielle* may be more show than substance, we are nonetheless aware of the overriding significance of events in a culture born of the violent penetration of early European capitalism.

It may be argued, endlessly no doubt, that it was the *political economy* of the region which generated *zonbi, wanga, makandal,* and sent sickness.[4] The second strand of this analysis must itself be historical, but the overwhelming impact on Haiti of plantation slavery, a component of international economies centered in Europe, cannot be overemphasized. Haiti, the world's first "underdeveloped" nation, was born of this template. Similarly, Haiti's place in the West Atlantic system, an international economy centered in the United States, helped to determine the current epidemiology of HIV. Such, at least, is the thesis advanced in chapter 14, which placed the advent of HIV in the context of larger forces—the push of rural poverty and the pull of urban factories and tourism catering to North Americans.

An interpretive anthropology of AIDS in Haiti would push us toward a "responsible materialism" sadly lacking in many ventures in symbolic anthropology. As noted at the outset, Marcus and Fischer (1986:86) put the challenge succinctly: "An interpretive anthropology fully accountable to its historical and political-economy implications thus remains to be written." Without previous awareness of history and political economy, the ethnographer may detect only the empty shells of meaning, since so much that is rich will be misunderstood or missed altogether. So will the most critical implications of such an anthropology. When an informant such as Dieudonné refers to *sida* as a "jealousy sickness," one "caused by poverty," he is unwittingly reminding us to explore the notion of "sent sickness" in its full symbolic register. This is especially true in Latin America and, of all countries, in Haiti, where the hard surfaces of life seem to underpin so much of experience. For contemporary Haiti is a place best described as "the parish of the poor," a place where bullets from abroad rain down on demonstrators and market women, where walls are sprayed with not-too-cryptic messages: "We all have AIDS: International Monetary Fund = AIDS," read the graffiti of 1987; "AIDS—it had to happen."

The West Atlantic Pandemic

Throughout the world, but particularly in what is termed the "Third World," much of human suffering is caused or aggravated by social forces, and social forces should be studied by medical anthropologists. Suffering is a legitimate subject of ethnographic investigations, with important intellectual and ethical provisos. One of these provisos, as stated at the outset, is that the *lived experience* of the disorder is paramount.

A second is that, when the subject is sickness, epidemiology should be another component of responsible materialism. Although repeatedly termed a "complete mystery" by North American academics, the epidemiology of AIDS and its silently transmitted precursor, HIV, is only superficially random. Careful review of existing data and critical assessment of the validity of certain studies allow us to conclude that the Haitian epidemic is a tragic but unsurprising component of a much larger pandemic. In the various theaters of this international scourge, whether New York or Port-au-Prince, HIV has become what Sabatier (1988) has termed a "misery-seeking missile." It has spread along the paths of least resistance, rapidly becoming a disorder disproportionately striking the poor and vulnerable.

Much is made in the public health literature of the similarities between the Haitian and the African AIDS epidemics, but the Caribbean epidemic is of this hemisphere. Current understandings of the epidemiology of HIV in the region suggest that the virus came to the Dominican Republic, Jamaica, Trinidad and Tobago, and the Bahamas in a manner similar to that documented in Haiti—from the United States, and perhaps especially through tourism. Caribbean tourism stands increasingly as an index of dependence on North America. This trade is also emblematic of the striking economic disparity between the poor periphery and the rich center.[5] The relation between the degree of "insertion" in the West Atlantic system and prevalence of AIDS was suggested by an exercise comparing AIDS attack rates to U.S.-Caribbean trade indices reflecting involvement in the West Atlantic system. The five countries with the largest number of cases by 1986 were as follows: the Dominican Republic, the Bahamas, Trinidad/Tobago, Mexico, and Haiti. In terms of exports, which are the five countries most dependent on the United States? In both 1983 and 1977, the same five countries held that honor—precisely those with the largest number of cases of AIDS. Haiti, the country with the most cases, is also the most economically dependent vis-à-vis the United States.

But it is unnecessary to posit a causal link based on mere association with trade patterns. In several of these countries, at the outset of the epidemic, seropositivity to HIV was correlated most strongly with a history of sexual contact with North Americans. For this and other reasons, it was suggested, the terminology deployed by the World Health Organization's Global Program on AIDS is somewhat obscurantist. The epidemiology of AIDS in the Caribbean is described as "Pattern II," as it is in sub-Saharan Africa. Pattern II is held to differ from Pattern I, seen in North America and Europe, "in that heterosexual intercourse has been the dominant mode of HIV transmission from the start. Blood transfusion, the reuse of contaminated needles, and intravenous drug use contribute to a variable degree, but homosexuality generally plays a minor role in this pattern" (Osborn 1989:126). And yet what is known of "the start" of AIDS in the Caribbean suggests that the epidemics there were introduced through international prostitution, same-sex sexual contacts, and bisexuality. Blood tranfusion also played a role. These island epidemics are not in all likelihood "direct descendants" of the African pandemic. They are American.

A historical understanding of the worldwide spread of HIV is of some significance, and I have attempted to postulate the trajectory of the virus in the Caribbean basin. Leibowitch (1985:57) offers a speculative history of another retrovirus, HTLV, which is endemic to parts of the Caribbean: "The map of HTLV in the New World is that of the African diaspora." Because that "diaspora" refers to the massive dislocations of Africans through the slave trade, another way of phrasing this would be that the map of HTLV in the New World is the map of European imperial expansion. Given that unequal relations between the Caribbean and North America have contributed to the current epidemiology of HIV, an analogous exercise leads to a somewhat analogous observation: the map of HIV in the New World reflects to an important degree the geography of U.S. neocolonialism.

Recourse to crude formulations—for example, "imperialism causes AIDS"—is unnecessary. But exhaustive exploration of AIDS as a "sent sickness," when conducted in tandem with careful study of the local epidemiology of HIV, emboldens us at least to discuss important correlations such as those made above. That such considerations have been important in the lineaments of the American epidemics is suggested by comparing Haiti with Cuba, where only 0.01 percent of persons tested were found to have antibodies to HIV. In most other parts of the Caribbean, seroprevalence among apparently healthy urban adults is two to three orders of magnitude higher than that registered in Cuba. As noted in chapter 14, the fact that HIV made its advent in the last decades of the century, rather than earlier, determined to no small extent the spread of HIV infection in the Caribbean.

Such assertions are a long way from the meaning-laden realm of sexuality, an understanding of which is necessary for a thorough understanding of the world AIDS pandemic. But here too it is impossible for long to steer clear of the hard surfaces of life. Here are the observations of Dr. Bernard Liautaud, who in 1979 identified the first documented case of Kaposi's sarcoma in a Haitian: "There are two groups of homosexuals. There are those who do it for pleasure and those who do it for economic reasons. In Haiti, we have economic homosexuals: poor people making love for money."[6] Certainly, the formula is simplistic. And yet it reminds us that few realms of human experience are beyond the reach of the social forces I have emphasized in this study of AIDS.

Finally, the history of HIV in Haiti suggests that, although non-Haitians were important in the early part of the epidemic, they no longer play a major role in HIV transmission on the island. The history of HIV, when read against the stories told in the ethnographic chapters, helps to demonstrate the means by which AIDS has become a heterosexually spread disorder. Poverty puts young adults at risk of exposure to HIV, and high rates of seroprevalence have already been registered throughout urban Haiti. The preceding chapters all demonstrate the salience of rural Haiti's ties to Port-au-Prince and the

United States, and the intimacy of these links is further suggested by the short doubling time of the Haitian epidemic. Together, these findings suggest that, if a disaster is to be averted in rural Haiti, vigorous and effective prevention campaigns must be initiated at once. And although such efforts must begin, the prospects of stopping the steady march of HIV are slim. AIDS is far more likely to join a host of other sexually transmitted diseases—including gonorrhea, syphilis, genital herpes, chlamydia, hepatitis B, lymphogranuloma venereum, and even cervical cancer—that have already become entrenched among the poor.[7]

AIDS, Anthropology, and Cultural Critique

Anthropology has much to offer those who seek a full and rich understanding of AIDS—which is of no small importance to efforts to halt the spread of HIV. One of the enduring strengths of the discipline is fieldwork, which helps to distinguish ethnographic texts from the often arid analyses of economists, policy specialists, or epidemiologists. In the past few years, however, many anthropologists have been asked to reduce their findings to "the bottom line," or to perform "rapid ethnographic assessments" of populations held to be at risk for exposure to HIV.[8] Perhaps the inevitable result of such bowdlerization is indicated by the observations of a person with AIDS: "Anthropologists of our *tristes tropiques* have accumulated a considerable store of information and conclusions about our genes and our mores, our mode of socialization and our myths, but in so doing, they've lost sight of our humanity" (Dreuilhe 1988:4).

One way to avoid losing sight of the humanity of those with AIDS is to focus on experience and insights of those who are afflicted. This study has attempted to link the large-scale events and structures of the world AIDS pandemic to the lived experience and commentary of people like Manno, Anita, and Dieudonné, and also of those who lived with them. In so doing, we see more than differences in culture, more than differences between the well and the sick. Listening to these stories offers us privileged insight into what it means to be sick and poor and aware of the causes of their suffering:

The oppressed are more than what social analysts—economists, sociologists, anthropologists—can tell us about them. We need to listen to the oppressed themselves. The poor, in their popular wisdom, in fact "know" much more about poverty than does any economist. Or rather, they know in another way, in much greater depth. (Boff and Boff 1987:30)

The understandings of rural Haitians take on a relevance far beyond their immediate ethnographic significance. What does it mean for a literate, English-speaking audience to read that AIDS is an affliction that is "not simple" and may be willfully sent by an enemy? What of the other evoked associations, those drawn from the larger political-economic context, those that speak of North American imperialism, a lack of class solidarity among the poor, or the corruption of the ruling Haitian elite? What results from an exercise in reading Haitian conspiracy theories with a hermeneutic of generosity? Seen in its full symbolic register, "sent sickness" is about historically given conditions that put people at risk for AIDS and the other afflictions that beleaguer them. It is, in short, about the victims' moral readings of the sources of their suffering. Such readings underline once again both local and large-scale connections, confronting the North American ethnographer (or reader) with a cultural critique that seems, at times, too perfectly crafted to have been intended for any other audience.

In a recent overview of anthropology, Marcus and Fischer remark that "the potential for developing a distinctive anthropological critique of American society is inherently linked to the . . . traditional arena of research abroad" (1986:4). The authors suggest that by juxtaposing familiar middle-class life with culturally different lifeways, a profound epistemological critique of the former could be fashioned. In researching AIDS in Haiti, no such metaphoric exercises are called for. The boundaries between "home" and "abroad," between "exotic" and "familiar" have been called into question by a virus that has had little difficulty relegating such boundaries to a secondary status.

The challenge of these readings to an anthropology of suffering is a daunting one, for the questions raised by many of the voices cited here seem to regard the frame of reference and scope of analysis appropriate to a subject such as AIDS in Haiti. The anthropological literature on Haiti has tended toward the exotic, with lurid treatises on ritual sacrifice and possession, potent poisons, and zombiism. As we have seen, AIDS slips all too neatly into this symbolic network, if theoretical precautions are not taken. The Haitians may be exotic to "us" (as that symbolic structure defines "us"), but "we" are not in the least exotic to Haitians like the inhabitants of Do Kay. We should pose once again Eric Wolf's (1982:4) pointed query: "If there are connections everywhere, why do we persist in turning dynamic, interconnected phenomena into static, disconnected things?" For AIDS in Haiti is about proximity rather than distance. AIDS in Haiti is a tale of ties to the United States, rather than to Africa; it is a story of unemployment rates greater than 70 percent. AIDS in Haiti has far more to do with the pursuit of trade and tourism in a dirt-poor country than with, to cite Alfred Métraux again, "dark saturnalia celebrated by 'blood-maddened, sex-maddened, god-maddened' negroes."

Notes

Chapter 1: Introduction

1. Dr. Bruce Chabner of the National Cancer Institute, cited in the *Miami News*, 2 December 1982, p. 8A.

2. The physicians also made the following, apparently offhand, comment: "If the syndrome originates in rural people, *and it seems likely that it does*, it occurs among those who have had little or no direct or indirect contact with Port-au-Prince or other urban areas" (Moses and Moses 1983:565; emphasis added).

3. The nature of such folk models and the long history of Haiti's "bad press" have been chronicled by Robert Lawless of the University of Florida. Unfortunately, his research has not yet been published.

4. The first of these two qualifiers is in Allman (1989:81). The second is in the 12 February 1990 edition of the *U.S. News and World Report*, p. 34.

5. Some speakers presciently warned that, regardless of the nature of its introduction to Haiti, AIDS had the potential to become "just another sexually transmitted disease."

6. *New York Times*, 31 July 1983.

7. The French acronym for *syndrome d'immuno-déficience acquise* is commonly rendered as S.I.D.A., SIDA, or Sida; *sida* is the Creole orthography. The latter is preferred here in order to reflect the substantial difference between the terms as used in different settings.

8. All names of ethnographic informants are pseudonymous as are "Do Kay" and "Ba Kay." Other geographical names are as cited.

9. My argument follows that of Moore, who has persuasively argued that the "issue of the day is how to address the fieldwork enterprise in a poststructuralist period, how to understand the fieldwork time as a moment in a se-

quence, how to understand the place of the small-scale event in the large-scale historical process, how to look at part-structures being built and torn down" (Moore 1987:730).

10. The expression is a paraphrase of that coined by Bateson and Goldsby (1988:3).

11. These voices may also contribute to a deepening of the shallow and stereotypic "Third World point-of-view" that has predominated in much First World journalistic coverage of AIDS in Haiti and in sub-Saharan Africa. In a trenchant essay, Treichler has done much to outline the "institutional forces and cultural precedents in the First World [that] prevent us from hearing the story of AIDS in the Third World as a complex narrative" (Treichler 1989:37).

12. Furthermore, it may be that only intense and prolonged exposure permits us to fulfill a commemorative role, serving as witness to those who have died of AIDS. For a discussion of methodological and ethical questions raised by ethnographic research on AIDS among the poor, see Farmer (1991a; 1991b).

13. Writing of AIDS in Zaire, Schoepf (1988:639) underlines "the importance of understanding how the macro-level political economies affect the socio-cultural dynamics at the micro-level—including the spread of disease and social response to epidemics."

14. Browner et al. (1988) advocate instead studies that employ "replicable methodologies" when investigating sickness. Theories must be falsifiable; external referents will be afforded by the "objective procedures" of modern "bioscience." See Janzen's (1988:695) and other incisive responses to the position of Browner and colleagues.

15. Anastos and Marte (1989:9, 10) continue by noting that address alone seems to put women at risk for exposure to HIV: "Breakdown of New York City data by zip code area also reveals that the most socially and economically devastated inner-city areas are those with the most HIV disease. . . . This means again that poor black and Latina women are at unduly high risk for infection, whatever their life-style, because poverty and lack of resources and opportunity keep them in areas of high HIV seroprevalence."

16. In February 1990, "local radio stations announced . . . that for the first time, the drug AZT is available in Haiti. It might as well have been on Mars. A bottle of 100 capsules costs $343—more than most Haitians make in a year" (Lief 1990:36).

Chapter 2: The Water Refugees

1. These narratives are complemented by other data, gathered during the last five years in an annual census conducted with the help of a small group of community health workers from Kay. In all households with members who were displaced by the reservoir, we conducted structured interviews using a rather crude questionnaire. Although these data are clearly of limited value,

enough was learned from the questionnaires to discern a few modal patterns of relocation leading eventually to Do Kay. I am grateful to Ophelia Dahl for her insights to these patterns.

2. A *karo* (from the French, *carreaux*) is equal to 1.29 hectares or 3.19 acres.

3. The 1861 founding of this church by an African-American is recounted by Romain (1986) in his history of Haitian Protestantism. See also Hayden (1987) and Heinl and Heinl (1978).

4. There he met the same fate as many other politically active and independent-minded individuals. Moreau was arrested and never seen again. His successor as pastor of Mirebalais maintains that he was taken to the palace and shot in the head—while pleading on his knees to be spared. "His executioner," observes Père Alexis, "was rumored to have been none other than François Duvalier."

5. In an interview conducted in 1987, Melifèt Fardin recalled a movement to go and *dechouke*, or "uproot," the administrators of the ODVA, and make them release the waters of the Lac de Peligre. Other water refugees denied that any such movement was significant. "Just talk," said Absalom, laughing. "We didn't even know where the ODVA headquarters were." As for the "docility" of the displaced peasants, it is interesting to note the commentary of Kethly Millet in her study of peasant revolts during the U.S. occupation: "In his struggle to hang onto his little bit of land and win a measure of well-being, the peasant has always shown a deep respect for the sanctity of human life. Threats, the destruction of agricultural implements, and the 'sit-down' characterize the beginnings of revolt. Violence usually comes from the adversary. [Full revolt] is thus a reaction to repression from the governmental and [North] American authorities" (Millet 1978:137).

6. During the dry season, however, many peasants of the region still run the risk of planting corn, tobacco, beans, yams, and other crops below the high watermark. They often lose bountiful harvests to early rains, which fill the reservoir just as the crops are ripening.

Chapter 3: The Remembered Valley

1. Scott encountered similar rhetoric among poor Malay villagers who had become even poorer after a decade of "successful" double-cropping served to widen the gap between the haves and the have-nots. His poor informants "have collectively created a *remembered* village and a *remembered economy* which serve as an effective ideological backdrop against which to explore the present" (Scott 1984:205; see also Scott 1985).

2. A *digo* is a hand-held agricultural implement used to weed gardens.

3. "Outside confirmation" of their descriptions comes from French geographer Paul Moral, who studied the area before the dam was erected. In describing the area, Moral (1961:134–135) writes "here, in the humid depths of

the valley, sugarcane, cotton, corn, and bananas are grown together in relatively fertile gardens that relegate livestock to secondary importance." Similarly, a report on Petit-Fond itself described the region as "a mountainous area with very fertile soil in the valleys" (Moore 1956:495). But surrounding these fertile valleys were the dry hills and "savanes" that constitute, continues Moral, "un milieu particulièrement hostile au petit défricheur isolé." It is of course in the same hills that the residents of the valley were obliged to take refuge.

4. On the decline of *lakou*, see also d'Ans (1987); Larose (1976); Murray (1977, 1980).

5. A *konbit* is a cooperative effort by which peasants help a covillager complete a large project (for example, clearing a fallow field). Trouillot (1986) suggests there is widespread nostalgia for these cultural institutions, which may have been of less importance than contemporary recollections would imply. See also Barthélemy (1989), Bastien (1985), Laguerre (1977).

6. "Haitian-African ceremonies are held in this area. Some of the people are familiar with private services ordered by the loas. On a date arranged by the head of the family, the relatives gather together and have a kind of meal offering" (Moore 1956:496).

7. More than one of the refugees noted that this *houngan* "became crazy" and left the region, never to be heard from again.

Chapter 4: The Alexis Advantage

1. Père Alexis was actually reestablishing the school attached to the Episcopal mission, as there had been a school in Petit-Fond. Church records claim that of 350 schoolage children, 25 students attended the parish school in 1955, and 60 attended a "public elementary school" (Moore 1956:496). Curiously, neither of these institutions is mentioned by the water refugees.

2. The pronoun "he" is clearly not intended to imply that the ambition is held most dearly by fathers; a mere two pages earlier, Métraux observes that "countless families depend upon the commercial acumen of the woman in order to make both ends meet. More than one middle-class Haitian owes his rise in society to some peasant woman who has toiled ceaselessly and worked miracles of ingenuity to pay for his studies."

3. An exception to the deplorable record of community organization is to be found in the efforts of the ecclesial base communities organized by progressive Catholics. See Wilentz (1990) for a discussion of these communities, and Aristide (1990) for an understanding of the philosophy that has galvanized their formation.

4. It is important to note that the word "development" is readily used by "specialists" to describe both the current activities of the community and the project that displaced them over thirty years ago. The people of Kay make finer distinctions.

5. Alexis also began a campaign to bring electricity to the village. He ap-

proached Électricité d'Haiti with the argument that "giving the people of Kay electricity is the least you could do, after all they lost." He has so far been unsuccessful, and recounts with indignation the response of the company's director: "Why on earth would those peasants want electricity?" Such attitudes help to explain why Alexis does not seek governmental aid. He states, too, that he mistrusts USAID, the dominant institution in the foreign-aid enclave of Haiti. The Alexis team currently receives most of its funding from private American donors (through a public charity), the Église Épiscopale d'Haiti and its North American cognate, and progressive funding organizations. Over the past five years, a single individual, a North American, has supported the bulk of the community development programs.

6. In 1987, a single case of enteric fever was registered with Projè Veye Sante. In the subsequent two years, the sole case in Do Kay was in a young man who was working as a gravedigger in Port-au-Prince. He returned to Do Kay when he became ill, and was treated there for typhoid.

7. That the pigs were accustomed to such luxury is clear from Diederich's (1985:16) description of the nucleus breeding centers from which they were shipped to Kay and other secondary centers: The pigs "lie on clean concrete, under roofed pens that keep the hot sun off their light skins, while a mist of water sprays down from a sprinkler to help them adjust to the 90-degree heat of the Haitian summer. Two teams of workers give them a morning bath before hosing out the stys. Some pigs suckle water from a special faucet (a blatant luxury in Haiti where only the rich have running water in their homes)."

8. The standard mechanism of action is offered by Sonson: "The pig eats the *kola*, it reaches the heart, and then its *fyèl* [organ thought to 'hold the heart']. The *kola* makes the *fyèl* burst, and the beast dies."

Chapter 5: The Struggle for Health

1. At this writing, Projè Veye Sante serves sixteen villages (between 25,000 and 30,000 persons), and a laboratory has been added to Clinique Saint-André, which is now staffed by three doctors, two auxiliary nurses, two medical technologists, two archivists, and a large ancillary staff. The health care team is completed by twenty-seven community health workers representing Do Kay and fifteen surrounding villages.

2. Malaria in Haiti is caused almost exclusively by *Plasmodium falciparum*, the species responsible for most cases of fatal malaria, and the only species to cause cerebral malaria. Research in Thailand, where mortality despite treatment is 22 percent, suggests that Dr. Pierre's prognosis was overly pessimistic (White and Warrell 1988:866).

3. Herskovits (1975 [1937]:240) notes that "the term *mange moun*, in Haiti as in Africa, is idiomatic for sending a fatal illness or bringing about an accidental death."

4. "A *bagi* is a veritable junk shop: jars and jugs belonging to the spirits

and the dead, platters sacred to the twins, carrying-pots belonging to the *hunsi*, 'thunder stones' or stones swimming in oil belonging to the *loa*, playing cards, rattles, holy emblems beside bottles of wine and liqueur—all for the gods" (Métraux 1972 [1959]:80). Tonton Mèmè hid some of the more sacred items—*govi* pitchers serving as receptacles for the *lwa*, his bell and rattle—under the altar.

5. The work of Hess (1984) shows the importance of home-based care in Haiti, and suggests that it endures even after emigration to Canada, a country with a radically different health-care infrastructure.

6. Two of the founding members of Projè Veye Sante were themselves felled by typhoid and malaria in their twenties. The project's first archivist died of infectious complications of childbirth.

7. The term "structures of feeling" is used following Raymond Williams (1980).

Chapter 6: 1986 and After: Narrative Truth and Political Change

1. Another irony of the era: the "food riots" that shook Cap Haitien in May 1984 consisted of hungry citizens raiding warehouses full of "spoiled food" destined for the newly arrived Iowa pigs.

2. Journalistic accounts of the downfall of the Duvaliers may be found in Abbott (1988); Desinor (1988); Ferguson (1987); and Rotberg (1988).

3. The important role of secrecy in rural Haiti is discussed by Chen and Murray (1976).

4. "The success or failure of a Haitian government is always ultimately determined by relations with the U.S." (Ferguson 1987:42).

5. Cited in Ferguson (1987:94).

6. For one of the chief mechanisms by which such claims are called in by those *laba* ("down there," i.e., still in Haiti), see Karen Richman's study of Haitian "cassette-discourse" (paper presented at the American Anthropological Association meeting, November 1989). Tape-recorded correspondence is perhaps the most important means of communication between rural Haiti and the urban United States.

7. "It was a good job," said Mme. Sonson a week after he lost it following an argument with the plant manager. "When Frico cut his finger off cutting the glass, they gave him fifteen days off with pay." There were plenty of able-bodied young men and women to take Frico's place, and so he was reduced to buying cigarettes in bulk and reselling them, one by one, on the streets of Port-au-Prince.

8. They would, in fact, be regarded as uninteresting by many political anthropologists. And yet the significance of these same sorts of changes have exercised social theorists since well before Marx, even if they are still poorly understood. Bloch (1975:2, 3), deploring "the lack of a clear theory for relating words to 'politics,'" notes that, "the political anthropologist, when he is analys-

ing and theorising about his data, rapidly abandons the reality of social intercourse, people saying things to each other, people coming into contact with
each other, and instead he 'imagines' the political which is taking place in a
hazy, artificially constructed area of hidden conflicts and alliances. By contrast
what is observed is simply dismissed as a front for this 'real' political activity."

Chapter 7: Manno

1. Saut d'Eau is the site of a waterfall at which the Virgin is said to have
appeared. Although Saut d'Eau is visited annually by thousands of Catholic
pilgrims, it is also sacred to adherents of voodoo, which draws heavily on
Catholicism.

2. Tuberculin skin tests such as the PPD or Mantoux tests may be negative
in persons with AIDS, who are often anergic.

3. It should be noted that Manno gave me identical accounts on three different occasions. On "promiscuity" and AIDS in Haiti, see Pape et al. (1986),
and also the review of this literature in chapter 13.

4. Père Jacques' assessment recalls that of Métraux, who reminds us that
"beliefs and 'folklore' practices are not only harmless superstitions. For many
they are a source of anxiety and a cause of serious expense. They sow discord
between relations and neighbors, foster chronic hatreds and sometimes end in
murder" (Métraux 1972:268). But Métraux was of two minds in his assessment of Haitian sorcery. See chapter 18 for a more thorough discussion of
AIDS-related sorcery.

5. Other ethnographers have documented widespread acceptance of such a
model of illness throughout Haiti. One of Hurbon's (1987a:194) informants
explains that "one can send a zombie on someone; he will die the same death
as the [zombified] person. There are some dead whose bodies cannot be taken.
One takes the zombie only. But if part of the body is there, it can still be used."

6. Tonton Mèmè states that he is the sole "real gangan" in Vieux Fonds.
Another man there is termed bokor by most, as he is thought to specialize in
maleficent magic. There are, however, two manbo in the area.

7. In translating the term voye yon mò tebe, I have used the less accurate "send
a tuberculous death" rather than the more cumbersome "send a dead person
who has died from TB." A similar rephrasing is used when translating voye yon
mò sida.

8. The ambience of the brutal summer of 1987 is well captured by Wilentz
(1989:95–101).

9. Saul later confessed that "I knew that you can't get sida by touching
someone with the disease; that's why I shook Manno's hand, so that he
wouldn't be discouraged. But afterwards it occurred to me several times that
I had been the only person to take his hand; if there were a possibility of transmission, I alone would fall ill. That frightened me. But later, I said to myself,
it's not true. Shaking hands is harmless."

10. A week after the funeral, Alourdes privately accused Fritz and his accomplices of having zombified her husband. "I know they raised him (*leve li*), because someone told me they saw Manno yesterday." She continued with a threat: "Well, we'll see: what a person does is what a person [later] sees."

11. Tonton Mèmè had much more to say about current Haitian politics, which seemed to be what was distracting him from our discussion of *sida*. He went off on a long tirade about the Haitian bourgeoisie. "They don't really want elections," he said vehemently, "because they don't want us to have a say in anything. If you have nine bourgeois Haitian brothers, and one of them is poor, the other eight won't try to raise him up. They'll make him their lackey (*tchoul*)." We were sitting near his little porch, upon which someone had painted a mangled version of "*Dechouke* every four years." *Kafou* had not been forgotten by the graffitist, nor had the word "love." Mèmè had also placed a large poster on his house. "Election 1987," it read. "Go register!"

12. A more thorough study of the elaboration over time of a collective representation of *sida* is offered in Farmer (1990c).

Chapter 8: Anita

1. It is not unusual for poor families to have (even poorer) servants. Laguerre's (1982:69) study of Belair would suggest that such arrangements have long been common there. He relates the history of one Sauveur, who had a regular job netting him twenty dollars per month; "the domestic was provided board and room and in addition earned $1.50 per month."

2. The slum was named, with poetic justice, for François Duvalier's wife. Following the departure of Duvalier *fils*, residents of the settlement rechristened it Cité Soleil.

3. On sexual unions in contemporary Haiti, see Allman (1980), Lowenthal (1984), Neptune-Anglade (1986), Simpson (1942), and Vieux (1989).

4. Mme. Sonson, who was not consulted until well after Anita's death, tells a different story. "I should know," she adds, "as I know the house she was staying in before she met the boy. . . . He was already ill. People already knew about *sida*, and they told her not to go with him. This is what I later heard."

5. This expression "put me in treatment" (*mete-m nan remèd*) usually refers to treatment with herbal remedies concocted to prevent illness in newly bereaved persons.

6. Luc, in 1985 the abusive boyfriend of a woman with *move san*, is described in less charitable terms in a previous study (Farmer 1988a).

7. In her study of illness stories in urban Ecuador, Price (1987) refers to such closing lines as "codas."

8. Note that in a previous interview, Anita had informed Dr. Constant and me that Vincent's coworkers had sent a *mò sida* on him.

9. Compare to 2 Timothy 4:5–6.

10. As Desinor (1988:172) observes, the country was "indifferent to the

February 7, 1988, inauguration of the new president, Leslie Manigat. The general feeling was that this was merely a change in titles and functions."

11. For consideration of the significance of dreams in rural Haiti, see the brief discussion by Romain (1959:197–199), and that of Métraux (1972:143–146). It is not uncommon to have treatments revealed in dreams. Métraux (1972:143) tells of a young woman of Marbial to whom Ogu came in a dream. Although she dreamed of her own brother, the woman knew that it was the warrior *lwa* because he was uniformed. In the dream, Ogu "led her out of the house by the hand and showed her plants which she must use in the preparation of a magic bath. When she woke up she faithfully followed the god's prescriptions and never had cause to regret it."

12. As noted in the next chapter, rural Haitian women often *mare vant yo*—tie up their bellies—"after the death of someone dear to them," as one of my informants put it. It is less usual behavior in a man.

13. Data suggest that rural Haitians have long spent exorbitant amounts on funerals. Noting a decline in the amount spent on these rituals, Bastien (1985 [1951]:190–191) cites an informant who held forth on these changes: "In the old days, the dead 'killed' the living, and the latter allowed themselves to be killed because of fear of what others might say. The cost of burials turned houses upside down! These days, we suffer enough with poverty that the dead shouldn't augment it. Remember the proverb, *Moun mouri pa konnen pri sèkèy*: the dead man never knows the price of his coffin!"

Chapter 9: Dieudonné

1. For an excellent portrayal of the resiliency of Haitian kinship in the face of land loss, the dissolution of *lakou*, and resulting migration, see Laguerre (1978).

2. Several people from Kay stated flatly that she had died from *sida*; two were sure that she had been shot while crossing a Carrefour street after a curfew. In 1986, her mother, who lived in Ba Kay, informed me that her daughter was working in a hotel, cleaning rooms.

3. Dieudonné, who was free only on Saturday afternoons, later recounted that his cousin's godmother eventually left her post because her employers would not let her attend church: she had to be present on Sundays "so that everything would be ready when they returned from mass."

4. The term is from *mort bossale*, as deployed in Saint-Domingue two hundred years earlier. And as Moreau de Saint-Méry (1984:543) shows, it meant precisely the same thing then: he wrote of "a wooden cross called 'Croix bossale' because for some time it had been the custom to bury unbaptised slaves around [this cross]."

5. And also, according to a certain M. Courtain, a judge in 1758 of the Siege Royal du Cap Français, *makandal* is a term for a sorcery bundle made popular by the Maroon of the same name (Courtain 1989:137).

6. Many of these projects were in fact quietly underwritten by Mme. Alexis, who often worked independently of her husband.

7. Dr. Roumain of the Clinique Saint-André documented the presence of the malaria parasite, *Plasmodium falciparum*, in her blood approximately one month before her death. In the months following Dieudonné's death, which was widely attributed to *sida*, I asked if the mother of his child might have had the new disorder. The majority of the twenty persons interviewed said no, and often added, "She had no diarrhea, and no sores."

8. I later asked Mme. Sonson if Dieudonné's illness might not have been sent by the woman's father. She thought that, no, the young rival in Port-au-Prince had sent it. When I persisted with, "Why did it take Dieudonné so long to succumb?" she responded with an oft-cited proverb: *Se pa jou fèy tonbe nan dlo a pou l pouri* ("A leaf doesn't rot as soon as it hits the water"). She reminded me, too, that Tonton Mèmè had revealed that the sickness had been sent from "a man in the city."

9. When pressed to speak of his own experience, he once replied rather sharply "that [politics] is my experience!"

10. Weise (1971:100–102) notes that the term *grippe* may correspond with "a common cold or primary tuberculosis, depending on duration of symptoms." In a study of forty-five Clinique Saint-André patients whose chief complaint was *grippe* with cough productive of sputum, two persons did indeed show bacteriologic evidence of active pulmonary tuberculosis.

11. The lesions, which recalled Kaposi's sarcoma, were in fact strikingly dissimilar from Manno's, whose skin lesions were documented superficial mycoses. As noted in chapter 11, Kaposi's sarcoma has become rare in Haitians with AIDS.

12. For a moving journalistic account of the destruction of Saint-Jean Bosco, and of the events and forces leading to it, see Wilentz (1989). The significance of the *ti legliz* movement is examined by Aristide (1990), the movement's most important proponent, and by Hurbon (1989), Midy (1989a; 1989b), and Wilentz (1989).

13. Recorded by Lerneus Joseph, to whom I am grateful. Compare the inspired Haitian adaptation to Isaiah 1:16–18.

14. "Before *sida*," observed Père Jacques referring to someone else with the disorder, "no one would have readily admitted to having TB. It's been upstaged." Although the majority of the persons with tuberculosis who were part of the Projè Veye Sante study were treated with compassion by their family members, many recalled tuberculosis as "the little house disease (*maladi ti kay*)," a reference to the separate quarters of the afflicted. Some older informants actually apologized before using the term *tibèkiloz*. Weise, who conducted fieldwork in Haiti's southern peninsula in the 1960s, offers case histories similar to the following: "Sometimes there is a separate room for the patient in the house. This is not necessarily a more agreeable situation than the 'ti tonnelle' [separate lean-to]. One family interviewed had one child, a boy of eighteen, living at home. They had a two-room wattle and daub house with an attached storage room. When the boy developed a cough and was diagnosed "tuberculose" by the local leaf doctor, the parents bedded him down on a rush

mat in the windowless storeroom. It was considered an ideal room, as tuberculosis is a cold disease; therefore one avoids drafts. The door to the storeroom was secured from the outside. The mother ministered to the boy daily, but his condition deteriorated steadily. He died, locked in his airless storeroom" (Weise 1971:97).

15. As Dieudonné's doctor observed, the international network in which Haitians now find themselves is "a semipermeable barrier through which we share the diseases, but not the treatments."

16. Still, Boss Yonèl's feelings about the matter had changed substantially over the years. In 1987, he stated that he "didn't really believe that [*sida*] exists. I think they just made it up to defame Haitians." Although such comments were common early in the Haitian epidemic, they were exceedingly rare by 1987.

17. In Creole, *Se yon lot bay pou rann pèp la fèb. Se yon maladi youn voye sou lòt. Sida desann, men li pa monte. . . . Se yon bay pou fè moun domi, kou wè "Vive la nation haitienne à tout jamais unie!" Sak te pase Sen Jan Bosko, se sak vre batay la, pa tout kont sa yo, pa tout madichon sa yo.* My content translation would read, "It's another burden to weaken the people. It's a sickness one poor person sends on another: AIDS goes down the social ladder, but does not go back up. It's a distraction, as is the false nationalism of the military leaders. The real struggle is not related to these intraclass squabbles, but rather to the struggle manifest in what happened at Saint-Jean Bosco."

18. Based on the observations of Saul Joseph. As a student at the Mirebalais *lycée*, Saul was one of those most inconvenienced by the report.

19. Stories about zombies abound when a young person dies, although their significance may easily be exaggerated. Few thought that Dieudonné had been raised, but I did register one dissenting opinion. It came from Jean-Jacques Fardin: "He was too hardy (*li te vanyan trop*), they thought he'd make a good *zonbi*. He would do a lot of work for the person [who zombified him]. . . . The person sent someone to his house in order to take his measurements while he was sleeping: his height and his width."

20. Tilibèt's addendum is one of the few references to a humoral classificatory system that Weise (1971:130) found to underlie the "health beliefs" of her informants: "The basic concept in rural Haitian health beliefs was found to be the maintenance of the delicate equilibrium of hot and cold elements." Her informants termed tuberculosis "the coldest of all diseases." The inhabitants of Do Kay, in contrast, rarely spoke of the disorder *per se* as hot or cold. Tuberculosis was held to cause hot states, such as fever or some night sweats, and cold states, such as chills or cold night sweats. Some termed these latter sweats *chofrèt*—"hotcold." In several years of research, it was not possible to uncover a coherent system of humoral classification with either high interindividual agreement or detectable relation to behavior (for example, diet, use of one therapeutic agent over another, avoidance of certain activities). Many of those in the Saint-André cohort (over twenty persons with active pulmonary tuberculosis) ate the foods that Weise's informants designated as proscribed to persons with tuberculosis (see Weise 1971:91, 107), and few made reference to such a framework in interviews spanning six years. Those who did invoke

such qualifiers tended to do so in a manner that justified their own courses of action. It has recently been suggested that humoral frameworks in Mexico play a similar validating role: "In Spanish-American popular therapies the role of humoral theories is not, as has been generally assumed, to provide guidelines for treatment, but rather to validate or legitimize empirical healing practices" (Foster 1988:133).

21. A term often translated as "common-law wife," but in reality describing a much more complicated state of affairs. See the brief review by J. Allman (1980) or the recent monograph by Vieux (1989).

Chapter 10: "A Place Ravaged by AIDS"

1. As Métraux (1972:266–267) notes, "Crossroads are favorite sites for the 'works' of magicians; handfuls of earth taken from them are an ingredient of many beneficent or harmful spells."

2. Intravenous drug abuse is unknown among rural Haitians, who are by all reports a remarkably abstemious people. There is, however, indiscriminate use of needles for intramuscular injections of antibiotics and vitamins, and it was for this reason that Projè Veye Sante began distributing single-use syringes. There had been, it was acknowledged, a disappointing response to the free condom program.

3. *Mwen pa nan politik anko; se tè m'ap travay.*

4. "It's a good thing we did cancel," Alexis joked the next morning. "The power went out shortly after midnight. Had the church been full of people, there would have been panic, a stampede. We would have been waiting for the soldiers' fire!"

5. Not everyone discerned a symbiotic relationship between AIDS and heightened concern with politics: "The political situation distracts the people's attention," says Dr. Bernard Liautaud, a member of a national commission on AIDS. "It's as if people think AIDS has gone away" (quoted in *U.S. News and World Report*, 12 February 1990).

6. In many ways, it was becoming increasingly difficult for the poor of the lower Plateau Central to find care elsewhere.

7. When later interviewed himself, the correspondent denied that he had attributed to the inhabitants of Kay high rates of the disorder: "I didn't say that Kay people had *sida*. I said that two or three people *from Port-au-Prince* who had been exposed to the germ (*jèm nan*) had come to live in Kay. I said that people should take many precautions. . . . The people misinterpreted what I said." He could not say what would lead residents of the capital to relocate to a tiny, impoverished village in the central plateau.

8. When I expressed surprise that the drivers would be so responsive to an erratum posted by Radio Soleil, the journalist replied with some heat that, at the height of the station's popularity, "three or four million of the six million [Haitians] listen to Radio Soleil."

9. *Doulè anba kè-m*: a chronic complaint in rural Haiti, "pain below the heart" seems to correlate with hyperacidity and reflux.

10. For research conducted between October and December 1988, I am grateful to Saul Joseph, who continued this research during my unexpectedly protracted absence from Do Kay.

11. Père Jacques later echoed, perhaps unwittingly, the message of Boss Yonèl. In a November sermon, he reminded his parishioners that "Kay is not for us alone. It is a center, it has been built to serve the rural poor, and you are their hosts."

12. A term suggested to me by Dr. Steven Nachman.

13. That some of these sicknesses are caused by magic in no way undermines this realism. It is, rather, a distinctly Haitian brand of realism, what has been termed the "marvelous realism" of the Haitian peasantry. Although the Cuban writer Alejo Carpentier is credited with its "discovery," marvelous realism describes an aesthetic that is most deeply embedded in rural Haitian culture. Carpentier acknowledges this by noting that the significance of the term was revealed to him in Haiti (see Taussig 1987:166).

Chapter 11: A Chronology

1. Some oncologists suspect that Kaposi's is somehow related to previous infection with cytomegalovirus. For a review of these data, see the article by Groopman (1983). For a study revealing a lack of association of cytomegalovirus with endemic Kaposi's, see Ambinder et al. (1987).

2. Stephen Murray (personal communication; see also Murray and Payne 1988; Payne 1987) poses sharp questions about the statistics used in various publications coming from Haitian researcher-physicians, including Pape and his GHESKIO coworkers. For example, Murray notes that it is not possible to go from an N of 34, of whom 13 are bisexual, to an N of 38, of whom 19 are said to be bisexual (compare Pape et al. 1984 and 1986). Dr. Murray's queries, which concern the relevance to the epidemic of bisexuality, deserve careful consideration and a reply in the scholarly literature. It should be noted, however, that the GHESKIO group worked with a gradually enlarging pool of ill informants, some of whom later and reluctantly revealed a history of bisexuality. In many countries, early reports on the AIDS epidemic were equally tentative and subject to revision (see Altman 1986; Oppenheimer 1988; Panem 1988; Shilts 1987).

3. In another review, Pape and Johnson (1988a:32) state that "in 1983, the majority of male patients with AIDS were bisexuals who had at least one sexual encounter with visiting North Americans or Haitians residing in North America."

4. The Collaborative Study Group of AIDS in Haitian-Americans (1987) was similarly unable to find a single Haitian with AIDS having a history of residence or travel in Africa.

5. Although the two populations are by no means comparable vis-à-vis established risk factors for HIV infection, it is instructive to compare these findings to contemporary studies from North America. In one study of 6,875 "male homosexuals and bisexuals," 4.5 percent were already seropositive in 1978 (Jaffe et al. 1985).

6. For example, in a letter response to the 1983 article by Pape and coworkers in the *New England Journal of Medicine*, two researchers from Yale University suggest that "Pape et al. do not convincingly exclude malnutrition as a cause of immune deficiency and opportunistic infection in the patients described" (Mellors and Barry 1984:1119). An earlier letter to the same journal suggested that "malnutrition is likely to be present in Haitians recently immigrated to Europe, Canada, or the United States," which might explain AIDS in Haitian infants (Goudsmit 1983:554). The theory was echoed by Beach and Laura (1983) in the *Annals of Internal Medicine*. The advent of antibody tests put an end to suggestions that malnutrition or some other disorder was masquerading as AIDS: among the GHESKIO patients, fully 96 percent of those diagnosed with AIDS on clinical grounds were found to be seropositive for HIV.

7. This is the thesis of Leibowitch's (1985) review, and is reiterated in Shilts's (1987) best-selling account of the pandemic.

Chapter 13: Haiti and the "Accepted Risk Factors"

1. In a recent colloquium held at Harvard University, Dr. Andrew Moss, director of the Department of AIDS Epidemiology at San Francisco General Hospital, observed that women are ten times as likely to become infected as men upon sexual exposure to HIV: "It worries me that the number of sexual partners is a risk factor for transmission [even among those who use intravenous drugs], and it worries me that the rate is twice as high in women as in men because this indicates that heterosexual transmission, not needle sharing, is responsible for new infections" (cited in the *Harvard AIDS Institute Monthly Report*, May 1990, p. 5).

2. In Haiti, the decreasing *relative* significance of same-sex contacts in the spread of HIV is the cause, it seems, for a decreasing incidence of Kaposi's sarcoma. Among North Americans with AIDS, Kaposi's sarcoma is seen most frequently among gay men (rather than among intravenous drug users, for example), especially those with histories of repeated exposure to cytomegalovirus.

3. It is not my intention to suggest that homosexuality is more stigmatized in Haiti than in other parts of Latin America. In fact, there are some ethnographic studies that would suggest the opposite (see the review in Murray 1987). It is nonetheless true that homosexuality remains stigmatized among Haitians, wherever they live.

4. The persistent conception of women as "AIDS transmitters," due in large

part, as Anastos and Marte (1989:10) note, to "deeply ingrained societal sexism as well as racism and classism," has skewed readings of U.S. epidemiology as well: women with HIV disease "are regarded by the public and studied by the medical profession as vectors of transmission to their children and male sexual partners rather than people with AIDS who are themselves frequently victims of transmission from the men in their lives." The tendency of North Americans to "blame the victims" will be further examined in chapter 21. For comprehensive studies of misreadings of HIV epidemiology among women, see the work of Paula Treichler.

Chapter 14: AIDS in the Caribbean

1. Studies of U.S. press coverage of AIDS suggest some of the reasons for public perceptions of Caribbean AIDS as a largely Haitian problem. When on July 25, 1985, CBS news ran a story about HIV transmission in Australia, "it was the network's first mention of AIDS outside the United States, Africa, or Haiti" (Kinsella 1989:144).

2. Such has also been the case in Denmark, where sexual contact with a North American gay man, rather than "promiscuity" per se, was an important risk factor in the first cases of AIDS (Gerstoft et al. 1985).

3. When questioned by Payne (1987) regarding the ethnographic validity of their observations of homosexuality in the Dominican Republic, Koenig and coworkers replied that their "information on the Dominican Republic does come from on-site visits to hotels that cater to the gay tourist trade. These places are frequented often by visitors from the United States and Caribbean countries" (Koenig, Brache, and Levy 1987:47). In a retrospective assessment seeming to support Koenig's argument, Garcia (1991:2) writes that "in the 1970s, [Puerta Plata] was favored by gay tourists and is considered to be one of the initial ports of entry for HIV in the Dominican Republic. During the 1970s, tourists were predominantly gay, over-sixty males who engaged in sex with local teenaged male prostitutes."

4. Haitians, notes Métraux (1972:359), are "irritated—understandably—by the label 'Voodoo-land' which travel agencies have stuck on their home."

5. The protagonist of Graham Greene's The Comedians is a Port-au-Prince hotelier who in 1961 remembers fondly the days when tourists flocked to his bar and made love in the pool. "The drummer's fled to New York, and all the bikini girls stay in Miami now," he explains to two prospective clients. "You'll probably be the only guests I have" (Greene 1966:11).

6. Although the lawsuit seemed ridiculous to most non-Haitian commentators, the effects of the CDC classification were probably apparent to some of the agency's operatives before the March 1983 announcement of the risk grouping. Requesting anonymity, one public-health officer made the following observations, cited in a front-page story in the New York Times of July 31, 1983: "It's a working definition. If there turned out to be a large national or ethnic

group, you would single that group out. But when you translate a working definition to a small, poverty-struck country like Haiti, it is devastating. It destroys one of their main cash industries—tourism."

7. Payne (1987:47) had previously observed that "several gay travel guides, such as the *Bob Damron Guidebook* for 1982, contain as many as ten entries for the Bahamas, but only four for the Dominican Republic and one for Haiti." It is important to note, as did Lange and Jaffe (1987), that the AIDS attack rate in the Bahamas was then even higher than that in Haiti.

8. It is not clear how such a misreading might have occurred. Ostensibly, however, d'Adesky has abandoned this tack, as her more recent essay underlines the sex-for-money exchanges that took place between tourists and poor Haitian men (see d'Adesky 1991:31).

9. See the International Monetary Fund's summaries of "Directions of Trade Statistics" in that organization's *Yearbook 1984*.

Part IV: AIDS, History, Political Economy

1. In regard to the logic underlying her Bolivian informants' ways of construing sickness, Libbet Crandon-Malamud makes the following, incisive claim: "As anthropology has propounded for all other forms of human behavior, medical practices and behaviors are also logical, regardless of their divergence from the opinion of the chiefs of staff at Presbyterian or Massachusetts General hospitals. History, social change, and political process, however, are essential to an understanding of them" (Crandon-Malamud 1991:210).

Chapter 15: Many Masters

1. Estimates of the indigenous population of Hispaniola vary widely. This variation reflects the controversy currently raging among physical anthropologists, archaeologists, and ethnohistorians: although all agree that the European discovery touched off devastating epidemics (of smallpox, measles, typhus, scarlet fever, and other highly contagious diseases) in previously unexposed native populations, there is no agreement about the size of pre-Columbian populations (see Roberts 1989 for a review of the debate). The figure of one million is often cited, but has been questioned by Anglade (1969:3053), who suggests the figure of 250,000. Francisque (1986), citing Las Casas ("une source digne de foi"), suggests 300,000. Cook and Borah (1971) have reviewed all contemporary sources at length, and have settled on the tragic figure of 8,000,000 as the aboriginal population of Hispaniola in 1492. There is, in contrast, more widespread agreement on the 1510, 1520, and 1530 figures. Using the figure of 1,000,000 and the role of imported infectious disease, Leibowitch (1985:56) observed that "scarlet fever, measles, smallpox, yellow fever, and other

Spanish-borne microbes will have transformed these lost pagans into 996,000 Christians saved for eternity."

2. It is held by some that Batholome de Las Casas, the lionized "Savior of the Indians," was reponsible for beginning the African slave trade. In order to spare the Indians, he suggested to Charles V that each white settler be issued a license to import twelve African slaves. As James acridly puts it, "In 1517, Charles V authorised the export of 15,000 slaves to San Domingo, and thus priest and King launched on the world the American slave-trade and slavery" (James 1980:4). Rout (1976:24) suggests that "it is more than likely that this decision would have been made even if Charles's friend, Las Casas, never suggested the importation of blacks to Hispaniola." Patterson would agree, for Africans, he asserts, "were literally the only source of labour that was politically weak enough, geographically accessible enough, epidemiologically suitable enough and (quite simply) known enough to be captured, transported and enslaved in the New World" (Patterson 1979:57). Other students of New World slavery underline the importance of diseases and immunity: "Had the Caribbean Indians not proved so susceptible to foreign pathogens, and had Europeans not proved so susceptible to African pathogens, it is doubtful that anywhere near the estimated 4.5 million, mostly West African, blacks would have been wrenched from their homeland and delivered to the islands of the Caribbean—all of which serves to illustrate the profound role that disease has played in the history of the West Indies" (Kiple 1984:4).

3. Wallerstein's (1974:88) dictum, "Slavery followed sugar," might be qualified by the more reasoned view held by Hirschman: "Obviously it was not sugarcane that created [American] slavery, but it is fairly safe to suggest that slavery would not have become as extended as it did after the sixteenth century without that particular staple and its peculiar bundle of characteristics" (cited in Mintz 1977:270 n. 54).

4. There is an enormous literature on slavery in the Caribbean, and several studies are cited in the text. Other key works include Gisler's (1981) study of slavery in the French Antilles and Pluchon's (1980) study of the mechanisms of the French trade. Klein's (1986) recent review includes much data, and Hargreaves (1969) has made important historical documents available. Sala-Molins (1987) offers commentary and interpretation of *Le Code Noir*.

5. If Schoelcher (1982:2) is correct, "the colony accounted for almost two-thirds of all French commercial interests."

6. As is suggested by Dieudonné Gracia's comments, the story of Macandal, the *grand empoisonneur* of Saint-Domingue, is relevant to an understanding of AIDS in contemporary Haiti.

7. See, for example, Auguste and Auguste (1985), Boisrond-Tonnerre (1804), Bryan (1984), Césaire (1981), Heinl and Heinl (1978), James (1980), Métral (1985), Nicholls (1985), Pamphile de Lacroix (1819), Schoelcher (1982). An exciting recent development has been the republication, by Imprimerie Deschamps, of Thomas Madiou's nine-volume history of the revolution and of the republic's first few decades. For studies examining the international context of the Haitian revolution, see Benot (1988), Blackburn (1988), Duffy (1987), and Murat (1976).

8. There is disagreement about the population of the colony in 1789. The figures offered by Williams are from Moreau de Saint-Méry. Malenfant, cited in Schoelcher (1982:1), suggests that, "only 500,000 slaves were declared in 1789, but as taxes were calculated per capita . . . neither children nor adults older than forty-five were declared; the number in these two groups approached 200,000."

9. The figures vary, of course; most of these come from British historian Bryan Edwards (1797), an eyewitness to the sack of Cap Français.

10. The reasons for the British invasion are treated fully by Williams, who cites the letter from a British army officer to Prime Minister Pitt: "The advantages of St. Domingo to Great Britain are innumerable—and would give her a monopoly of sugar, indigo, cotton and coffee. This island, for ages, would give such aid and force to industry as would be most happily felt in every part of the empire" (Williams 1970:249).

11. Toussaint's biographers, including the nineteenth-century French abolitionist Victor Schoelcher, maintain that Toussaint was an accomplished autodidact. "Having read and re-read the long volume by Abbé Raynal on the East and West Indies," notes James (1980:91), "he had a thorough grounding in the economics and politics, not only of San Domingo, but of all the great empires of Europe which were engaged in colonial expansion and trade."

12. Schoelcher notes approvingly the successes of Toussaint as the ruler of the colony. The former slaves, "more and more proud of him," were brought back to the cane fields. It is likely that the abolitionist is interpreting the historical record in a kindly light. There is ample evidence that the return to the plantation system was unpopular with the *nouveaux libres*, many of whom had already adopted a more "peasant" mode of farming. And although they may have obeyed Toussaint, the return to the large plantations was a move future Haitians would be reluctant to make under any conditions.

13. There is, of course, much confusion about the actual number of troops dispatched with Leclerc. Auguste and Auguste (1985:27–28) cite five prominent French and Haitian historians, each advancing a different total. These estimates range from 12,000 to 35,000. And many more soldiers were yet to come. General Rochambeau, Leclerc's second-in-command, reported that a total of 43,039 troops had arrived, in three waves, within the space of fifteen months. But as the Haitian historian Thomas Madiou and others have noted, these figures do not include the navy, itself active in combat, and numbering almost as many troops. Offering sober enough calculations, Auguste and Auguste (1985:29) reach the conclusion that a grand total of 80,000 men reached the shores of Saint-Domingue between February 1802 and November 1803. Even when counting both regular troops and popular militias, Toussaint's army numbered, at the time of Leclerc's arrival, some 33,000 troops. "We are lost," Toussaint was said to have murmured on seeing the French armada as it approached the colony's northern shore; "all France has come to St. Domingue" (Heinl and Heinl 1978:102).

14. At the close of his study, Davis (1975:557–558) summarizes these contributions as follows: "Toussaint's achievements had stunned the world. They had ensured British dominance in the Caribbean, had allowed Americans to

expand westward into Louisiana and Missouri, and had tautened the nerves of slaveholders from Maryland to Brazil. The repercussions continued to unfold. Early in 1816, Simon Bolivar made his historic pledge to Alexandre Pétion, then one of the rulers of Haiti, having first tried to win aid from slaveholding Jamaica. In return for the arms and provisions given by Pétion, Bolivar promised that, if his cause were successful, he would free the slaves of Venezuela. Back on South American soil, Bolivar issued his decree to all Negro males from the age of fourteen to sixty: fight or remain in bondage." Furthermore, there is also the undeniable fact that it was the Haitian insurrection that destroyed Napoleon's American dream. Louverture barred the Mississippi to the French. It is for this reason that Henry Adams (1947:151) observes that "the story of Toussaint Louverture has been told almost as often as that of Napoleon, but not in connection with the United States, although Toussaint exercised on their history an influence as decisive as that of any European ruler."

15. "I have given the French cannibals blood for blood," proclaimed Dessalines (Geggus 1989:47). "I have avenged America."

Chapter 16: The Nineteenth Century

1. Trouillot (1986: 78–79) suggests that "it is possible that the impression of a total disaster is a late and revisionist exaggeration." More important, he feels, was the absence of capital and, most important, the resistance of the nascent peasantry, which tenaciously "held on to its control over the work process and rejected militaristic [production] formulas."

2. On the vexed question of race, class, and color in Haiti, see the overviews by Trouillot (1986, 1990). After the revolution, practically speaking, there were no more *blancs, grands* or *petits*. This radical alteration has led some scholars to amplify the importance of one factor: "race." In Saint-Domingue, whites exploited blacks; in Haiti, the argument goes, mulattoes exploit blacks. For example, Leyburn's (1966) central assertion is that Haitian society is sharply divided into two segments, and that the division is so rigid that the term "caste" is wholly appropriate to the Haitian groupings. In one corner, the black peasantry, making up more than 90 percent of the population. In the other, the mulatto "elite," which dominates the state bureaucracy and other governmental institutions. These two factions of Haitian society differ, insists Leyburn, in all important regards: level of income, place of residence, education, language, religion, kinship structure, values and attitudes, and—above all—phenotypic characteristics. Such "angles" on Haiti carry substantial risks, as Trouillot notes: "The danger of this formulation—or of the elite/masses, rural/urban, mulatto/black dichotomies—lies in the risk of masking the economic mechanisms underlying these oppositions, especially that of rural versus urban. The danger is that one can miss classes and sub-classes within the peasantry and outside of it, and neglect the dynamic of social reproduction" (Trouillot 1986:89–90).

3. The planter added for good measure his assessment of the Haitian lead-

ers: "As for Haiti now you see that it is a stupid, insignificant, impotent government of orangutans which in two kicks fly to the mountains to eat *jobos* [a Cuban fruit] and guava" (Paquette 1988:180).

4. During the massacre of the French, often erroneously referred to as the massacre of the whites, Dessalines carefully picked out and spared the Polish and some other non-French members of Leclerc's expeditionary force. These men were held to be victims of Napoleon's imperial designs. Thus Article 13 of the 1805 constitution adds that the "Allemands et Polonais naturalisés par le Gouvernement" are exempt from the prohibition set forth in Article 12, which prohibited land ownership by non-Haitians.

5. John W. Eppes of Virginia set the tone for congressional debate: "Some gentlemen will declare St. Domingo free; if any gentleman harbors such sentiments let him come forward boldly and declare it. In such case, he will cover himself with detestation. A system that will bring immediate and horrible destruction on the fairest portion of America" (Jordan 1974:148–149).

6. Foreign currencies were important throughout the nineteenth century. In 1890, observes Castor (1988b:22), three different currencies were used in Haiti: the gourde, the dollar, and the Mexican peso. These last two were simply imposed by government fiat.

7. Under the stipulations of the treaty, "Louis XVIII was granted the right to regain all his American possessions. A secret article, agreed to by Great Britain, specifically recognized Haiti or Saint-Domingue as a French colony" (Lacerte 1981:500).

8. In his study of Haitian coffee cultivation, Girault (1982:57) underlines the central importance of the retention, by independent Haiti's leaders, of the colonial economy: "There is no doubt that the political and military thought of the leaders of Haitian liberation was very advanced for their era. One may cite their progressivism (struggle against racism), their new [military] strategies (guerilla warfare), their internationalism (aid to Latin-American independence movements). As regards economic theory, however, their concepts were indebted to the era's dominant models. They had no alternative economic model. And that was the tragedy of the young Haiti."

9. Nicholls recounts the following anecdote: "When it was suggested to Dessalines that the fierce policy he pursued toward the former French colonists would jeopardise his trade relations with other white countries, the emperor replied: 'Such a man does not know the whites. Hang a white man below one of the pans in the scales of the customs house, and put a sack of coffee in the other pan; the other whites will buy the coffee without paying attention to the body of their fellow white man'" (Nicholls 1985:89–90).

10. Brisk trade by no means assured equal relations between Haiti and the imperial powers. As early as 1827, these countries had taken to sending uninvited gunboats into Haitian waters. These surprise visits not only "served . . . to produce in the minds of the natives a favourable impression towards the whites," attested one British subject, "they also tended to ensure a continuance of their peaceful and respectful behaviour" (Nicholls 1985:92).

11. One North American diplomat reported that Soulouque's plan was to establish a nation of "pure black race," which would serve as the nucleus of a

"black empire" encompassing all the Antilles. An even more detailed (and impassioned) account of the strife of this period is given by Price-Mars, who concludes, "The Haitian-Dominican dispute was invested with a significance far beyond the issue of the territorial indivisibility of the island or the Dominican community's right to national independence; it grew, taking on dramatic proportions as a racial antagonism that pitted the tiny group of some six or seven hundred thousand black and mulatto Haitians against hundreds of millions of white Europeans and Americans" (Price-Mars 1953, vol. 2:180).

12. The production and marketing of coffee reveals the structures underpinning the economic crisis. The majority of Haitian coffee has long been planted, tended, and harvested by peasants; very often, it was processed and bulked by peasants as well. Peasants involved in coffee production lost up to 40 percent of their income to federal taxes. Because there were many links in the chain leading to the coastal cities where the coffee was prepared for export, and even more distance between the peasants and those who regulated prices on an international market, the producers were often far removed from those who benefited most from their labor (Girault 1984; Tanzi 1976).

13. "Because of corruption, promises of political support . . . the authorities closed their eyes to foreigners' illegal schemes, which completely controlled the import-export trade as well as retail commerce. The bank was regulated by them, as was the financing of foreign debts. And thus, inexorably and little by little, were accumulated the millions of floating debt concentrated in the hands of those abroad" (Castor 1988a:23).

14. The "Affaire Luders," an even more flagrant example of imperialist diplomacy, is the story of one Emile Luders, who, born in Haiti of a Haitian mother and a German father, was by Haitian law a Haitian citizen. In September 1897, Luders was arrested for assaulting two police officers, and sentenced to prison. The German emperor's chargé d'affaires set the cogs of imperial retribution in motion: although Luders had already been released from prison, by December a threat was published in a government newspaper in Berlin. Not surprisingly, it was not read by any Haitians, and the emperor sent another of his warships to exact reparations. The Haitian secretary of state received a "brutal, vulgar, and monstrous ultimatum," which included an indemnity of $20,000, a letter of apology to His Majesty the Emperor, a twenty-cannon salute to the German flag then flapping in the bay, and a "gracious reception" for the German envoy by the Haitian president. The emperor himself publicly referred to Haiti as "a despicable band of negroes, lightly tinted by French civilization" (Menos 1986:375). The Haitian statesmen were given four hours in which to consider these terms. They mulled it over. The stakes, it was concluded, were high: they were faced with the loss of the Haitian navy, both boats of it, as well as the country's coastal fortifications, much of which were over a century old. They also knew that cities built largely of wood burn quickly when bombarded. Four hours was not enough time in which to evacuate the civilian population. The Haitians capitulated.

15. "It is prophetic," comments Williams (1970:219), "that the appearance of North America in the Caribbean was marked, almost from the beginning, by a disregard of national boundaries."

Chapter 17: The United States and the People with History

1. Cited in the 12 March 1990 edition of the *International Business Chronicle*, p. 14. The same source notes that Florida exported $289 million worth of goods to Haiti in 1988.

2. In his study of the rise of the United States to world power, Dulles (1954:76) does not mince words: "The virtual protectorates the United States set up over the Dominican Republic, Haiti, and Nicaragua, in conjunction with possession of Puerto Rico and the Canal Zone, and the semiprotectorate over Cuba, consequently transformed the Caribbean into a [North] American lake from which all trespassers were rigidly barred."

3. His dismemberment has been described in great detail by several foreign historians. As Castor (1988b:54–55) notes somewhat defensively, "This event was much discussed as an example of Haitian savagery. Yet the people's anger had legitimate foundations. By killing those directly responsible for the odious prison massacre, people wished to revenge themselves and at the same time to show their determination to break with a past dominated by those ubiquitous satraps who, having committed their crimes, left [Haiti] to peacefully enjoy their money stolen from the country."

4. Heinl and Heinl (1978:441 n. 24) explain: "In a speech at Butte, Montana, on 18 August 1920, Roosevelt, then running for the vice-presidency, expansively remarked, 'You know, I have had something to do with running a couple of little republics. The facts are that I wrote Haiti's Constitution myself and, if I do say it, I think it's a pretty good Constitution.' Warren Harding, soon to be elected on the opposing ticket, took Roosevelt at face value and rejoined, 'I will never empower an assistant secretary of the Navy to draft a constitution for helpless neighbors in the West Indies and jam it down their throat at the point of bayonets.' Both politicians were wide of the mark: Sumner Welles, *éminence grise* of Latin American policy, put the facts straight in 1927: 'Although Franklin Roosevelt claimed . . . the Constitution had been written by him, his statement was not accurate, since it was drafted in the Department of State.' In the same letter Welles added that the Constitution 'was practically forced upon the Haitian Congress in a manner which was unwise and undoubtedly open to criticism.'"

5. Castor (1988b) also argues that the occupation aggravated the misery of the peasantry, leading to massive out-migration—some 250,000 Haitians emigrated to Cuba alone during the occupation.

6. Heinl and Heinl (1978:463, 470) attempt to counter what they see as the "strident, unbridled, and ashamedly partisan" accounts offered by nationalist Haitians and their North American sympathizers and insist that the "Caco rebellion at most involved no more than one quarter of Haiti and a fifth of its population." To appreciate the significance of the Caco rebellion, which never received outside funding, compare even these conservative figures to the more

recent struggles in Nicaragua, where even hundreds of millions of dollars and the most modern weapons could not muster more than 10,000 *contras*.

7. It was further suggested, perhaps first by British diplomat R. S. F. Edwards, that many of the North American servicemen had been recruited from the southern states on the notion that Southerners were better equipped to "handle coloured people." This is hotly contested by Colonel and Mrs. Heinl (1978:487–490), who suggest this was propaganda floated by non-Haitians, such as Edwards, who were hostile to the occupation. Regardless of the actual proportion of Southerners in the occupying force, the marines were first brought ashore by one Colonel Littleton W. T. Waller of Virginia. "I know the nigger and how to handle him," he wrote in 1916 to a superior officer (Heinl and Heinl 1978:489). In another commentary, Colonel Walker qualifies the Haitians as "real niggers and no mistake—there are some very fine looking, well educated polished men here but they are real nigs beneath the surface." It seems odd that the Heinls would reduce this to a purely demographic affair: a few Wallers, especially in top positions, can go a long way. On the question of Southerners, see also Millet (1978:71–73).

8. Lowenthal (1976:663) puts it mordantly: "Nine-tenths of the population still manages to produce nine-tenths of the total value of national exports *in addition to* their own needs, by working an inadequate amount of worn-out land, with an archaic technology, in the absence of functioning credit services, so that the other one-tenth of the population may continue to consume nine-tenths of all imported goods and the finest agricultural products, from fresh eggs to scotch whiskey."

9. See the report from the Institut Haitien de Statistique et d'Informatique, *Recueil des Statistiques de Base* (Port-au-Prince: Division des Statistiques Générales, 1986), p. 68. This government office keeps important statistics, many of which are irregularly published in report form.

10. In spite of the decline of the world sisal market, continues Francisque, "fiber production assures substantial profits to two large [North] American companies: The Haytian Américan Development Co. (HAYDCO) and the Societé Haitiano-Americain de développement agricole (SHADA), which occupy more than 11,000 hectares and employ almost 50,000 persons at starvation wages (less than four dollars for ten hours of work)." Also worthy of mention are essential oils: from World War II until recently, Haiti was the world's largest producer of vetiver (extract of *citron vert*), the sole producer of amyris, and an important exporter of other essential oils (Francisque 1986:125).

11. On slavery charges, see Plant (1987), Corten (1986), and Lemoine (1985). In June 1991, Dominican President Joaquin Balaguer ordered the expulsion of thousands of Haitian laborers.

12. In their consideration of unequal exchange and the urban informal sector, Portes and Walton (1982:74) designate Haiti as the most rural of all Latin American nations: in 1950, it was held to be 88 percent rural; in 1960, 85 percent; in 1970, 81 percent.

13. In 1984, Girault (1984:178) was able to complain that "Port-au-Prince

with 17–18 percent of the national population consumes as much as 30 percent of all the food produced in the country and a larger share of imported food." Government statistics reveal that the "Port-au-Prince agglomeration" consumed, in 1979, 93 percent of all electricity produced in the country. More recently, and more eloquently, Trouillot (1986:201) brings us up to date: "Monstrous capital, prisoner of its own contradictory tentacles—filthy shantytowns, ostentatious suburbs—Port-au-Prince houses 20 percent of the national population, but consumes 80 percent of all state expenditures."

14. Smith (1978:576), writing from Guatemala, notes that such malevolent neglect characterizes much of Latin America: "Rural people, rather than being directly exploited as in the [earlier economic system] are simply marginalized—left to fend for themselves in the depopulating rural hinterlands. The economic growth that takes place in the . . . urban centers of Latin America is, of course, funded for the most part by foreign investors, who also take most of the profits. But the most serious problem with this kind of dependency is that it deprives many . . . of the means for achieving even a peasant standard of living."

15. "Haitian soil was so exhausted and poor, it could produce only .90 units of rice per hectare whereas the Dominican Republic produced 2.67, Mexico 3.28, the U.S. 5.04, and wonderfully fertile Spain 6.04. Haiti could grow .67 units of corn to the Dominican Republic's 2.10, Canada's 5.38, the U.S.'s 6.35. Its sugarcane grew at 49 units compared to the Dominican Republic's 62.35, the U.S.'s 80.51, and Spain's 100. And coffee, Haiti's chief export crop, grew only .25 units whereas the Dominican Republic grew .31, Guadeloupe .95, and Mexico .75, statistics as dry as the eroded land that was starving the Haitians" (Abbott 1988:275).

16. Migration specialists, lulled by the accepted wisdom of Haiti's overwhelming rurality, were puzzled by the demographic picture presented by the "boat people" who reached the United States in significant numbers between 1972 and 1982. Commenting on "the shift away from agriculture," Stepick writes, "Over 40 percent of the migrants were either born in or had lived in Port-au-Prince; 34.2 percent were born or lived in a medium-size city and only 25.4 percent have spent all their lives in villages. The migrants are largely one generation removed from their peasant roots. Over 61 percent of the migrants' fathers were engaged in agriculture, but only 4.5 percent of the migrants themselves. Almost 21 percent of the migrants' fathers had semiskilled occupations, but 67.2 percent of the migrants had semiskilled occupations. Most frequent were tailors, but there were nearly as many teachers and mechanics. In both generations there were small numbers of unskilled, nonagricultural workers (5 percent in the fathers' and 4.5 percent in the migrants')" (Stepick 1984:346; paragraphing altered).

17. Using data from IHSI (1987), Locher (1984:325–336), Prince (1985).

18. There is a growing literature treating the Haitian diaspora in North America. See the studies by Chierici (1987), Conway and Buchanan (1985), DeWind and Kinley (1988), Laguerre (1984), Magloire (1984), Stepick (1984), and Stepick and Portes (1986). On transnationalism and Haitians, see the incisive study by Glick-Schiller and Fouron: "Transnationals are migrants

who are fully encapsulated neither in the host society nor in their native land but who nonetheless remain active participants in the social settings of both locations. They construct their identities in relation to both societies" (Glick-Schiller and Fouron 1990:331).

19. Commenting more on the violent atmosphere (and on the increasing boldness of Haitian death squads), Massing (1987) has recently written of the "salvadorization" of Haiti. Violent deaths have become rarer since the installation of a democratic government in early 1991.

20. In 1978, well before any impressive surge of organizing, "in an open letter to the government, a group of industrialists demanded that limits be placed on workers' organizing because of the 'wrongs' it has inflicted on their 'businesses'" (Hector 1989:177). For a report on violations of labor rights in the past decade, see Compa (1989).

21. In an unattributed cable that was circulated around "the U.S. mission" in 1988, the USAID health officer noted that "rumors abound that concern about AIDS among the American public led to the discontinuation of the production of 'Care Bears' in Haiti and that the same fear threatens the market for foods grown in Haiti that will be exported to the U.S."

22. Some estimates of Haitian unemployment are even higher. Boodhoo (1984:81) remarks that in 1978 "unemployment remained (almost unbelievably) in the 70–80 percent range."

Chapter 18: AIDS and Sorcery

1. Cited in Herskovits (1975 [1937]:247).

2. I later asked Saul why Étienne might choose not to answer. Looking somewhat impatient, Saul replied, "After dark, you don't have to answer just anyone who calls you."

3. In case anyone had any doubt as to the nature of the sacrifice, the Oxford English Dictionary (vol. XII, p. 310) adds the following sentence, ostensibly to illustrate usage: "As generally understood, Voodoo means the persistence, in Hayti, of abominable magic, mysteries, and cannibalism, brought originally by the negroes from Africa."

4. On the antisuperstition campaigns, see Bellegarde (1953), Dayan (1977), and Métraux (1972). There have been more indigenous attempts, also without success, to extirpate voodoo. More recently, the flight of Jean-Claude Duvalier (whose father, at least, was seen as an ally of voodoo), has led to the expression of much antivoodoo sentiment. In 1986 alone, several *houngan* were murdered, and scores of temples were destroyed. This violence illustrates the marked cultural and religious heterogeneity of Haiti, and calls into question the pat conclusions of Leyburn (1966) and many others who divide Haiti into two internally homogenous groups: the small wealthy elite, and the large, poor majority. See Hurbon (1987b) for a discussion of this persecution, which was inextricably bound up in popular associations of voodoo with *macoutisme*.

5. Weise (1971:130) asserts that "any illness which defies natural medicine is, by definition, supernatural in nature." Fieldwork in the Kay area does not support this contention. My informants recognize illnesses that demand immediate "supernatural" intervention, and also many "natural" illnesses that are difficult to cure (for example, chronic leg ulcers), or that are unresponsive to biomedical intervention (for example, malignancy in an aged person, or *move san*).

6. The speed with which his informants attributed illness to human agency, together with the high cost of "treatment," again strain Métraux's (1972: 269) relativism: "Unfortunately rural society has plenty of neurotics or simply troubled and downcast spirits who are quick to suggest that an illness is not 'from God,' that an accident is surrounded with suspicious circumstances and that a death was not due to natural causes."

7. As Maximilien (1945:185–191) explains, *pakèt* are more often "talismans crafted for therapeutic purposes."

8. In the course of a discussion of *maji*, one often hears Creole speakers state in French that *le mal existe*: evil exists. The expression is invoked most frequently by those professing a faith other than that in the *lwa*, and is meant to imply, "You ascribe to what you want, I'll ascribe to what I want. But let neither of us foolishly question the existence of evil forces such as aggressive magic." Furthermore, there are no doubt "subtypes" of sorcery. That deployed in voodoo is slightly different from that feared by the rural Haitian equivalents of "born-again Christians." Mabille (in Maximilien 1945:xix) makes this point obliquely when he observes that "European magic has profoundly marked not only voodoo, but all rural Haitian sorcery."

9. The preceding discussion is not meant to suggest that the beliefs of my informants are internally consistent and without a great deal of fuzziness. The ambivalence is real. The point is that ambivalence about responses to misfortune need not lead us to question the "authenticity" of chosen religious affiliation. One of Lowenthal's informants put it this way: "I don't really believe in the lwa, but when they come to me or to someone else it doesn't matter if you believe in them or not—there they are!" (in Lowenthal 1978:405).

10. In this regard, is is useful to return to the ethnographic materials presented in previous chapters. Recall the example offered by the Protestant pastor who came to perform Anita's burial rites. He recounted the story of the distraught *houngan* who, following the death of his son, knew that he had been killed through sorcery and that his murderers would later try to zombify the child. The *houngan* went to the cemetery and "raised the child." He then took him to Hinch to "Pastor Daniel," a well-known Evangelical Christian. When "the devil's people" later found the grave empty, they were of course thwarted in their efforts to zombify the boy. Pastor Daniel, meanwhile, "lay his body upon that of the dead child, saying, 'Get up, I say, and join the living.'" The child stirred. Once the child was "protected" against zombification he was free to die a natural death, and was promptly reburied. The lesson was that the powers of a Pastor Daniel are greater than the powers of those who engage in sorcery.

11. Pig poisoning, like so many other phenomena in Haiti, may be "sim-

ple," that is, due to a toxic substance alone, or "not simple." In the latter case, the effects of the magic are the cause of death. A survey of over three-fourths of all adult villagers revealed that 100 percent of those questioned cited *kola* as a common cause of death of their pigs. More often than not, the *kola* was not simple, and this was revealed through the afflicted pig's agonal movements. Witnesses would report that these pigs went through bizarre contortions before expiring.

12. Brown, who describes the rural Haitian ethic as an "intensely contextual one," observes that "another moral force is the belief that only in extreme circumstances may one use sorcery to harm another, and only if one is absolutely just in doing so" (Brown 1989a:54–55).

13. In their most extreme forms, these concerns may contribute to the formation of voodoo secret societies, termed *chanpwel* or *bizango*. Davis (1988: 278) writes of the "Bizango judicial process," which considers as grave offense the following transgressions: "1. Ambition—excessive material advancement at the obvious expense of family and dependents; 2. Displaying lack of respect for one's fellows; 3. Denigrating the Bizango society; 4. Stealing another man's woman; 5. Spreading loose talk that slanders and affects the well-being of others; 6. Harming members of one's family; 7. Land issues—any action that unjustly keeps another from working the land."

14. In her classic study of kuru in the New Guinea highlands, Lindenbaum (1979) concludes that "in the absence of alternative methods of settling disputes, sorcery may serve to regulate relations between individuals who must cooperate and also compete. . . . Sorcery seems designed not to interrupt, but to modulate the process."

15. The proverb is literally translated as "Your amount of money is your amount of *wanga*."

16. Taussig (1987:282) writes of poor black migrants to the town of Puerto Tejado, "alert to the slightest infraction of sharing and equality. Reciprocity was their code. 'Here on the coast,' went one expression, 'one hand washes the other.' And they feared and mustered the weapon of *maleficio* if that code was denied." It must be noted, however, that in village Haiti there are many other reasons to fear having more than others. "In certain villages," observed Hurbon (1987b:14), "the development of *macoutisme* leads some merchants and small producers to reduce the volume of their production to avoid working solely for the macoutes' benefit. . . . The macoute always begins by suspecting and accusing of opposition to the government those whose belongings he covets." In rocky and infertile Do Kay, however, these forces are less important than in more functional agricultural settlements: poverty in the Kay area is so extreme that there is less chance of attracting the attention of the macoutes.

17. The mother died "well before her date," explained Mme. Sonson, of a wasting illness that "took away her appetite." During a postmortem divination session, one of Fardin's relatives learned that he was the culprit.

18. See also Herskovits (1975 [1937]), Métraux (1972), and Romain (1959:206–208). A similar dynamic accounts for the mottoes that are painted on the trucks and buses used for public transportation. Because such an acquisi-

tion is one of the few means by which an unlettered person may accumulate wealth, it is necessary to certify the origin of the vehicle: "Gift from God," "Fruit of My Prayer," "Praise God From Whom All Blessings Flow," and "Thank You, Papa" are emblazoned on the vehicles that cross the central plateau. Alternatively, the vehicle might display mottoes meant to forestall speculations of shady dealings with the devil ("Say What You Will"), or pre-emptively dismiss such comments as drivel ("You Jabber, I'll Work"). Similar themes are prominent in Haitian popular music (see Courlander 1960).

19. Of course, somewhat different conditions may also give rise to struc-tures of feeling similar to those encountered in rural Haiti. Among peasants in a Mysore village in India, "witchcraft acts as a moralising agent by condemning socially undesirable traits in individuals" (Epstein 1967:154), most notably greediness.

Chapter 19: AIDS and Racism

1. Hurbon (1987b:25) underlines this point when he asserts that "with the exception of the 4,000 families with annual incomes of more than $90,000, all social classes in Haiti are consumed with the desire to leave."

2. One of the victims, twenty-six-year-old Solange Eliodar, died in Jackson Memorial Hospital in Miami, but had been one of those held in Krome Avenue detention camp as an illegal entrant. See the *Miami Herald*, 30 June 1983, p. 58.

3. Furthermore, epidemiologists knew that cases of AIDS had also occurred in Haiti, which might have changed the denominator to well over 6 million (Olle-Goig 1984:124).

4. Writing in the *Miami Times*, Dr. Robert Auguste of the Haitian Coali-tion on AIDS remarked that "in the annals of medicine, this categorization of a nationality as a 'risk group' is unique."

5. As Treichler (1988a:198) has observed, "This list structured the collec-tion of evidence for the next several years and contributed to the view that the major risk factor in acquiring AIDS was being a particular kind of person rather than doing particular things."

6. Although the Haitian studies were published in refereed scientific jour-nals, they were to a large extent ignored. "By decree of (Western) arrogance," observes Leibowitch (1985:62) wryly, "the dating of the disease in Haiti can-not rest on the testimonies of Third World doctors."

7. Others have noted that during the polio epidemic in New York City, blame *was* assessed in predictable ways: "Ethnic minorities and the powerless poor had been stigmatized in the name of established public health dogma" (Risse 1988:56). See chapter 21 for a more thorough discussion of patterns of blame and accusation in North America and Haiti. It is also important to note the importance of mode of transmission. That HIV is sexually transmitted,

while polio is not, is highly significant, as Brandt's (1987) study of syphilis in the United States would suggest.

8. Reported in the *Miami Herald,* 20 August 1983, p. 1B.

9. Cited in the *Miami News,* 30 May 1983, p. 5A.

10. "Diaspora, the newest formulation of 'community,' remains an ideology that masks real divisions in experience and outlook and obscures the existence of differing political goals and strategies" (Glick-Schiller and Fouron 1990:341). Since these words were written, a new term has replaced "diaspora." Recently inaugurated President Jean-Bertrand Aristide observes that, although Haiti is ostensibly divided into nine *départements,* a tenth *département* exists in the hearts of most Haitians. This *dixième département,* he says, is constituted by all Haitians living outside the homeland.

11. It is important to acknowledge the deep political divisions within these coalitions (see Nachman and Dreyfuss 1986; Saint-Gérard 1984), with more "moderate" individuals grouped around Haitian-American physicians. Progressive community leaders, who have been heard to accuse the physician-dominated collectives of "collaborationism," have opted for a more sweeping critique of North American society. Glick-Schiller and Fouron (1990) offer the most incisive analysis of these divisions, although they do not speak explicitly of the anti-AIDS coalitions.

12. *Tampa Tribune,* Thursday, 15 February 1990, p. 9.

13. In a 29 April 1990 editorial, the *New York Times* termed the Haitian complaint "arcane."

14. A similar point was made by Saint-Gérard (1984:72), who cautioned, "To understand this emotional trauma one must examine the source of all episodes termed 'national embarrassments': the boat-people phenomenon, the drama of Cayo Lobos, the enslavement of Haitians in the *bateys* of the Dominican Republic. . . . So many unforeseen situations closely linked to the country's decline. The affective importance [of these events] for Haitians in the diaspora is even more significant, because it is reinforced by the difficulties associated with emigration." Writing of anti-Americanism in contemporary Haiti, Massing (1987:49) makes a similar observation: "To understand the depth of Haitian feelings about these matters, one must remember that Haitians have accumulated a huge backlog of complaints against the United States."

15. Cited in the *Boston Globe,* 5 Apr. 1990, p. 27.

16. From the *Boston Globe,* 11 May 1990, p. 25.

17. Quoted in the *Boston Globe,* 11 May 1990, p. 25.

18. Cited in *Haiti Progrès,* 25 Apr.–1 May 1990, p. 13.

19. Cited in the *New York Daily News,* 25 Apr. 1990, p. 23.

20. From the *New York Times,* 21 Apr. 1990, p. 10.

21. The article appeared in the *New York Daily News,* 25 Apr. 1990, p. 23 .

22. It is important to recognize, however, that important divisions persist within this movement. That these are fundamental, and thus likely to limit the effectiveness of such organizing, is suggested in an important essay by Glick-Schiller and Fouron: "Large numbers of immigrants may decide to identify publicly with their country of origin and may respond to efforts to mobilize

them in short-term actions. They may come together in activities that express publicly their pride in their country of origin. Such actions or activities may be precipitated by events in either society: a hurricane at home, a blatant case of discrimination abroad. However, a political leader interested in developing a constituency will generally try to shape a transnational population into an organized political base vis-à-vis the system of either the home or the host society. It is at this point that the interests of leaders and those of the general immigrant population may well diverge, with much of the immigrant population having no interest in the political status quo of either polity. Consequently, no sustained joint pattern of action emerges" (Glick-Schiller and Fouron 1990:342).

23. In 1986, one Haitian physician prominent in AIDS research complained about the journalists that had been haranguing him for over two years: "Americans are never interested in Haiti unless there's some disaster to report. Now they have AIDS in Haitians, and all they want to know is 'How do they get it from voodoo?' When we tell them that Haitians contract AIDS the same way that Americans get it, they just don't believe us. They simply go and find someone who will tell them what they want to hear, some story about blood sacrifice."

24. As for the mechanisms by which "magic rituals sometimes transfer blood and secretions from person to person," Viera (1987:122) adds that "worshippers of Eurzulie, a benign deity, engage in rituals during which the houngan, or priest, may engage in intercourse with other male worshippers."

25. The authors are quick to abandon even the conditional tenor of their speculations: "The subsequent spread of the epidemic to Western populations was through international gay tourism to Haiti, not central Africa, which has comparatively little tourism" (Moore and LeBaron 1986:77–78).

26. Such conceptual distancing is by no means reserved for Haitians, as Treichler (1989) suggests: "The Third World typically enters First World discourse more or less unconsciously as a stereotypically reliable explanatory figure for the exotic and alien." It should be noted, however, that the "Black Republic" of Haiti served throughout the nineteenth century as a sort of prototypical Third World nation, the first of its type.

27. The term "semantic network" is used following Good (1977) and Good and Good (1982).

28. Accordingly, these exotic theories had their echoes in the popular sector. In a returned examination, a Haitian pupil at a Boston public school was informed by her white, North American teacher that AIDS had originated in Haiti. This commentary, proferred in a written evaluation of the student's essay about AIDS, read as follows: "You answered the question very well. I don't think homosexuals spread AIDS. My doctor told me that Haitians created AIDS because they have sexual intercourse with monkeys." British researchers were also guilty of floating such theories, although their target was the much larger continent of Africa. In 1986, the following words appeared in The Lancet: "Monkeys are often hunted for food in Africa. Once caught, monkeys are often kept in huts for some time before they are eaten. Dead monkeys are often used as toys by African children" (Sabatier 1988:62).

29. For example, a research proposal drafted in 1983 by top researchers in

Miami contained a long questionnaire to be administered to Haitian patients. The questionnaire read, "Do you consider yourself (check one) ____ heterosexual ____ homosexual." The questionnaire was "to be translated into French." When an anthropologist noted that most Haitians did not speak French, the investigators conceded that, given this fact, Creole should be the language in which interviews would be conducted (see Farmer 1990a:83–87).

30. From the *Miami News,* 1 Nov. 1986. The man, who was being held in the INS detention center in South Dade, was later deported on charges of drug trafficking.

31. See "Some Haitian AIDS victims are gay, U[niversity of] M[iami] study shows," in the 19 May 1984 issue of the *Miami Herald,* p. 1B.

32. For the latest contribution to the literature drawing on this symbolic network, see Palmer's (1991) *Extreme Measures*—"a novel of medical suspense." The novel is set in a Boston teaching hospital, but in it one finds crazy Haitians, zombies, mention of "goddam cannibals" and AIDS, and yet another hero who is young and white and male.

33. The fact that this comment could come from an Australian does indeed underline the significance of race and class in the structuring of an international gay "community."

34. In May 1983, one Florida bathhouse owner "brushed off questions of the baths' role in the epidemic by insisting that most of Florida's AIDS cases were Haitians, and it wasn't a problem for gays. This was not accurate" (Shilts 1987:306). See also the articles that appeared in 1983–84 in the New York-based *Native,* or Kinsella's (1989) discussion of these essays.

Chapter 20: AIDS and Empire

1. The term "American plan for Haiti" was heard frequently in 1987, when a document by the same name was floated to the local press (see Wilentz 1989:269–279).

2. "FDA WANRAGE" is copyrighted by Ansy and Yole Dérose. Used with permission.

3. See Treichler's (1989:39–48) important reading of this article and of the larger corpus of "third world AIDS in first world media."

4. From an editorial first published in *Haiti Progrès,* 17–23 Aug. 1983, and reprinted in the edition of 25 Apr.–1 May 1990.

5. The *New York Times,* 21 Apr. 1990, p. 10.

6. Dalton (1989:220) explains that African-Americans' frequent use of the term *genocide* "reflects the genuine suspicion of many that the AIDS virus was developed in a government laboratory for the express purpose of killing off the unwanted." See also the commentary of Kinsella (1989:245), who finds in the *Amsterdam News,* "the granddaddy of the black media," a great deal of enthusiasm for tracking down conspiracy theories "such as the idea that AIDS is a product of a CIA experiment run afoul in the Congo." Borneman analyzes similar assertions as advanced in Europe, including East Germany and the Soviet Union. "Coverage of the conspiracy theory of AIDS," he concludes, "is

only a variant of the Western press's tendency to sensationalize the AIDS crisis" (Borneman 1988:234). Shilts (1987:228) notes the straight world's incredulity that often greeted gay men's fears of internment in camps. In Johnson's *Plague: A Novel About Healing* (1987), we are introduced to a gay psychiatrist who helps to uncover the truth about AIDS: the virus was in fact disseminated by right-wing weapons consultants to the armed forces. Although the protagonist and his lover hope that they will wake up from a "paranoid nightmare," the sad fact, they observe, is that "it'd be perfectly consistent with history." The book's hero is well schooled in the history of discrimination against gay men, but he finds it difficult to apply his persecution theory to others: "As for the Haitians, I don't know. Chance, I guess" (T. Johnson 1987:189). See also S. Murray (1987).

7. Drs. Gallo's and Montagnier's letter is in response to one addressed to the editors of *Scientific American*. Both are published on pp. 10–11 of the June 1989 issue of the journal.

8. Shilts continues: "Campbell's role in the gay community, however, illuminated one reason the gay political leadership would be reluctant to get stern with bathhouses. Campbell, for example, served on the board of five major national gay organizations. Without dispute, he was the most powerful gay leader in Florida. No Miami gay leader and no liberal politician out to curry favor with Florida's sizable gay community would drop a word about bathhouse closure."

9. Banner headline in *Miami News*, 27 Oct. 1979.

10. In the *Miami Herald*, 27 Mar. 1981, p. 1C.

11. Reported in *Miami Herald*, 2 July 1982, p. 1C.

12. In addition to the legendary Dominican hatred for Haitians are the less well-known prejudices of many Bahamians: "The ongoing hostility of Bahamian citizens and authorities had provoked two concerted attempts to rid the Commonwealth of Haitians, once in 1974 and again in 1978 when they were hunted down in the streets like dogs, imprisoned, beaten, then deported. At any given time in Nassau's Fox Hill prison, 900 to 1,500 Haitians occupied cells designed for 600, and as fast as inmates were deported, new ones took their places. Even for Haitians resident for as long as twenty-five years, there was no security" (Abbott 1988:234). In 1991, the Population Reference Bureau in Washington estimated that the per capita GNP of Haiti was $400. In the Bahamas, GNP was pegged at $11,370.

13. Many infectious diseases are indeed endemic to Haiti, but that a socially constructed stereotype is at play is suggested by Leyburn (1966:275), who in a strange melding of the folk concepts of black promiscuity and contagion observed that in Haiti, "tuberculosis progresses rapidly when it appears. The people have never developed a specific immunity to it, and promiscuous sex relations play their part in spreading the disease by contagion."

14. In the San Francisco *Sunday Punch*, 31 Mar. 1991.

15. Saint-Gérard (1984:108) declares the principal beneficiary to have been a certain Joseph Gorinstein.

16. "Cambronne also dealt in cadavers, in almost as much demand. To save the living, medical students must dissect the dead, and obtaining corpses in sufficient quantity is the perennial problem of medical schools. Haitian cadav-

ers, readily available once Cambronne entered the business, had the distinct advantage of being thin, so the student had no layers of fat to slice through before reaching the object of the lesson. Cambronne, using the refrigerated container service recently introduced into Haiti, supplied these corpses on demand. When the General Hospital failed to provide him with enough despite the $3.00 he paid for each body, he simply stole them from various funeral parlors" (Abbott 1988:171).

17. The *Albuquerque Journal,* 14 Oct. 1985.

18. The Africa-to-Haiti-to-the-United States theory is still widely circulated, even in more critical quarters. Randy Shilts writes that the epidemiological story "was fairly easy to piece together. A remote tribe may have harbored the virus. With the rapid urbanization of [equatorial Africa] after colonization, the virus may have only recently reached the major cities, such as Kinshasa. From Africa, the virus jumped to Europe, where AIDS cases were appearing regularly by the late 1970s, and to Haiti, through administrators imported from that island to work in Zaire throughout the 1970s. From Europe and Haiti, the virus quickly made its debut in the United States" (Shilts 1987:459).

19. Those who would dismiss persistent rumors of medical experimentation on disempowered black people should read accounts of the "Tuskegee Experiment," in which treatment for syphilis was withheld from some four hundred black sharecroppers in Alabama in order to chart the "natural history" of the disease. See the accounts by Brandt (1978, 1987) and by Jones (1981). As for suggestions that AIDS came to Haiti via a CIA-sponsored plot to destroy Cuban livestock, it is true that such theories have always been feeble. But before dismissing the Haitian speculations as "rubbish," we should note with humility that the very same theory was entertained by many North American scientists: "An epidemic of deadly fevers ravaged the Cuban swine-stocks, beginning in 1975. At its source, an African strain of virus whose first victims had been hogs from the Kenya plateaus. Kenya-Angola-Cuba-AIDS, such might have been the chain of importation, either through contaminated animals or else, according to the testimony of former members of the famous 'agency,' by the direct and malicious contamination of the Cuban hogs financed by the CIA. Despite its seductive exotico-historical features, however, this outsider virus is neither retro-, nor humanophiliac, nor T4-trope, nor present in Japan. *Yet it briefly took the lead among the virus-candidates for AIDS,* in the highly imaginative period of the first quarter of 1983" (Leibowitch 1985:69–70; emphasis added).

Chapter 21: Blame, Cause, Etiology, and Accusation

1. This evaluation should be tempered by another assessment by Métraux, in which he warns that "beliefs and 'folklore' practices are not only harmless superstitions. For many they are a source of anxiety and a cause of serious expense. They sow discord between relations and neighbors, foster chronic hatreds and sometimes end in murder" (Métraux 1972:268).

2. In fact, poor women in general have been to some extent scapegoated, as Anastos and Marte (1989:12) have noted: "Sexism feeds on itself with the false perception of women as vectors rather than victims of HIV transmission. When classism and racism join with sexism, as they do for inner-city women, the impact of AIDS is devastating."

3. For an overview of "biblical" justifications of slavery, see Smith (1972). Fascinating documents treating *La Traite des Noirs au Siècle des Lumières* have recently been presented by Vissière and Vissière (1982:7) who explain that "the system's profiteers had no need to orchestrate propaganda campaigns: there was, at the base of the trade and of slavery, such a chain of events that this vicious exploitation of one man by another seemed necessary, inevitable, written in the very nature of things." The finest study of the question, however, is David Brion Davis's magisterial *Problem of Slavery in the Age of Revolution, 1770–1823* (1975).

4. For an important study of the "humanitarian" justifications of North American imperialism, see Weinberg (1963:434–435). That blaming-the-victim readings of Haitian history are still uncritically accepted is suggested by a recent essay by Martha Gellhorn: "The unlucky ignorant people of Haiti never understood that they had to take an interest in politics while they still had the chance. I think their brains were fuddled by three hundred years of voodoo. They were too busy propitiating a gang of demented malevolent gods to notice that men, not gods, were running their country and themselves into the ground. If they know now, it is late" (Gellhorn 1984:103).

5. See the excellent 1981 report, *Socialization for Scarcity*, submitted by Maria Alvarez and Gerald Murray to USAID in Port-au-Prince, Haiti.

6. "The stigma that marks the victim and accounts for his victimization is an acquired stigma, a stigma of social, rather than genetic, origin. But the stigma, the defect, the fatal difference—though derived in the past from environmental forces—is still located *within* the victim, inside his skin. With such an elegant formulation, the humanitarian can have it both ways. He can, all at the same time, concentrate his charitable interests on the defects of the victim, condemn the vague social and environmental stresses that produced the defect (some time ago), and ignore the continuing effect of victimizing social forces (right now). It is a brilliant ideology for justifying a perverse form of social action designed to change, not society, as one might expect, but rather society's victim" (Ryan 1971:7).

7. Cited in Abbott (1988:235).

Chapter 22: Conclusion

1. This is not meant to suggest that investigation of illness representations is not a key task for medical anthropology. For such studies, see Farmer (1990c) and Farmer and Good (1991).

2. Webster (1981) defines temporality as "concern with time, process, and

overt mundane events as more real or significant than timeless or external forms, structures, or patterns: emphasis is on change rather than permanence."

3. Earlier in this century, historians were taken to task by their colleagues Bloch, Febvre, Braudel, and other representatives of the *Annales* school. All too often, claimed the innovators, historians had been seduced by documents treating flashy diplomacy, regal pageantry, and spectacular battles. The product was a facile and superficial *histoire événementielle,* a "history of brief, rapid, nervous fluctuations, by definition ultra-sensitive; the least tremor sets all its antennae quivering" (Braudel 1972:21). The leaders of the *Annales* movement encouraged their students to examine *la longue durée* and to attempt to discern underlying structures with explanatory efficacy.

4. Such has been persuasively argued by Depestre (1980), Hurbon (1987a, 1987c), and other thoughtful students of Haitian cultural phenomena.

5. The 1991 "World Population Data Sheet" of the Population Reference Bureau (Washington, D.C.) suggests the dimensions of this economic disparity: Haitian per capita GNP is estimated at $400 per annum; that of the United States at $21,100.

6. Cited in the *Houston Chronicle,* 1 Nov. 1987, p. 8 (section 9).

7. In their recent review of "Sexually Transmitted Diseases in the AIDS Era," Aral and Holmes (1991:69) reach a similar conclusion: "By themselves, the medical solutions to the prevention and control of STDs and AIDS are not enough: they must be coupled with the identification and correction of the societal factors reponsible for the global pandemic."

8. A critique of the use of such "quick-and-dirty" anthropology in AIDS research is elaborated in Farmer (1991a).

Bibliography

Abbott, Elizabeth
  1988   *Haiti: The Duvaliers and Their Legacy.* New York: McGraw-Hill.
Adams, H.
  1947 [1889] *The Formative Years: History of the United States of America During the First Administration of Thomas Jefferson.* Vol. 1. Cambridge, MA: The Riverside Press.
Adelaide-Merlande, J.
  1982   Introduction. In V. Schoelcher, *Vie de Toussaint Louverture,* pp. v–xxiii. Paris: Éditions Karthala.
  1985   Introduction. In A. Métral, *Histoire de l'Expédition des Français à Saint-Domingue,* pp. v–xxxiii. Paris: Éditions Karthala.
Albert, Edward
  1986   Illness and Deviance: The Response of the Press to AIDS. In *The Social Dimensions of AIDS: Method and Theory,* Douglas Feldman and Thomas Johnson, eds., pp. 163–178. New York: Praeger.
Allen, John
  1930   An Inside View of Revolutions in Haiti. *Current History* 32:325–329.
Allman, James
  1980   Sexual Unions in Rural Haiti. *International Journal of Sociology of the Family* 10:15–39.
  1981   Estimates of Haitian International Migration: Some Policy Considerations. Paper presented at the meetings of the Population Association of America. Washington, D.C., March 26–28.
Allman, T. D.
  1989   After Baby Doc. *Vanity Fair* 52(1):74–116.
Altéma, Reynald, and Leslie Bright
  1983   Only Homosexual Haitians, Not All Haitians. *Annals of Internal Medicine* 99(6):877–878.

301

Altman, Dennis
    1986   *AIDS in the Mind of America*. Garden City, NY: Anchor Books.
Alvarez, Maria, and Gerald Murray
    n.d.   *Socialization for Scarcity: Child Feeding Beliefs and Practices in a Haitian Village*. Report submitted 28 August 1981 to USAID/ Haiti, Port-au-Prince.
Ambinder, R. F., C. Newman, G. S. Hayward, R. Biggar, M. Melbye, L. Kestens, E. Van Marck, P. Piot, P. Gigase, P. B. Wright, et al.
    1987   Lack of Association of Cytomegalovirus with Endemic African Kaposi's Sarcoma. *Journal of Infectious Disease* 156(1):193–197.
Ambursley, F., and R. Cohen, eds.
    1983   *Crisis in the Caribbean*. New York: Monthly Review Press.
American Public Health Association
    1983   Avoiding the Public Health Consequences of Anti-Immigrant Racism. *American Journal of Public Health* 73(3):345–346.
Anastos, Kathryn, and Carola Marte
    1989   Women —The Missing Persons in the AIDS Epidemic. *Health/ PAC Bulletin* (Winter):6–13.
Anglade, Georges
    1969   *Contribution à l'étude de la population d'Haiti; évolution démographique et répartition géographique*. Services des thèses, Institut de géographie appliquée, Université de Strasbourg.
    1974   *Mon Pays d'Haiti*. Port-au-Prince: Imprimerie Le Natal.
Antoine, L. B., L. Pierre, and J. B. Page
    1990   Exclusion of Blood Donors by Country of Origin and Discrimination against Black Foreigners in the USA [letter]. *AIDS* 4:818.
Aral, Sevgi, and King Holmes
    1991   Sexually Transmitted Diseases in the AIDS Era. *Scientific American* 264(2):62–69.
Archer, Marie-Thérèse
    1987   *La Créolologie Haitienne: Latinité du Créole d'Haiti*. Port-au-Prince: Imprimerie Le Natal.
Aristide, Jean Bertrand
    1989   *La Verité! En Verité! Dossier de Défense présenté à la Sacrée Congrégation pour les Religieux et les Instituts Séculiers*. Port-au-Prince: Imprimerie Le Natal.
    1990   *In the Parish of the Poor: Writings from Haiti*. New York: Orbis.
Asad, Talal
    1975   Introduction. In *Anthropology and the Colonial Encounter*, T. Asad, ed., pp. 9–19. London: Ithaca Press.
Augé, Marc
    1974   Les croyances à la sorcellerie. In *La Construction du monde (Collection "Dossiers africains")*, M. Augé, ed., pp. 52–74. Paris: Éditions Maspéro.
Auguste, C., and M. Auguste
    1985   *L'Expédition Leclerc 1801–1803*. Port-au-Prince: Imprimerie Henri Deschamps.

Auguste, M., and C. Auguste
   1980   *La Participation Étrangère à l'Expédition Française de Saint-Domingue.* Privately published in Canada.
Auguste, Yves
   1987   *Haiti & Les États Unis.* Port-au-Prince: Imprimerie Henri Deschamps.
Balch, Emily, ed.
   1927   *Occupied Haiti.* New York: The Writers Publishing.
Balibar, Etienne
   1988   The Vacillation of Ideology. In *Marxism and the Interpretation of Culture,* Cary Nelson and Lawrence Grossberg, eds., pp. 159–209. Urbana: University of Illinois Press.
Barros, J.
   1984   *Haiti de 1804 à nos jours.* 2 vols. Paris: Éditions l'Harmattan.
Barthélemy, Gérard
   1989   *Le Pays en Dehors.* Port-au-Prince: Imprimerie Henri Deschamps.
Bartholemew, Courtenay, Carl Saxinger, Jefferey Clark, Mitchell Gail, Ann Dudgeon, Bisram Mahabir, Barbara Hull-Drysdale, Farley Cleghorn, Robert Gallo, and William Blattner
   1987   Transmission of HTLV–1 and HIV Among Homosexual Men in Trinidad. *Journal of the American Medical Association* 257(19): 2604–2608.
Bastien, Rémy
   1961   Haitian Rural Family Organization. *Social and Economic Studies* 10(4):478–510.
   1985 [1951] *Le Paysan Haitien et sa Famille: Vallée de Marbial.* Paris: Éditions Karthala.
Bateson, Mary Catherine, and Richard Goldsby
   1988   *Thinking AIDS: The Social Response to the Biological Threat.* Reading, MA: Addison-Wesley.
Beach, Richard, and Peter Laura
   1983   Nutrition and the Acquired Immune Deficiency Syndrome. *Annals of Internal Medicine* 99(4):565–566.
Beghin, Ivan, William Fougere, and Kendall King
   1970   *L'Alimentation et la Nutrition en Haiti.* Paris: Presses Universitaires de France.
Bellegarde, Dantes
   1953   Alexandre Pétion: The Founder of Rural Democracy in Haiti. *Caribbean Quarterly* 3:167–173.
Bellow, Saul
   1989   *A Theft.* New York: Penguin Books.
Benot, Yves
   1988   *La Révolution Française et la Fin des Colonies.* Paris: Éditions La Découverte.
Berggren, Warren, Douglas Ewbank, and Gretchen Berggren
   1981   Reduction of Mortality in Haiti through a Primary Health Care Program. *New England Journal of Medicine* 304(22):1324–1330.

Berreman, Gerald
    1981   *The Politics of Truth: Essays in Critical Anthropology*. New Delhi: South Asian Publishers.
Bing, Fernande
    1964   Entretiens avec Alfred Métraux. *l'Homme* 4(2):20–32.
Blackburn, Robin
    1988   *The Overthrow of Colonial Slavery 1776–1848*. London: Verso.
Blaser, Martin
    1983   Acquired Immunodeficiency Syndrome Possibly Arthropod-Borne. *Annals of Internal Medicine* 99(6):877.
Bloch, M., ed.
    1975   *Political Language and Oratory in Traditional Society*. New York: Academic Press.
Boff, Leonardo, and Clodovis Boff
    1987   *Introducing Liberation Theology*. Paul Burns, trans. Maryknoll, NY: Orbis Press.
Boisrond-Tonnerre, Félix
    1804   *Mémoires Pour Servir à l'Histoire d'Hayti*. Port-au-Prince: Imprimerie Centrale du Gouvernement.
Bonnardot, M. L., and G. Danroc
    1989   *La Chute de la Maison Duvalier*. Paris: Éditions Karthala.
Boodhoo, Kenneth
    1984   The Economic Dimension of U.S. Caribbean Policy. In *The Caribbean Challenge: U.S. Policy in a Volatile Region*, H. Erisman, ed., pp. 72–91. Boulder, CO: Westview Press.
Bordes, Ary
    1979   *Évolution des Sciences de la Santé et de l'Hygiène Publique en Haiti*. Tome 1. Port-au-Prince: Centre d'Hygiène Familiale.
    1989   *Un Médecin Raconte*. Port-au-Prince: Imprimerie Henri Deschamps.
Borneman, John
    1988   AIDS in the Two Berlins. In *AIDS: Cultural Analysis/Cultural Activism*, D. Crimp, ed., pp. 223–235. Cambridge, MA: MIT Press.
Bourdieu, Pierre
    1972   *Esquisse d'une Théorie de la Pratique (Précédé de Trois Études d'Ethnologie Kabyle)*. Genève: Librairie Droz.
    1984   *Questions de Sociologie*. Paris: Éditions de Minuit.
Brandt, Allan
    1978   Racism and Research: The Case of the Tuskegee Syphilis Study. *Hastings Center Report* 8:21–28.
    1987   *No Magic Bullet: A Social History of Venereal Disease in the United States Since 1880* (expanded ed.). New York: Oxford University Press.
    1988   AIDS: From Social History to Social Policy. In *AIDS: The Burdens of History*, E. Fee and D. Fox, eds., pp. 147–171. Berkeley: University of California Press.

Braudel, Fernand
    1972   *The Mediterranean and the Mediterranean World in the Age of Philip II*. Sian Reynolds, trans. New York: Harper & Row.
Brown, Karen McCarthy
    1989a   Afro-Caribbean Spirituality: A Haitian Case Study. *Second Opinion* 11:36–57.
    1989b   Systematic Remembering, Systematic Forgetting: Ogou in Haiti. In *Africa's Ogun: Old World and New,* Sandra Barnes, ed., pp. 65–89. Bloomington: Indiana University Press.
Browner, C. H., Bernard R. Ortiz de Montellano, and Arthur J. Rubel
    1988   A Methodology for Cross-Cultural Ethnomedical Research. *Current Anthropology* 29(5):681–702.
Brunet, J. B., and R. A. Ancelle
    1985   The International Occurrence of the Acquired Immunodeficiency Syndrome. *Annals of Internal Medicine* 103(5):670–674.
Brutus, Jean-Robert
    1989a   Problèmes d'éthique liés au dépistage du virus HIV–1. Congrès des Médecins Francophones d'Amérique. Fort-de-France, Martinique, 12–16 June, 1989.
    1989b   Séroprévalence de HIV Parmi Les Femmes Enceintes à Cité Soleil, Haiti. Fifth International Conference on AIDS. Montreal, Canada, 5–7 June, 1989.
Bryan, Patrick
    1984   *The Haitian Revolution and Its Effects*. Kingston, Jamaica: Heinemann.
Burbach, Roger, and Marc Herold
    1984   The U.S. Economic Stake in Central America and the Caribbean. In *The Politics of Intervention: The United States in Central America,* Roger Burbach and Patricia Flynn, eds., pp. 190–211. New York: Monthly Review Press.
Butler, Samuel
    1970   *Erewhon*. Harmondworth: Penguin Books.
Campbell, Mavis
    1975   *The Dynamics of Change in a Slave Society: A Socio-Political History of the Free Coloured of Jamaica 1800–1865*. London: Associated Universities Press.
Carduso, F., and E. Faletto
    1979   *Dependency and Development in Latin America*. M. Urquidi, trans. Berkeley: University of California Press.
Carpenter, Frank
    1930   *Lands of the Caribbean*. Garden City, NY: Doubleday, Doran and Co.
Casper, Virginia
    1986   AIDS: A Psychosocial Perspective. In *The Social Dimensions of AIDS: Method and Theory,* Douglas Feldman and Thomas Johnson, eds., pp. 197–209. New York: Praeger.

Castor, Suzy
    1988a   *Le Massacre de 1937 et les Rélations Haitiano-Dominicaines.* Port-au-Prince: Imprimerie Henri Deschamps.
    1988b   *L'Occupation Américaine d'Haiti.* Port-au-Prince: Imprimerie Henri Deschamps.

Cauna, Jacques
    1984   L'État Sanitaire des Esclaves sur une Grande Sucrérie (Habitation Fleuriau de Bellevue 1777–1788). *Revue de la Société Haitienne d'Histoire et de Géographie* 42(145):18–78.

Centers for Disease Control
    1982a   Opportunistic Infections and Kaposi's Sarcoma among Haitians in the United States. *Morbidity and Mortality Weekly Report* 31:353–354, 360–361.
    1982b   Update on Kaposi's Sarcoma and Opportunistic Infections in Previously Well Persons—United States. *Morbidity and Mortality Weekly Report* 31:294, 300–301.
    1983   Acquired Immunodeficiency Syndrome Update. *Morbidity and Mortality Weekly Report* 32:465–467.
    1990   AIDS in Women—United States. *Morbidity and Mortality Weekly Report* 39:845–846.

Césaire, Aimé
    1981   *Toussaint Louverture: La Révolution Française et le Problème Colonial.* Paris: Présence Africaine.

Chaisson, R. E., G. F. Schechter, C. P. Theuer, G. W. Rutherford, and D. F. Echenberg
    1987   Tuberculosis in Patients with the Acquired Immunodeficiency Syndrome. *American Reviews in Respiratory Disease* 136(3):570–574.

Chaze, William
    1983   In Haiti, a View of Life at the Bottom. *U.S. News and World Report* 95(18):41–42.

Chen, Kwan-Hwa, and Gerald Murray
    1976   Truths and Untruths in Village Haiti: An Experiment in Third World Survey Research. In *Culture, Natality, and Family Planning,* John Marshall and Steven Polgar, eds., pp. 241–262. Chapel Hill: University of North Carolina Press.

Chierici, Rose-Marie
    1987   Making it to the Center: Migration and Adaptation among Haitian Boat People. *New York Folklore* 13(1–2):107–116.

Chinchilla, Norma, and Nora Hamilton
    1984   Prelude to Revolution: U.S. Investment in Central America. In *The Politics of Intervention: The United States in Central America,* Roger Burbach and Patricia Flynn, eds., pp. 214–249. New York: Monthly Review Press.

Chittester, Joan
    1989   Haiti: Voices of Misery, Voices of Promise. *Pax Christi USA* 14(3):4–9.

Chlebowski, R. T., M. B. Grosvenor, N. H. Bernard, L. S. Morales, and
L. M. Bulcavage
    1989   Nutritional Status, Gastrointestinal Dysfunction, and Survival in
              Patients with AIDS. *American Journal of Gastroenterology* 84(10):
              1288–1293.
Choi, Keewhan
    1987   Assembling the AIDS Puzzle: Epidemiology. In *AIDS: Facts
              and Issues,* Victor Gong, ed., pp. 15–24. New Brunswick, NJ:
              Rutgers.
Clarke, Loren, and Malcolm Potts, eds.
    1988   *The AIDS Reader: Documentary History of a Modern Epidemic.* Bos-
              ton: Branden Publishing Co.
Clérismé, Calixte
    1979   *Recherches sur la Médecine Traditionelle.* Port-au-Prince: Éditions
              Fardin.
Clumeck, N., M. Carael, D. Rouvroy, and D. Nzaramba
    1985   Heterosexual Promiscuity among African Patients with AIDS.
              New England Journal of Medicine 313(3):182.
Collaborative Study Group of AIDS in Haitian-Americans
    1987   Risk Factors for AIDS Among Haitians Residing in the United
              States: Evidence of Heterosexual Transmission. *Journal of the
              American Medical Association* 257(5):635–639.
Comaroff, Jean
    1983   The Defectiveness of Symbols or the Symbols of Defectiveness?
              On the Cultural Analysis of Medical Systems. *Culture, Medicine
              and Psychiatry* 7:3–20.
Comhaire, Suzanne, and J. Comhaire Sylvain
    1959   Urban Stratification in Haiti. *Social and Economic Studies* 8(2):
              179–189.
Compa, Lance
    1989   *Labor Rights in Haiti.* Washington, D.C.: International Labor
              Rights Education and Research Fund.
Conner, Steve, and Sharon Klingman
    1988   *The Search for the Virus.* London: Penguin Books.
Conway, Frederick, and Susan Buchanan
    1985   Haitians. In *Refugees in the United States,* David Haines, ed., pp.
              95–110. Westport, CT: Greenwood Press.
Cook, Sherburne, and Woodrow Borah
    1971   *Essays in Population History: Mexico and the Caribbean.* Berkeley:
              University of California Press.
Coreil, Jeannine
    1980   Traditional and Western Responses to an Anthrax Epidemic in
              Rural Haiti. *Medical Anthropology* 4:79–105.
    1983a   Allocation of Family Resources for Health Care in Rural Haiti.
              Social Science and Medicine 17(11):709–719.
    1983b   Parallel Structures in Professional Folk Health Care: A Model
              Applied to Rural Haiti. *Culture, Medicine and Psychiatry* 7:131–
              151.

1988   Innovation Among Haitian Healers: The Adoption of Oral Re-
hydration Therapy. *Human Organization* 47(1):48–57.

Cornevin, R.
1982   *Haiti*. Paris: Presses Universitaires de France.

Corten, André
1986   *Port-au-Sucre: Prolétariat et Prolétarisations: Haiti et République
Dominicaine*. Montreal: CIDIHCA.
1989   *L'État Faible: Haiti et République Dominicaine*. Montreal:
CIDIHCA.

Corvington, Georges
1984   *Port-au-Prince au Cours des Ans: La Capitale d'Haiti sous l'Occupation 1915–1922*. Port-au-Prince: Imprimerie Henri Deschamps.
1987   *Port-au-Prince au Cours des Ans: La Capitale d'Haiti sous l'Occupation 1922–1934*. Port-au-Prince: Imprimerie Henri Deschamps.

Courlander, Harold
1960   *The Drum and the Hoe: Life and Lore of the Haitian People*.
Berkeley: University of California Press.

Courtain, M.
1989   Mémoire sommaire sur les prétendues pratiques magiques et em-
poisonnements prouvés au procès instruit et jugé au Cap contre
plusieurs nègres et négresses dont le chef, F. Macandal, a été con-
damné au feu et exécuté le 20 janvier 1758. *Chemins Critiques*
1(1):136–142.

Craighead, J., A. Moore, H. Grossman, W. Ershler, U. Frattini, C. Saxinger,
U. Hess, and F. Ngowi
1988   Pathogenetic Role of HIV Infection in Kaposi's Sarcoma of
Equatorial East Africa. *Archives of Pathology and Laboratory Medicine* 112(3):259–265.

Crandon-Malamud, Libbet
1991   *From the Fat of Our Souls*. Berkeley: University of California Press.

Crouse, N.
1966   *The French Struggle for the West Indies 1665–1713*. New York:
Octagon Books.

d'Adesky, Anne-Christine
1991   Silence + Death = AIDS in Haiti. *The Advocate* 577:30–36.

Dalton, Harlon
1989   AIDS in Blackface. *Daedalus* 118(3):205–228.

Danner, Mark
1989   A Reporter at Large: Beyond the Mountains I. *The New Yorker*,
27 November:55–100.

d'Ans, André-Marcel
1985   Rémy Bastien et l'ethnologie haitienne. Introduction. In R. Bastien. *Le Paysan Haitien et sa Famille*, pp. 7–18. Paris: Éditions
Karthala.
1987   *Haiti: Paysage et Société*. Paris: Éditions Karthala.

Darwin, Charles
1989 [1839] *Voyage of the Beagle*. London: Penguin Books.

Davies, K. G.
   1974   *The North Atlantic World in the Seventeenth Century.* Minneapolis:
           University of Minnesota Press.
Davis, David Brion
   1975   *The Problem of Slavery in the Age of Revolution, 1770–1823.* Ithaca:
           Cornell University Press.
Davis, Wade
   1988   *Passage of Darkness: The Ethnobiology of the Haitian Zombie.* Chapel
           Hill: University of North Carolina Press.
Dayan, Joan
   1977   Introduction. In R. Depestre, *Rainbow for the Christian West.*
           Amherst: University of Massachusetts Press.
Debien, Gabriel
   1962   Plantations et esclaves à Saint Domingue: Sucrérie Cottineau.
           Notes d'Histoire Coloniale 66:9–82.
DeCock, Kevin
   1984   AIDS: An Old Disease from Africa? *British Medical Journal*
           289(6440):306–308.
DeHovitz, Jack, Jean Pape, Madeleine Boncy, and Warren Johnson
   1986   Clinical Manifestations and Therapy of *Isospora belli* Infection in
           Patients with the Acquired Immunodeficiency Syndrome. *The
           New England Journal of Medicine* 315:87–90.
Delince, Kern
   1979   *Armée et Politique en Haiti.* Paris: Éditions l'Harmattan.
de Mattéis, Arthur
   1987   *Le Massacre de 1937: Une Succession Immobilière Internationale.*
           Port-au-Prince: l'Imprimeur II.
Depestre, René
   1980   *Bondieu et Adieu à la Négritude.* Paris: Laffont.
Deschamps, Marie-Marcelle, Jean Pape, Rose Verdier, Jack DeHovitz, Franck
Thomas, and Warren Johnson
   1988   Treatment of *Candida* Esophagitis in AIDS Patients. *The Amer-
           ican Journal of Gastroenterology* 83(1):20–21.
Desinor, Carlo
   1988   *De Coup d'État en Coup d'État.* Port-au-Prince: l'Imprimeur II.
   1989   *Il Était Une Fois: Duvalier, Bosch & Kennedy, 1963.* Port-au-
           Prince: l'Imprimeur II.
Detienne, Marcel
   1986   *The Creation of Mythology.* Margaret Cook, trans. Chicago: Uni-
           versity of Chicago Press.
DeWind, Josh, and David Kinley
   1988   *Aide à la Migration: L'Impact de l'Assistance Internationale à Haiti.*
           Montreal: CIDIHCA.
Diederich, Bernard
   1985   Swine Fever Ironies: The Slaughter of the Haitian Black Pig.
           Caribbean Review 14(1):16–17, 41.

Diederich, Bernard, and Al Burt
1986   *Papa Doc et les Tontons Macoutes*. Henri Drevet, trans. Port-au-Prince: Imprimerie Henri Deschamps.

Douglass, Frederick
1955   *The Life and Writings of Frederick Douglass*. Vol. 4. Philip Foner, ed. New York: International Publishers.

Dreuilhe, Emmanuel
1988   *Mortal Embrace: Living With AIDS*. New York: Hill and Wang.

Duffy, Michael
1987   *Soldiers, Sugar and Seapower: The British Expeditions to the West Indies and the War against Revolutionary France*. Oxford: Oxford University Press.

Dulles, John Foster
1954   *America's Rise to World Power 1898–1954*. New York: Harper Torchbooks.

Dundes, Alan
1987   At Ease, Disease—AIDS Jokes as Sick Humor. *American Behavioral Scientist* 30(1):72–81.

Dunn, Richard
1972   *Sugar and Slaves: The Rise of the Planter Class in the English West Indies, 1624–1713*. Chapel Hill: University of North Carolina Press.

Edstrom, Lars
1988   AIDS Virus Epidemic in Haiti: Projecting Its Likely Future Impact and Assessing the Potential for Intervention. M. Phil. diss., Development Studies, University of Sussex, England.

Edwards, Bryan
1797   *A Historical Survey of the French Colony of the Island of St. Domingo*. London: J. Stockdale.

Efferen, L. S., D. Nadarajah, and D. S. Palat
1989   Survival Following Mechanical Ventilation for *Pneumocystis carinii* Pneumonia in Patients with the Acquired Immunodeficiency Syndrome: A Different Perspective. *American Journal of Medicine* 87(4):401–404.

ENDA-Panos
1987   SIDA et Tiers Monde. *Environnement Africain* (Série Études et Recherches) 118–119:1–140.

Epstein, T. Scarlett
1967   Sociological Analysis of Witch Beliefs in a Mysore Village. In *Magic, Witchcraft, and Curing*, John Middleton, ed., pp. 135–154. Garden City, NY: Anchor Books.

Erikson, Kai
1976   *Everything in Its Path: Destruction of Community in the Buffalo Creek Flood*. New York: Simon & Schuster.

Ernst, P., M. F. Chen, N. S. Wang, and M. Cosio
1983   Symbiosis of *Pneumocystis carinii* and Cytomegalovirus in a Case of Fatal Pneumonia. *Canadian Medical Association Journal* 128:1089–1092.

Fabian, Johannes
  1983   *Time and the Other: How Anthropology Makes Its Object*. New York: Columbia University Press.
Farmer, Paul
  1988a   Bad Blood, Spoiled Milk: Bodily Fluids as Moral Barometers in Rural Haiti. *American Ethnologist* 15(1):62–83.
  1988b   Blood, Sweat, and Baseballs: Haiti in the West Atlantic System. *Dialectical Anthropology* 13:83–99.
  1990a   AIDS and Accusation: Haiti and the Geography of Blame. In *AIDS and Culture: The Human Factor,* Douglas Feldman, ed., pp. 67–91. New York: Praeger.
  1990b   The Exotic and the Mundane. Human Immunodeficiency Virus in the Caribbean. *Human Nature* 1(4):415–445.
  1990c   Sending Sickness: Sorcery, Politics, and Changing Concepts of AIDS in Rural Haiti. *Medical Anthropology Quarterly* 4(1):6–27.
  1991a   New Disorder, Old Dilemmas: AIDS and Anthropology in Haiti. In *Social Analysis in the Time of AIDS,* G. Herdt and S. Lindenbaum, eds., Beverly Hills: Sage Publications.
  1991b   The Power of the Poor in Haiti. *America* 164(9):260–267.
Farmer, Paul, and Byron Good
  1991   Illness Representations in Medical Anthropology: A Critical Review and a Case Study of the Representation of AIDS in Haiti. In *The Mental Representation of Health and Illness,* J. Skelton and R. Croyle, eds., pp. 131–167. New York: Springer-Verlag.
Farmer, Paul, and Jim Yong Kim
  1991   Anthropology, Accountability, and the Prevention of AIDS. *The Journal of Sex Research* 28(2):203–221.
Farmer, Paul, and Arthur Kleinman
  1989   AIDS as Human Suffering. *Daedalus* 118(2):135–160.
Farmer, Paul, Simon Robin, St. Luc Ramilus, and Jim Yong Kim
  1991   Tuberculosis, Poverty, and "Compliance": Lessons from Rural Haiti. *Seminars in Respiratory Infections* 6(4):373–379.
Fass, Simon
  1978   Port-au-Prince: Awakening to the Urban Crisis. In *Latin American Urban Research,* W. Cornelius and R. Kemper, eds., pp. 115–180. Beverly Hills: Sage Publications.
  1988   *Political Economy in Haiti: The Drama of Survival*. New Brunswick, NJ: Transaction.
Fee, Elizabeth
  1988   Sin versus Science: Venereal Disease in Twentieth-Century Baltimore. In *AIDS: The Burdens of History,* E. Fee and D. Fox, eds., pp. 121–146. Berkeley: University of California Press.
Feilden, Rachel, James Allman, Joel Montague, and Jon Rohde
  1981   *Health, Population and Nutrition in Haiti: A Report Prepared for the World Bank*. Boston: Management Sciences for Health.
Ferguson, James
  1987   *Papa Doc, Baby Doc: Haiti and the Duvaliers*. Oxford: Basil Blackwell.

FIC (Frères de l'Instruction Chrétienne)
    1942   *Histoire d'Haiti*. Port-au-Prince: Imprimerie Henri Deschamps.
Fombrun, Odette
    1983   *Résumé de Moreau de Saint-Méry*. Port-au-Prince: Le Natal.
Foster, C., and A. Valdman, eds.
    1984   *Haiti—Today and Tomorrow: An Interdisciplinary Study*. Lanham,
            MD: University Press of America.
Foster, George
    1988   The Validating Role of Humoral Theory in Spanish-American
            Therapeutics. *American Ethnologist* 15(1):120–135.
Francisque, Édouard
    1986   *La Structure Économique et Sociale d'Haiti*. Port-au-Prince: Impri-
            merie Henri Deschamps.
Frank, André Gunder
    1979   *Dependent Accumulation and Underdevelopment*. New York:
            Monthly Review Press.
Frank, Elliot, Stanley Weiss, John Compas, Jessica Benstock, John Weber, Ann
Bodner, and Sheldon Landesman
    1985   AIDS in Haitian-Americans: A Reassessment. *Cancer Research*
            suppl. 45:4619s–4620s.
Friedman, Y., C. Franklin, E. C. Rackow, and M. H. Weil
    1989   Improved Survival in Patients with AIDS, *Pneumocystis carinii*
            Pneumonia, and Severe Respiratory Failure. *Chest* 96(4):862–
            866.
Fuller, John
    1991   *AIDS and the Church: A Stimulus to Our Theologizing*. Cambridge,
            MA: Weston School of Theology.
Gail, Mitchell, Philip Rosenberg, and James Goedert
    1990   Therapy May Explain Recent Deficits in AIDS Incidence. *Journal
            of the Acquired Immune Deficiency Syndromes* 3:296–306.
Gaillard, Roger
    1974   *Les Cent-jours de Rosalvo Bobo, ou une Mise à Mort Politique*. Port-
            au-Prince: Imprimerie Le Natal.
    1981a   *Premier Ecrasement du Cacoisme*. Port-au-Prince: Imprimerie Le
            Natal.
    1981b   *La République Autoritaire*. Port-au-Prince: Imprimerie Le Natal.
    1982a   *Charlemagne Péralte le Caco*. Port-au-Prince: Imprimerie Le Natal.
    1982b   *Hinche Mise en Croix*. Port-au-Prince: Imprimerie Le Natal.
    1983   *La Guerilla de Batraville*. Port-au-Prince: Imprimerie Le Natal.
    1984   *La République Exterminatrice I: Une Modernisation Manquée*. Port-
            au-Prince: Imprimerie Le Natal.
    1988   *La République Exterminatrice II: L'État Vassal*. Port-au-Prince:
            Imprimerie Le Natal.
Gaines, Atwood, and Paul Farmer
    1986   Visible Saints: Social Cynosures and Dysphoria in the Mediterra-
            nean Tradition. *Culture, Medicine and Psychiatry* 11:295–330.

Garcia, Rafael
  1991   Tourism and AIDS—A Dominican Republic Study. *AIDS and Society* 2(3): infold, 1–3.
Geggus, David
  1989   The Haitian Revolution. In *The Modern Caribbean,* Franklin Knight and Colin Palmer, eds., pp. 21–50. Chapel Hill: University of North Carolina Press.
Gellhorn, Martha
  1984   White into Black. *Granta* 10:93–106.
Georges Adams, A.
  1982   *Une Crise Haitienne 1867–1869: Sylvain Salnave.* Port-au-Prince: Imprimerie Henri Deschamps.
Gerstoft, J., J. Nielsen, E. Dickmeiss, T. Ronne, P. Platz, and L.Mathiesen
  1985   The Acquired Immunodeficiency Syndrome (AIDS) in Denmark. *Acta Med Scand* 217:213–224.
GHESKIO (Boncy et al.)
  1983   Acquired Immunodeficiency in Haitians. *New England Journal of Medicine* 308(23):1419–1420.
Gibson, C.
  1966   *Spain in America.* New York: Harper & Row.
Gilman, Sander
  1988a   AIDS and Syphilis: The Iconography of Disease. In *AIDS: Cultural Analysis/Cultural Activism,* Douglas Crimp, ed., pp. 87–107. Cambridge, MA: MIT Press.
  1988b   *Disease and Representation: Images of Illness from Madness to AIDS.* Ithaca: Cornell University Press.
Girault, Christian
  1982   *Le Commerce du Café en Haiti: Habitants, Spéculateurs et Exportateurs.* Paris: Éditions CNRS.
  1984   Commerce in the Haitian Economy. In *Haiti—Today and Tomorrow: An Interdisciplinary Study,* C. Foster and A. Valdman, eds., pp. 173–179. Lanham, MD: University Press of America.
Gisler, Antoine
  1981   *L'Esclavage aux Antilles Françaises (XVIIe–XIXe siecle).* Paris: Éditions Karthala.
Glick-Schiller, Nina, and Georges Fouron
  1990   "Everywhere We Go, We Are in Danger": Ti Manno and the Emergence of a Haitian Transnational Identity. *American Ethnologist* 17(2):329–347.
Good, Byron
  1977   The Heart of What's the Matter: The Semantics of Illness in Iran. *Culture, Medicine and Psychiatry* 1:25–58.
Good, Byron, and Mary-Jo DelVecchio Good
  1982   Toward a Meaning-Centered Analysis of Popular Illness Categories: "Fright Illness" and "Heart Distress" in Iran. In *Cultural Conceptions of Mental Health and Therapy,* A. J. Marsella and G. M. White, eds., pp. 141–166. Boston: Reidel.

Gorman, E. Michael
   1986   The AIDS Epidemic in San Francisco: Epidemiological and An-
            thropological Perspectives. In *Anthropology and Epidemiology,*
            C. Janes, R. Stall, and S. Gifford, eds., pp. 157–172. Dordrecht:
            Reidel.

Gottlieb, Michael, Jerome Groopman, Wilfred Weinstein, John Fahey, and
Roger Detels
   1983   The Acquired Immunodeficiency Syndrome. *Annals of Internal
            Medicine* 99:208–220.

Goudsmit, J.
   1983   Malnutrition and Concomitant Herpesvirus Infection as a Possi-
            ble Cause of Immunodeficiency Syndrome in Haitian Infants [let-
            ter]. *New England Journal of Medicine* 309(9):554–555.

Greco, R. S.
   1983   Haiti and the Stigma of AIDS [letter]. *Lancet* 2:515–516.

Greene, Graham
   1966   *The Comedians.* London: The Bodley Head.
   1980   *Ways of Escape.* London: The Bodley Head.

Greenfield, William
   1986   Night of the Living Dead II: Slow Virus Encephalopathies and
            AIDS: Do Necromantic Zombiists Transmit HTLV-III/LAV
            During Voodooistic Rituals? *Journal of the American Medical As-
            sociation* 256:2199–2200.

Greenwood, Davydd, Shirley Lindenbaum, Margaret Lock, and Allan Young
   1988   Introduction to theme issue on medical anthropology. *American
            Ethnologist* 15(1):1–3.

Groopman, Jerome
   1983   Viruses and Human Neoplasia: Approaching Etiology. *American
            Journal of Medicine* 75(3):377–380.

Grunwald, J., L. Delatour, and K. Voltaire
   1984   Offshore Assembly in Haiti. In *Haiti—Today and Tomorrow: An
            Interdisciplinary Study,* C. Foster and A. Valdman, eds., pp. 231–
            252. Lanham, MD: University Press of America.

Guérin, J., R. Malebranche, R. Elie, A. Laroche, G. Pierre, E. Arnoux, T. Spira,
J. Dupuy, T. Seemayer, and C. Pean-Guichard
   1984   Acquired Immune Deficiency Syndrome: Specific Aspects of the
            Disease in Haiti. *Annals of the New York Academy of Sciences*
            437:254–261.

Guinan, Mary, Pauline Thomas, Paul Pinsky, James Goodrich, Richard Selik,
Harold Jaffe, Harry Haverkos, Gary Noble, and James Curran
   1984   Heterosexual and Homosexual Patients with the Acquired Im-
            munodeficiency Syndrome. *Annals of Internal Medicine* 100:213–
            218.

Gutierrez, Gustavo
   1987   *On Job: God-Talk and the Suffering of the Innocent.* Maryknoll, NY:
            Orbis Books.

Haitian Refugee Center
   1990   *Affidavits Concerning Conditions in INS Detention.* Miami: Haitian
           Refugee Center.
Hall, Robert
   1953   *Haitian Creole.* Philadelphia: American Folklore Society.
Halsey, N., R. Boulos, and J. Brutus, et al.
   1987   HIV Antibody Prevalence in Pregnant Haitian Women. Abstracts
           of the Third International Conference on AIDS, Washington,
           D.C., June, p. 174.
Hancock, Graham
   1989   *The Lords of Poverty: The Power, Prestige, and Corruption of the In-
           ternational Aid Business.* New York: Atlantic Monthly Press.
Hargreaves, John, ed.
   1969   *France and West Africa: An Anthology of Historical Documents.* New
           York: St. Martin's Press.
Haring, C. H.
   1957   *The Spanish Empire in America.* New York: Harcourt, Brace and
           World.
Harrison, Lawrence
   1985   *Underdevelopment is a State of Mind.* Lanham, MD: University
           Press of America.
Hayden, J. Carleton
   1987   Afro-Anglican Linkages, 1701–1900: Ethiopia Shall Soon Stretch
           Out Her Hands Unto God. *Journal of Religious Thought* 44(1):
           25–34.
Hazard, Samuel
   1873   *Santo Domingo, Past and Present; With a Glance at Hayti.* New
           York: Harper and Brothers.
Hector, Michel
   1989   *Syndicalisme et Socialisme en Haiti, 1932–1970.* Port-au-Prince: Im-
           primerie Henri Deschamps.
Heinl, Robert, and Nancy Heinl
   1978   *Written in Blood.* Boston: Houghton Mifflin Co.
Heise, Lori
   1988   AIDS: New Threat to the Third World. *World Watch* 1(1):
           19–43.
Henrys, Daniel
   1989   Propositions pour une Démocratisation de la Santé. *Forum Libre
           1 (Médicine, Santé et Démocratie en Haiti)*:29–37.
Herold, J. Christopher, ed. and trans.
   1955   *The Mind of Napoleon: A Selection from His Written and Spoken
           Words.* New York: Columbia University Press.
Herskovits, Melville
   1975 [1937] *Life in a Haitian Valley.* New York: Farrar, Straus and Giroux.
Hess, Salinda
   1984   Domestic Medicine and Indigenous Medical Systems in Haiti.
           Ph.D. diss., McGill University.

Hicks, Albert
   1946   *Blood in the Streets: The Life and Rule of Trujillo.* New York: Creative Press.

Holcomb, Richard
   1937   *Who Gave the World Syphilis? The Haitian Myth.* New York: Froben Press.

Hospedales, James
   1989   Heterosexual Spread of HIV Infection. *Reviews of Infectious Diseases* 11(4):663–664.

Hurbon, Laennec
   1979   *Culture et Dictature en Haiti: L'Imaginaire sous Contrôle.* Paris: Éditions l'Harmattan.
   1987a   *Le Barbare Imaginaire.* Port-au-Prince: Imprimerie Henri Deschamps.
   1987b   *Comprendre Haiti: Essai sur l'État, la Nation, la Culture.* Paris: Éditions Karthala.
   1987c   *Dieu dans le Vaudou Haitien.* Port-au-Prince: Imprimerie Henri Deschamps.
   1989   Enjeu politique de la crise actuelle de l'Église. *Chemins Critiques* 1(1):13–22.

Institut Haitien de la Statistique et de l'Informatique [IHSI]
   1987   *Recueil des Données de Base.* Port-au-Prince: Division des Statistiques Générales.

International Monetary Fund
   1984   Directions of Trade Statistics. In *Yearbook 1984.* Washington, D.C.: IMF.

Jaffe, Harold, Dennis Bregman, and Richard Selik
   1983   Acquired Immune Deficiency Syndrome in the United States: The First 1,000 Cases. *Journal of Infectious Diseases* 148(2):339–345.

Jaffe, Harold, et al.
   1985   The Acquired Immunodeficiency Syndrome in a Cohort of Homosexual Men. *Annals of Internal Medicine* 103:210–214.

James, C. L. R.
   1980   *The Black Jacobins.* London: Allison and Busby.

Janvier, L. J.
   1883   *La République d'Haiti et ses Visiteurs (1840–1882).* Tome 1. Paris: Marpon et Flammarion.

Janzen, John
   1978   *The Quest for Therapy: Medical Pluralism in Lower Zaire.* Berkeley: University of California Press.
   1988   Reply to Browner et al. *Current Anthropology* 29(5):695.

Jean-Louis, Robert
   1989   Diagnostic de l'État de Santé en Haiti. *Forum Libre 1 (Médicine, Santé et Démocratie en Haiti)*:11–20.

Joachim, Benoît
   1979   *Les Racines du Sous-Développement en Haiti.* Port-au-Prince: Imprimerie Henri Deschamps.

Johnson, Toby
1987   *Plague: A Novel About Healing.* Boston: Alyson Publications.
Johnson, Warren, and Jean Pape
1989   AIDS in Haiti. In *AIDS: Pathogenesis and Treatment,* Jay Levy,
        ed., pp. 65–78. New York: Marcel Dekker.
Jones, James
1981   *Bad Blood: The Tuskegee Syphilis Experiment.* New York: Free Press.
Jordan, Winthrop
1974   *The White Man's Burden: Historical Origins of Racism in the United
        States.* London: Oxford University Press.
Kajiyama, W., S. Kashiwagi, H. Ikematsu, J. Hayashi, H. Nomura, and
K. Okochi
1986   Intrafamilial Transmission of Adult T-Cell Leukemia Virus. *Jour-
        nal of Infectious Diseases* 154:851–857.
Kinsella, James
1989   *Covering the Plague: AIDS and the American Media.* New Bruns-
        wick, NJ: Rutgers University Press.
Kiple, Kenneth
1984   *The Caribbean Slave: A Biological History.* Cambridge: Cambridge
        University Press.
Klein, Herbert
1986   *African Slavery in Latin America and the Caribbean.* New York:
        Oxford University Press.
Kleinman, Arthur
1975   Explanatory Models in Health Care Relationships. In *Health of the
        Family,* pp. 159–172. Washington, D.C.: NCIH.
1980   *Patients and Healers in the Context of Culture.* Berkeley: Univer-
        sity of California Press.
1986   *Social Origins of Distress and Disease: Depression, Neurasthenia and
        Pain in Modern China.* New Haven: Yale University Press.
1988   *The Illness Narratives: Suffering, Healing, and the Human Condi-
        tion.* New York: Basic Books.
Kleinman, Arthur, Leon Eisenberg, and Byron Good
1978   Culture, Illness and Care: Clinical Lessons from Anthropologic
        and Cross-Cultural Research. *Annals of Internal Medicine* 88:251–
        258.
Kleinman, Arthur, and Joan Kleinman
1989   Suffering and Its Professional Transformation: Toward an Eth-
        nography of Experience. Paper presented at the First Conference
        of the Society for Psychological Anthropology. San Diego, Oc-
        tober 6–8.
Koenig, Ellen, L. Gonzalez Brache, and J. A. Levy
1987   Response to K. W. Payne. *Journal of the American Medical Associ-
        ation* 258:47.
Koenig, Ellen, Juan Pittaluga, Marie Bogart, Manolo Castro, Francisco
Nunez, Israel Vilorio, Luis Delvillar, Manuel Calzada, and Jay Levy
1987   Prevalence of Antibodies to Human Immunodeficiency Virus in

Dominicans and Haitians in the Dominican Republic. *Journal of the American Medical Association* 257(5):631–634.

Kreiss, Joan, et al.
1986   AIDS Virus Infection in Nairobi Prostitutes. *New England Journal of Medicine* 314(7):414–418.

Labat, Père
1970   *Mémoires, 1693–1705.* John Eaden, trans. London: Frank Cass.

Labelle, Micheline
1987   *Idéologie de Couleur et Classes Sociales en Haiti.* Montreal: CIDIHCA.

Lacerte, Robert
1981   Xenophobia and Economic Decline: The Haitian Case, 1820–1843. *The Americas* 37(4):499–515.

Laguerre, Michel
1977   Le coumbite haitien. *Actes du XLII Congrès International des Américainistes.* Vol. 1, pp. 341–357. Paris, 2–9 septembre 1976.
1978   Ticouloute and His Kinfolk: The Study of a Haitian Extended Family. In *The Extended Family in Black Societies,* Demitri Shimkin et al., eds., pp. 407–445. The Hague: Mouton.
1982   *Urban Life in the Caribbean.* Cambridge, MA: Schenkman.
1984   *American Odyssey: Haitians in New York City.* Ithaca: Cornell University Press.
1987   *Afro-Caribbean Folk Medicine.* South Hadley, MA: Bergin and Garvey.
1989   *Voodoo and Politics in Haiti.* New York: Saint Martin's Press.

Landesman, S. H., H. M. Ginzburg, and S. H. Weiss
1985   The AIDS Epidemic. *New England Journal of Medicine* 312:521–525.

Landesman, Sheldon
1983   The Haitian Connection. In *The AIDS Epidemic,* Kevin Cahill, ed., pp. 28–37. New York: St. Martin's Press.

Lange, W. Robert, and Elizabeth Dax
1987   HIV Infection and International Travel. *AFP* 36(3):197–204.

Lange, W. Robert, and Jerome Jaffe
1987   AIDS in Haiti. *New England Journal of Medicine* 316(22):1409–1410.

Langley, Lester
1989   *The United States and the Caribbean in the Twentieth Century* (4th ed.). Athens: University of Georgia Press.

Lappé, Frances, Joseph Collins, and David Kinley
1980   *Aid as Obstacle.* San Francisco: IFDP.

Larose, Serge
1976   *L'Exploitation Agricole en Haiti.* Montreal: Centre de Recherches Caraibes, Université de Montréal.
1977   The Meaning of Africa in Haitian Vodu. In *Symbols and Sentiments: Cross-Cultural Studies in Symbolism,* Joan Lewis, ed., pp. 85–116. New York: Academic Press.

Larrain, Jorge
    1983   *Marxism and Ideology*. London: Macmillan.
Laverdiere, Michel, Jacques Tremblay, René Lavallée, Yvette Bonny, Michel Lacombe, Jacques Boileau, Jacques Lachapelle, and Christian Lamoureaux
    1983   AIDS in Haitian Immigrants and a Caucasian Woman Closely Associated with Haitians. *Canadian Medical Association Journal* 129:1209–1212.
Lawless, Robert
    n.d.   Haiti's Bad Press. Unpublished MS. Collection of the Author.
LeBlanc, Robert, Marie Simard, Kenneth Flegel, and Norbert Gilmore
    1983   Opportunistic Infections and Acquired Cellular Immune Deficiency among Haitian Immigrants in Montreal. *Canadian Medical Association Journal* 129:1205–1209.
Léger, J.
    1907   *Haiti et ses Détracteurs*. New York: Neale.
Leibowitch, Jacques
    1985   *A Strange Virus of Unknown Origin*. Richard Howard, trans. New York: Ballantine Books.
Lemoine, Maurice
    1985   *Bitter Sugar: Slaves Today in the Caribbean*. Chicago: Banner Press.
Leonides, J. R., and N. Hyppolite
    1983   Haiti and the Acquired Immune Deficiency Syndrome. *Annals of Internal Medicine* 98:1020–1021.
Leyburn, James
    1966   *The Haitian People*. New Haven: Yale University Press.
Liautaud, B., C. Laroche, J. Duvivier, and C. Pean-Guichard
    1982   Le sarcome de Kaposi (maladie de Kaposi) est-il fréquent en Haiti? Presented at the 18ème Congrès des médecins francophones de l'hémisphere américain. Port-au-Prince, Haiti.
    1983   Le Sarcome de Kaposi en Haiti: Foyer méconnu ou récemment apparu? *Annals of Dermatological Venereology* 110:213–219.
Liautaud, B., J. Pape, and M. Pamphile
    1988   Le Sida dans les Caraibes. *Médecine et Maladies Infectieuses*. December:687–697.
Lief, Louise
    1990   Where Democracy isn't about to Break Out. *U.S. News and World Report* 12 February:34–36.
Lindenbaum, Shirley
    1979   *Kuru Sorcery: Disease and Danger in the New Guinea Highlands*. Palo Alto, CA: Mayfield.
    1981   Images of the Sorcerer in Papua New Guinea. *Social Analysis* 8:119–128.
Locher, Uli
    1984   Migration in Haiti. In *Haiti—Today and Tomorrow: An Interdisciplinary Study,* C. Foster and A. Valdman, eds., pp. 325–336. Lanham, MD: University Press of America.

320   BIBLIOGRAPHY

Logan, R.
1968   *Haiti and the Dominican Republic*. London: Oxford University Press.
Lowenthal, Ira
1974   *Catelogue de las Collection Mangones*. New Haven: Antilles Research Program.
1976   Haiti: Behind Mountains, More Mountains. *Reviews in Anthropology* pp. 656–669.
1978   Ritual Performance and Religious Experience: A Service for the Gods in Southern Haiti. *Journal of Anthropological Research* 34(3): 392–414.
1984   Labor, Sexuality and the Conjugal Contract in Rural Haiti. In *Haiti—Today and Tomorrow: An Interdisciplinary Study*, C. Foster and A. Valdman, eds., pp. 15–33. Lanham, MD: University Press of America.
Lundahl, Mats
1983   *The Haitian Economy*. New York: St. Martin's Press.
1984   The Roots of Haitian Underdevelopment. In *Haiti—Today and Tomorrow: An Interdisciplinary Study*, C. Foster and A. Valdman, eds., pp. 181–203. Lanham, MD: University Press of America.
Madiou, Thomas
1989   *Histoire d'Haiti*. 9 vols. Port-au-Prince: Imprimerie Henri Deschamps.
Magloire, Eddy
1984   *Regards sur la Minorité Ethnique Haitienne aux Etats-Unis*. Sherbrooke: Éditions Naaman.
Malebranche, R., E. Arnoux, and J. M. Guérin, et al.
1983   Aquired Immunodeficiency Syndrome with Severe Gastro-Intestinal Manifestations in Haiti. *Lancet* 2:873–878.
Marasca, G., and M. McEvoy
1986   Length of Survival of Patients with Acquired Immunodeficiency Syndrome in the United Kingdom. *British Medical Journal* 292(6537):1727–1729.
Marcus, George, and Michael Fischer
1986   *Anthropology as Cultural Critique: An Experimental Moment in the Human Sciences*. Chicago: University of Chicago Press.
Marshall, Dawn I.
1979   *"The Haitian Problem": Illegal Migration to the Bahamas*. Kingston, Jamaica: Institute of Social and Economic Research, University of the West Indies.
Massing, Michael
1987   Haiti: The New Violence. *The New York Review of Books* 34:45–52.
Maximilien, Louis
1945   *Le Vaudou Haitien: Rite Radas-Canzo*. Port-au-Prince: Imprimerie Henri Deschamps.

May, Robert, Roy Anderson, and Sally Blower
 1988   The Epidemiology and Transmission Dynamics of HIV-AIDS.
           Daedalus 118:163–201.
Mellors, John, and Michele Barry
 1984   Malnutrition or AIDS in Haiti? *New England Journal of Medicine*
           310(17):1119–1120.
Menos, Solon
 1986 [1898] *L'Affaire Luders*. Port-au-Prince: Les Editions Fardin.
Merino, Nhora, Ricardo Sanchez, Alvaro Munoz, Guillermo Prada, Carlos
Garcia, and B. Frank Polk
 1990   HIV–1, Sexual Practices, and Contact with Foreigners in Homo-
           sexual Men in Colombia, South America. *Journal of the Acquired
           Immune Deficiency Syndromes* 3:330–334.
Météllus, Jean
 1987   *Haiti: Une Nation Pathétique*. Paris: Denoel.
Métral, A.
 1985 [1825] *Histoire de l'Expédition des Français à Saint-Domingue*. Paris:
           Éditions Karthala.
Métraux, Alfred
 1953   Médecine et Vodou en Haiti. *Acta Tropica* 10(1):28–68.
 1960   *Haiti: Black Peasants and Voodoo*. Peter Lengyel, trans. New York:
           Universe Books.
 1972   *Haitian Voodoo*. Hugo Charteris, trans. New York: Schocken.
Midy, Franklin
 1989a   L'Affaire Aristide en perspective: Histoire de la formation et du
           rejet d'une vocation prophétique. *Chemins Critiques* 1(1):45–60.
 1989b   Haiti, la religion sur les chemins de la démocratie. *Chemins
           Critiques* 1(1):23–44.
Millet, Kethly
 1978   *Les Paysans Haitiens et l'Occupation Américaine 1915–1930*. La
           Salle, Quebec: Collectif Paroles.
Mills, C. Wright
 1959   *The Sociological Imagination*. London: Oxford University Press.
Mintz, Sidney
 1960   *Worker in the Cane*. New Haven: Yale University Press.
 1966   Forward to Leyburn, James, *The Haitian People*. New Haven: Yale
           University Press.
 1971   Toward an Afro-American History. *Cahiers d'Histoire Mondiale*
           13(2):317–332.
 1972   Introduction. In A. Métraux, *Voodoo in Haiti*, pp. 1–14. New
           York: Schocken.
 1974a   *Caribbean Transformations*. Baltimore: Johns Hopkins University
           Press.
 1974b   The Caribbean Region. In *Slavery, Colonialism, and Racism*,
           S. Mintz, ed., pp. 45–72. New York: Norton.
 1977   The So-Called World System: Local Initiative and Local Re-
           sponse. *Dialectical Anthropology* 2(4):253–270.

1985   *Sweetness and Power: The Place of Sugar in Modern History.* New York: Viking Penguin.

Moore, Alexander, and Ronald LeBaron
1986   The Case for a Haitian Origin of the AIDS Epidemic. In *The Social Dimensions of AIDS: Method and Theory,* Douglas Feldman and Thomas Johnson, eds., pp. 77–93. New York: Praeger.

Moore, Joseph
1956   *A Study of the Episcopal Church in the Missionary District of Haiti.* Evanston, IL: The National Council of the Protestant Episcopal Church.

Moore, Sally Falk
1975a   Selection for Failure in a Small Social Field: Ritual Concord and Fraternal Strife among the Chagga, Kilimanjaro, 1968–1969. In *Symbol and Politics in Communal Ideology: Cases and Questions,* Sally Falk Moore and Barbara Myerhoff, eds., pp. 109–143. Ithaca: Cornell University Press.

1975b   Uncertainties in Situations, Indeterminacies in Culture. In *Symbol and Politics in Communal Ideology: Cases and Questions,* Sally Falk Moore and Barbara Myerhoff, eds., pp. 211–239. Ithaca: Cornell University Press.

1986   *Social Facts and Fabrications: Customary Law on Kilimanjaro, 1880–1980.* Cambridge: Cambridge University Press.

1987   Explaining the Present: Theoretical Dilemmas in Processual Ethnography. *American Ethnologist* 14(4):727–736.

Moral, Paul
1959   *L'Économie Haitienne.* Port-au-Prince: Imprimerie de l'État.

1961   *Le Paysan Haitien.* Port-au-Prince: Les Éditions Fardin.

Moreau de Saint-Méry, M.-L.-E.
1984   *Description Topographique, Physique, Civile, Politique et Historique de la Partie Française de l'Isle Saint-Domingue (1797–1798).* 3 vols. (New ed., B. Maurel and E. Taillemite, eds). Paris: Société de l'Histoire des Colonies Françaises and Librairie Larose.

Moses, Peter, and John Moses
1983   Haiti and the Acquired Immune Deficiency Syndrome. *Annals of Internal Medicine* 99(4):565.

Moskowitz, Lee, Paul Kory, Joseph Chan, Harry Haverkos, Frances Conley, and George Hensley
1983   Unusual Causes of Death in Haitians Residing in Miami. *Journal of the American Medical Association* 250(9):1187–1191.

Murat, Inez
1976   *Napoleon and the American Dream.* F. Frenaye, trans. Baton Rouge: Louisiana State University Press.

Murphy, Edward, Peter Figeroa, William Gibbs, Alfred Brathwaite, Marjorie Holding-Cobham, David Waters, Beverly Cranston, Barrie Hanchard, and William Blattner
1989   Sexual Transmission of Human T-Lymphotropic Virus Type I (HTLV-I). *Annals of Internal Medicine* 111(7):555–560.

Murray, Gerald
    1976   Women in Perdition: Ritual Fertility Control in Haiti. In *Culture, Natality, and Family Planning,* John Marshall and Stephen Polgar, eds., pp. 59–78. Chapel Hill: Carolina Population Center, University of North Carolina.
    1977   The Evolution of Haitian Peasant Land Tenure: A Case Study of Agricultural Adaptation to Population Growth. Ph.D. diss., Columbia University.
    1980   *Population Pressure, Land Tenure and Voodoo.* New York: Academic Press.
    1984   The Wood Tree as a Peasant Cash-Crop: An Anthropological Strategy for the Domestication of Energy. In *Haiti—Today and Tomorrow: An Interdisciplinary Study,* C. Foster and A. Valdman, eds., pp. 141–160. Lanham, MD: University Press of America.

Murray, Gerald, and Maria Alvarez
    1975   Haitian Bean Circuits: Cropping and Trading Maneuvers Among a Cash-Oriented Peasantry. In *Working Papers in Haitian Society and Culture,* S. Mintz, ed., pp. 85–126. New Haven: Antilles Research Center.

Murray, Stephen
    1986   A Note on Haitian Tolerance of Homosexuality. In *Male Homosexuality in Central and South America,* Stephen Murray, ed., pp. 92–100. Gai Saber Monograph 5.
    1987   A Loaded Gun: Some Thoughts on American Concentration Camps and the AIDS Epidemic. *New York Native* 27 July:15–17.

Murray, Stephen, and Kenneth Payne
    1988   Medical Policy Without Scientific Evidence: The Promiscuity Paradigm and AIDS. *California Sociologist* 11(1–2):13–54.

Nachman, Steven
    n.d.   Wasted Lives: Tuberculosis and Other Health Risks of Being Haitian in a U.S. Detention Camp. Paper presented at the Southern Anthropological Society Meeting, Baton Rouge, 14 February 1983.

Nachman, Steven, and Ginette Dreyfuss
    1986   Haitians and AIDS in South Florida. *Medical Anthropology Quarterly* 17(2):32–33.
    n.d.   Haitians and AIDS in South Florida. Unpublished manuscript.

Neptune-Anglade, Mireille
    1986   *L'Autre Moitié du Développement: A Propos du Travail des Femmes en Haiti.* Pétion-Ville, Haiti: Éditions des Alizés.

Nicholls, David
    1979   *From Dessalines to Duvalier: Race, Colour, and National Independence in Haiti.* Cambridge: Cambridge University Press.
    1985   *Haiti in Caribbean Context: Ethnicity, Economy and Revolt.* New York: St. Martin's Press.

Nicolas, H.
    1957   *L'Occupation Américaine d'Haiti.* Madrid: Industrias Graficas Espana.

Olle-Goig, Jaime
  1984   Groups at High Risk for AIDS. *New England Journal of Medicine* 311:124.
Oppenheimer, Gerald
  1988   In the Eye of the Storm: The Epidemiological Construction of AIDS. In *AIDS: The Burdens of History*, E. Fee and D. Fox, eds., pp. 267–300. Berkeley: University of California Press.
Ortner, Sherry
  1984   Theory in Anthropology since the Sixties. *Comparative Studies in Society and History* 26:126–166.
Osborn, June
  1989   Public Health and the Politics of AIDS Prevention. *Daedalus* 118(3):123–144.
  1990   Policy Implications of the AIDS Deficit. *Journal of Acquired Immune Deficiency Syndromes* 3:293–295.
Packard, Randall
  1989   *White Plague, Black Labor: Tuberculosis and the Political Economy of Health and Disease in South Africa*. Berkeley: University of California Press.
Palmer, Michael
  1991   *Extreme Measures*. New York: Bantam Books.
Palmer, Ransford
  1979   *Caribbean Dependence on the United States Economy*. New York: Praeger.
Pamphile de Lacroix, F. J.
  1984 [1819] *Mémoires pour servir à l'Histoire de la Révolution de Saint-Domingue*. Port-au-Prince: Editiones Fardins.
Panem, Sandra
  1988   *The AIDS Bureaucracy*. Cambridge: Harvard University Press.
Pape, Jean
  1988   Treatment of Gastrointestinal Infections. *AIDS* 2(suppl.1): S161–S167.
Pape, Jean, et al.
  1983   Characteristics of the Acquired Immunodeficiency Syndrome (AIDS) in Haiti. *The New England Journal of Medicine* 309(16): 945–950.
  1984   Acquired Immunodeficiency Syndrome in Haiti (abstract). *Clinical Research* 32(2):379A.
  1985   The Acquired Immunodeficiency Syndrome in Haiti. *Annals of Internal Medicine* 103:674–678.
  1986   Risk Factors Associated with AIDS in Haiti. *American Journal of Medical Sciences* 29(1):4–7.
Pape, Jean, and Warren Johnson
  1988a   Epidemiology of AIDS in the Caribbean. *Baillière's Clinical Tropical Medicine and Communicable Diseases* 3(1):31–42.
  1988b   Perinatal Transmission of Human Immunodeficiency Virus. *Boletín de la Oficina Sanitaria Panamerican* 105(5–6):73–89.

Paquette, Robert
   1988   *Sugar is Made with Blood: The Conspiracy of La Escalera Conflict be-
             tween Empires over Slavery in Cuba*. Middletown, CT: Wesleyan
             University Press.
Parker, Richard
   1987   Acquired Immunodeficiency Syndrome in Urban Brazil. *Medical
             Anthropology Quarterly* 1(2):155–175.
Parkinson, Wenda
   1978   *"This Gilded African": Toussaint L'Ouverture*. London: Quartet.
Patterson, Orlando
   1967   *The Sociology of Slavery*. London: MacGibbon and Kee.
   1979   On Slavery and Slave Formations. *New Left Review* 117:31–67.
   1987   The Emerging West Atlantic System: Migration, Culture and Un-
             derdevelopment in the U.S. and Circum-Caribbean Region. In
             Population in an Interacting World, William Alonzo, ed., pp. 227–
             260. Cambridge, MA: Harvard University Press.
Paul, M.
   1984   Société et Histoire: Notes sur les Événements de 1902 à partir des
             Archives Allemandes. *Bulletin du Bureau National d'Ethnologie*
             2:85–96.
Payne, Kenneth W.
   1987   Response to Koenig et al. 1987. *Journal of the American Medical
             Association* 258(1):46–47.
Peterman, T. A., R. L. Stoneburner, J. R. Allen, H. W. Jaffe, and J. W. Curran
   1988   Risk of Human Immunodeficiency Virus Transmission from Het-
             erosexual Adults with Transfusion-Associated Infections. *Journal
             of the American Medical Association* 259:55–58.
Pitchenik, Arthur
   1984   Tuberculosis, Atypical Mycobacteria, and AIDS among Haitian
             and Non-Haitian Patients in South Florida. *Annals of Internal
             Medicine* 101:641–645.
Pitchenik, Arthur, Margaret Fischl, Gordon Dickenson, Daniel Becker, Arthur
Fournier, Mark O'Connell, Robert Colton, and Thomas Spira
   1983   Opportunistic Infections and Kaposi's Sarcoma Among Haitians:
             Evidence of a New Acquired Immunodeficiency State. *Annals of
             Internal Medicine* 98(3):277–284.
Pitman, Frank
   1967 [1917] *The Development of the British West Indies 1700–1763*. Hamden,
             CT: Archon Books.
Planson, Claude
   1978   *À la Découverte de Vaudou*. Vicence: Éditions de Vecchi.
Plant, Roger
   1987   *Sugar and Modern Slavery: A Tale of Two Countries*. London: Zed
             Books.
Pluchon, Pierre
   1980   *La Route des Esclaves: Négriers et Bois d'Ébène au XVIIIe Siècle*.
             Paris: Hachette.

1987   *Vaudou, sorciers, empoisionneurs: de Saint-Domingue à Haiti.* Paris: Éditions Karthala.

Plummer, Brenda Gayle
1988   *Haiti and the Great Powers, 1902–1915.* Baton Rouge: Louisiana State University Press.

Portes, A., and J. Walton
1982   *Labor, Class, and the International System.* New York: Academic Press.

Price, Hannibal
1900   *De la Réhabilitation de la Race Noire par la République d'Haiti.* Port-au-Prince: Imprimerie de l'État.

Price, Laurie
1987   Ecuadorian Illness Stories: Cultural Knowledge in Natural Discourse. In *Cultural Knowledge in Language and Thought,* Dorothy Holland and Naomi Quinn, eds., pp. 313–342. Cambridge: Cambridge University Press.

Price-Mars, Jean
1953   *La République d'Haiti et la République Dominicaine: Les Aspects Divers d'un Problème d'Histoire, de Géographie et d'Ethnologie.* 2 vols. Lausanne: Imprimerie Held.

Prince, Rod
1985   *Haiti: Family Business.* London: Latin American Bureau.

Quesenberry, C. P., B. Fireman, R. A. Hiatt, and J. B. Selby
1989   A Suvival Analysis of Hospitalization among Patients with Acquired Immunodeficiency Syndrome. *American Journal of Public Health* 79(12):1643–1647.

Rieder, Ines, and Patricia Ruppelt
1988   *AIDS: The Women.* Pittsburgh: Cleis Press.

Rigaud, Milo
1985   *Secrets of Voodoo.* Robert Cross, trans. San Francisco: City Lights Books.

Risse, Guenter
1988   Epidemics and History: Ecological Perspectives and Social Responses. In *AIDS: The Burdens of History,* E. Fee and D. Fox, eds., pp. 33–66. Berkeley: University of California Press.

Roberts, Leslie
1989   Disease and Death in the New World. *Science* 246:1245–1247.

Robertson, W.
1967 [1939] *France and Latin-American Independence.* New York: Octagon Books.

Romain, Charles-Poisset
1986   *Le Protestantisme dans la Société Haitienne.* Port-au-Prince: Imprimerie Henri Deschamps.

Romain, J. B.
1959   *Quelques Moeurs et Coutumes des Paysans Haitiens.* Port-au-Prince: Imprimerie de l'État.

Romelus, Marc
    1987   Transformations Foncières et Développement National: Le Cas d'Haiti. In *Enjeux Fonciers dans la Caraibe, en Amérique Centrale et à la Réunion: Plantations et Paysanneries,* Christian Deverre, ed., pp. 15–37. Paris: Éditions Karthala.

Rosenberg, Charles
    1988   What is an Epidemic? AIDS in Historical Perspective. *Daedalus* 118:1–17.

Rotberg, Robert
    1971   *Haiti: The Politics of Squalor.* Boston: Houghton Mifflin.
    1988   Haiti's Past Mortgages its Future. *Foreign Affairs* 67(1):93–109.

Rothenberg, R., M. Woelfel, R. Stoneburner, J. Milberg, R. Parker, and B. Truman
    1987   Survival with the Acquired Immunodeficiency Syndrome: Experience with 5833 Cases in New York City. *New England Journal of Medicine* 317(21):1297–1302.

Rout, Leslie
    1976   *The African Experience in Spanish America.* Cambridge: Cambridge University Press.

Ryan, William
    1971   *Blaming the Victim.* New York: Vintage.

Sabatier, Renee
    1988   *Blaming Others: Prejudice, Race, and Worldwide AIDS.* Philadelphia: New Society Publishers.

Said, Edward
    1987   *Orientalism.* New York: Vintage Books.

Saint-Gérard, Yves
    1984   *L'État de Mal: Haiti.* Toulouse: Eche.

St. John, R. K.
    1988   The Public Health Challenge of AIDS in Latin America and the Caribbean. In *AIDS in Children, Adolescents and Heterosexual Adults: An Interdisciplinary Approach to Prevention,* Raymond Schinazi and Andre Nahmias, eds., pp. 34–41. New York: Elsevier.

St. John, Spenser
    1884   *Hayti: Or the Black Republic.* London: Smith and Elder.

Sala-Molins, Louis
    1987   *Le Code Noir, ou le Calvaire de Canaan.* Paris: Presses Universitaires de France.

Sanchez, Thomas
    1989   *Mile Zero.* New York: Knopf.

Schmidt, Hans
    1971   *The United States Occupation of Haiti, 1915–1934.* New Brunswick, NJ: Rutgers University Press.

Schoelcher, Victor
    1982 [1889] *Vie de Toussaint Louverture.* Paris: Editions Karthala.

Schoepf, Brooke Grundfest
    1988   Women, AIDS, and the Economic Crisis in Central Africa. *Canadian Journal of African Studies* 29(3):625–644.
Scott, James
    1984   History According to Winners and Losers. *Senri Ethnological Studies* 13:161–210.
    1985   *Weapons of the Weak: Everyday Forms of Peasant Resistance.* New Haven: Yale University Press.
Selzer, Richard
    1987   A Mask on the Face of Death. *Life* 10(8):58–64.
Sencer, David
    1983   Tracking a Local Outbreak. In *The AIDS Epidemic,* Kevin Cahill, ed., pp. 18–27. New York: St. Martin's Press.
Service d'Hygiène
    1933   *Notes Bio-bibliographiques: Médecins et Naturalistes de l'Ancienne Colonie Française de Saint-Domingue.* Port-au-Prince: Imprimerie de l'État.
Shilts, Randy
    1987   *And the Band Played On: Politics, People, and the AIDS Epidemic.* New York: St. Martin's Press.
Siegal, Frederick P., and Marta Siegal
    1983   *AIDS: The Medical Mystery.* New York: Grove Press.
Simpson, George
    1942   Sexual and Family Institutions in Northern Haiti. *American Anthropologist* 44:655–674.
    1978   *Black Religions in the New World.* New York: Columbia University Press.
Sklar, Holly
    1988   *Washington's War on Nicaragua.* Boston: South End Press.
Smith, Carol
    1978   Beyond Dependency Theory: National and Regional Patterns of Underdevelopment in Guatemala. *American Ethnologist* 5(3):574–617.
Smith, H. Shelton
    1972   *In His Image, But . . . Racism in Southern Religion.* Durham, NC: Duke University Press.
Smith, Helen
    1983   AIDS: The Haitian Connection. *MD* (December):46–52.
Sontag, Susan
    1988   *AIDS and Its Metaphors.* New York: Farrar, Strauss, and Giroux.
Stehr-Green, J. K., R. C. Holman, and M. A. Mahoney
    1989   Survival Analysis of Hemophilia-associated AIDS Cases in the US. *American Journal of Public Health* 79(7):832–835.
Stepick, Alex
    1984   The Roots of Haitian Migration. In *Haiti—Today and Tomorrow: An Interdisciplinary Study,* C. Foster and A. Valdman, eds., pp. 337–349. Lanham, MD: University Press of America.

Stepick, Alex, and Alejandro Portes
    1986   Flight into Despair: A Profile of Recent Haitian Refugees in South Florida. *International Migration Review* 20(2):329–350.

Tanzi, Vito
    1976   Export Taxation in Developing Countries: Taxation of Coffee in Haiti. *Social and Economic Studies* 25:66–76.

Tardo-Dino, Frantz
    1985   *Le Collier de Servitude: La Condition Sanitaire des Esclaves aux Antilles Françaises du XVIIe au XIXe Siècle.* Paris: Éditions Caraibéennes.

Taussig, Michael
    1980   *The Devil and Commodity Fetishism in South America.* Chapel Hill: University of North Carolina Press.
    1987   *Shamanism, Colonialism, and the Wild Man: A Study in Terror and Healing.* Chicago: University of Chicago Press.

Teas, Jane
    1983   Could AIDS Agent Be a New Variant of African Swine Fever Virus? *The Lancet* 23 April:923.

Terry, P.
    1987   Acquired Immunodeficiency Syndrome in the Caribbean. Presentation at the First Teleconference on AIDS in the Americas, Quito, Ecuador.

Treichler, Paula
    1988a   AIDS, Gender, and Biomedical Discourse: Current Contests for Meaning. In *AIDS: The Burdens of History,* Elizabeth Fee and Daniel Fox, eds., pp. 190–266. Berkeley: University of California Press.
    1988b   AIDS, Homophobia, and Biomedical Discourse: An Epidemic of Signification. In *AIDS: Cultural Analysis/Cultural Activism,* D. Crimp, ed., pp. 31–70. Cambridge, MA: MIT Press.
    1989   AIDS and HIV Infection in the Third World: A First World Chronicle. In *Remaking History,* Barbara Kruger and Phil Mariani, eds., pp. 31–86. Seattle: Bay Press.
    1990   Uncertainties and Excesses. *Science* 248:232–233.

Trouillot, Henock
    1983   *Introduction à une Histoire du Vaudou.* Port-au-Prince: Éditions Fardin.

Trouillot, Michel-Rolph
    1986   *Les Racines Historiques de l'État Duvalierien.* Port-au-Prince: Imprimerie Henri Deschamps.
    1990   *Haiti, State Against Nation: The Origins and Legacy of Duvalierism.* New York: Monthly Review Press.

Turnier, Alain
    1985   *La Société des Baionnettes: Un Regard Nouveau.* Port-au-Prince: Imprimerie Le Natal.

Viaud, Leonce
    1984   Le Houmfor. *Bulletin du Bureau National d'Ethnologie* 2:29–33.

Viera, J., E. Frank, T. J. Spira, and S. H. Landesman
  1983   Acquired Immune Deficiency in Haitians: Opportunistic Infec-
          tions in Previously Healthy Haitian Immigrants. *New England
          Journal of Medicine* 308:125–129.
Viera, Jeffrey
  1985   The Haitian Link. In *Understanding AIDS: A Comprehensive
          Guide,* Victor Gong, ed., pp. 90–99. New Brunswick, NJ: Rut-
          gers University Press.
  1987   The Haitian Link. In *AIDS: Facts and Issues,* Victor Gong, ed.,
          pp. 117–123. New Brunswick, NJ: Rutgers University Press.
Vieux, Serge-Henri
  1989   *Le Plaçage: Droit Coutumier et Famille en Haiti.* Paris: Éditions
          Publisud.
Vissière, Isabelle, and Jean-Louis Vissière, eds.
  1982   *La Traite des Noirs au Siècle des Lumières.* Paris: A. M. Métaile.
Wallerstein, Immanuel
  1974   *The Modern World-System: Capitalist Agriculture and the Origins
          of the European World-Economy in the Sixteenth Century.* San
          Diego: Academic Press.
Weber, Jonathan
  1984   Is AIDS an Epidemic Form of African Kaposi's Sarcoma? *Journal
          of the Royal Society of Medicine* 77:572–576.
Weidman, Hazel
  1978   *Miami Health Ecology Project Report: A Statement on Ethnicity and
          Health.* Miami: University of Miami Press.
Weinberg, Albert
  1963   *Manifest Destiny: A Study of Nationalist Expansionism in American
          History.* Chicago: Quadrangle Books.
Weise, Jean
  1971   The Interaction of Western and Indigenous Medicine in Haiti in
          Regard to Tuberculosis. Ph.D. diss., Department of Anthropol-
          ogy, University of North Carolina, Chapel Hill.
  1976   Tuberculosis in Rural Haiti. *Social Science and Medicine* 8:359–
          362.
White, N. J., and D. A. Warrell
  1988   The Management of Severe Malaria. In *Malaria: Principles and
          Practice of Malariology,* W. M. Wernsdorfer and Sir I. McGregor,
          eds., pp. 865–886. Edinburgh: Churchill Livingstone.
Wilentz, Amy
  1989   *The Rainy Season: Haiti After Duvalier.* New York: Simon and
          Schuster.
  1990   Forward to Aristide, J. B., *In the Parish of the Poor: Writings from
          Haiti.* Maryknoll, N.Y.: Orbis Press.
Williams, Eric
  1970   *From Columbus to Castro: The History of the Caribbean 1492–1969.*
          London: Andre Deutsch.

Williams, Raymond
  1977   *Marxism and Literature*. Oxford: Oxford University Press.
  1980   *Problems in Materialism and Culture*. London: Verso.
Wolf, Eric
  1982   *Europe and the People Without History*. Berkeley: University of California Press.
Yonker, Dolores
  1985   Rara: A Lenten Festival. *Bulletin du Bureau National d'Ethnologie* 2:63–71.

Index

Gallo, Robert, 234
Garcia, Rafael, 144
Georges Adam, A., 172, 173
GHESKIO, 126, 128, 131, 134. *See also*
Pape, Jean
Gilman, Sander, 4, 223, 235
Girault, Christian, 183
Glick-Schiller, Nina, 4, 209–210, 215
Goedert, James, 15–16
Gonorrhea, 262
Good, Byron, xvi, 59, 294 n. 27
Good, Mary-Jo DelVecchio, xvi, 294
n. 27
Gracia, Dieudonné, 11–12, 95–109 pas-
sim; work in Port-au-Prince, 96–97;
political views of, 99, 106–107; sexual
history of, 99–100, 108; diagnosed
with tuberculosis, 101–102; diag-
nosed with AIDS, 105–106; "socio-
logical imagination" of, 242–243
Greene, Graham, 186
Greenwood, Davydd, 12
Grenada, 142
Grunwald, J., 188
Guadéloupe, 142
Guérin, Jean-Michel, 127, 147–148
Gutierrez, Gustavo, 61, 80, 95

Haiti: contemporary political unrest in,
6–7, 48–58 passim, 88, 102–103,
114–115, 255–256; links to United
States, 22, 48–49, 128, 146–150,
152, 161, 165, 166–167, 168, 169,
170–171, 173–190 passim, 249–250,
255–256, 263–264; effects of "AIDS
scare" on, 48, 146–147, 213; European destruction of indigenous population of, 153–154; pre-revolutionary
slavery in, 154–159; plantation economy as template of, 155, 163, 171–
172, 179–180, 184, 258; struggle for
independence of, 159–163; early trade
and commerce in, 166–172; struggle
of great powers to control, 170–176
passim; U.S. occupation of, 177–
183; armed resistance to U.S. occupation of, 180–181; contemporary
economy of, 183–190; role of Haitians abroad, 185–186
Haitian Medical Association. *See* Association Médicale Haitienne

Haitian Study Group on Kaposi's Sar-
coma and Opportunistic Infections.
See GHESKIO
Hamilton, Nora, 187
Hancock, Graham, 189
Harrison, Lawrence, 250
Heinl, Nancy, 155, 156, 159, 172, 175,
176, 181
Heinl, Robert, 155, 156, 159, 172, 175,
176, 181
Hepatitis, 214, 217, 234–235, 262
"Hermeneutic of generosity," 235, 243,
250, 263
Herold, Marc, 187
Herpes, 262
Herskovits, Melville, 156, 193, 199
Hicks, Albert, 182
History, role of in anthropological
studies, xiii, 9–10, 21, 151–152, 256–
258
Holcomb, Richard, 237
Homophobia, 208–209, 248
Homosexuality, 64, 78, 134–135, 136,
143–145, 146–148, 224, 225, 261.
See also Bisexuality
Hospedales, James, 145
Houngan: defined, 31; role in delivering
healthcare, 85, 90, 98, 197–198, 246.
See also Amatè; *Bokor*; Tonton Mèmè
Human Immunodeficiency Virus (HIV),
130–150 passim; prevalence as reflection of economic and historical forces,
10, 14, 15–16, 141–150 passim, 257,
258, 259–262; world epidemiology
of, 122–123, 260; seroprevalence in
asymptomatic Haitian adults, 130–
132; seroprevalence in Haitian children, 132–133; risk factors for, 134–
140; female-to-male transmission of,
136–140; increasing significance of
heterosexual transmission of, 139–
140; theories about origins of, 233–
235. *See also* AIDS; Poverty; West
Atlantic Pandemic
Human T-cell Lymphotropic Virus
(HTLV-1), 136, 143, 260–261
Hurbon, Laënnec, xvi, 48, 54, 57, 98,
119, 183, 196, 199, 202, 205, 206

Immigration and Naturalization Service
(INS), 1, 209–210, 224, 226

INDEX   337

Compositor: Prestige Typography
Text: 10/13 Galliard
Display: Galliard